Nursing Outcomes Classification (NOC)

Nursing Outcomes Classification (NOC)

Editors

Marion Johnson, PhD, RN

Meridean Maas, PhD, RN, FAAN

Authors
Iowa Outcomes Project

Marion Johnson, PhD, RN
Meridean Maas, PhD, RN, FAAN
Mary Aquilino, PhD, RN, CS, FNP
Sandra Bellinger, EdD, RN
Veronica Brighton, MA, RN
Ginette Budreau, MA, MBA, RN
Jeanette Daly, PhD, RN
M. Patricia Donahue, PhD, RN, FAAN
Joyce Eland, BSN, RN
Deborah Perry Jensen, PhD, RN
Kathleen Kelly, PhD, RN

Tom Kruckeberg, MS
Anne Lewis, MA, RN
Leslie Marshall, PhD, RN
Sue Moorhead, PhD, RN
Colleen Prophet, MA, RN
Margaret A. Rankin, PhD, RN
Elizabeth A. Swanson, PhD, RN
Bonnie L. Westra, PhD, RN
Marilyn Willits, MS, RN, CPHQ
George Woodworth, PhD

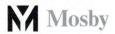 Mosby

St. Louis   Baltimore   Boston   Carlsbad   Chicago   Naples   New York   Philadelphia   Portland
London   Madrid   Mexico City   Singapore   Sydney   Tokyo   Toronto   Wiesbaden

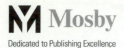

Mosby
Dedicated to Publishing Excellence

A Times Mirror Company

Vice President and Publisher: Nancy Coon
Senior Editor: Robin Carter
Developmental Editor: Liz Fathman
Project Manager: Deborah L. Vogel
Production Editor: Sarah E. Fike
Designer: Renée Duenow
Manufacturing Supervisor: Don Carlisle

Copyright © 1997 by Mosby–Year Book, Inc.

Printed in the United States of America
Composition by Top Graphics
Lithography/color film by Top Graphics
Printing/binding by R. R. Donnelley & Sons Company

Mosby–Year Book, Inc.
11830 Westline Industrial Drive
St. Louis, Missouri 63146

Library of Congress Cataloging-in-Publication Data
Nursing outcomes classification (NOC) : Iowa outcomes project /
   editors, Marion Johnson, Meridean Maas.
      p.   cm.
   Includes bibliographical references and index.
   ISBN 0-8151-4546-2
   1. Nursing audit.   2. Outcome assessment.   I. Johnson, Marion,
1936- . II. Maas, Meridean.
   [DNLM: 1. Nursing Methodology Research—standards. 2. Outcome
Assessment (Health Care)—standards. 3. Nursing Care—standards.
WY 20.5 N9734 1997]
RT85.5.N864 1997
610.73—dc21
for Library of Congress   96-50091
                                      CIP

97 98 99 00 01 / 9 8 7 6 5 4 3 2 1

Members of the Nursing-sensitive Outcomes Classification Research Team, 1996

CO-PRINCIPAL INVESTIGATORS

Marion Johnson, PhD, RN
Associate Professor
College of Nursing
The University of Iowa
Iowa City, Iowa

Meridean Maas, PhD, RN, FAAN
Professor
College of Nursing
The University of Iowa
Iowa City, Iowa

CO-INVESTIGATORS

Mary Aquilino, PhD, RN, CS, FNP
Postdoctoral Fellow
College of Nursing
The University of Iowa
Iowa City, Iowa

Sandra Bellinger, EdD, RN
Academic Dean
Trinity College of Nursing
Moline, Illinois

Veronica Brighton, MA, RN
Lecturer
College of Nursing
The University of Iowa
Iowa City, Iowa

Ginette Budreau, MA, MBA, RN
Advance Practice Nurse
The University of Iowa Hospital and Clinics
Iowa City, Iowa

Jeanette Daly, PhD, RN
Director of Nursing
Greenwood Manor Convalescent Center
Iowa City, Iowa

M. Patricia Donahue, PhD, RN, FAAN
Professor
College of Nursing
The University of Iowa
Iowa City, Iowa

Joyce Eland, BSN, RN
Performance Improvement Coordinator
VNA of Johnson County
Iowa City, Iowa

Deborah Perry Jensen, PhD, RN
Lecturer
College of Nursing
The University of Iowa
Iowa City, Iowa

Kathleen Kelly, PhD, RN
Associate Professor
College of Nursing
The University of Iowa
Iowa City, Iowa

Tom Kruckeberg, MS
Senior Computer Consultant
College of Nursing
The University of Iowa
Iowa City, Iowa

Anne Lewis, MA, RN
Neuro-Science Clinical Nurse Specialist
Genesis Medical Center, West
Davenport, Iowa

Leslie Marshall, PhD, RN
Associate Professor
College of Nursing
The University of Iowa
Iowa City, Iowa

Sue Moorhead, PhD, RN
Assistant Professor
College of Nursing
The University of Iowa
Iowa City, Iowa

Colleen Prophet, MA, RN
Director, Nursing Informatics
Nursing Director, Clinical Informatics
The University of Iowa Hospitals and Clinics
Iowa City, Iowa

Margaret A. Rankin, PhD, RN
Lecturer
College of Nursing
The University of Iowa
Iowa City, Iowa

Elizabeth A. Swanson, PhD, RN
Associate Professor, College of Nursing
Associate Vice President, Health Profes-
    sions Education-Office of the Vice Presi-
    dent for Health Sciences
The University of Iowa
Iowa City, Iowa

Bonnie L. Westra, PhD, RN
Director, Clinical Design and Support
    Services
Epsilon Systems
St. Paul, Minnesota

Marilyn Willits, MS, RN, CPHQ
Standards Nurse Specialist
Genesis Medical Center, East
Davenport, Iowa

George Woodworth, PhD
Professor
Department of Statistics and Actuarial
    Science
The University of Iowa
Iowa City, Iowa

TEAM MEMBERS

Mary Ann Anderson, PhD, RN
Assistant Professor
University of Illinois at Chicago
College of Nursing
Quad Cities Regional Program
Rock Island, Illinois

Judy Collins, MA, ARNP, CS
Clinical Nurse Specialist
Genesis Medical Center
Davenport, Iowa

Kala Minnick Dahms, MA, RN, CNA
Nurse Manager
Surgical/Urological Unit
Genesis Medical Center, East
Davenport, Iowa

Kris Davis, MA, RN, MSN
Advance Practice Nurse-HIV
Department of Nursing
The University of Iowa Hospitals and Clinics
Iowa City, Iowa

Susan Ellenbecker, MS, RN
Staff Nurse
Mayo Medical Center
Rochester, Minnesota

Vicky Fraser, RN
Assistant Director of Nursing
Oaknoll Retirement Residence
Iowa City, Iowa

Rose Gebhart, MS, RN
Associate Professor
Trinity College of Nursing
Moline, Illinois

Linda Guebert, MS, RN
Nurse Educator
Trinity Medical Center
Education Department
Rock Island, Illinois

Cheryl Hardison, MS, RN
Associate Professor
Black Hawk College
Associate Degree Nursing Program
Moline, Illinois

Jane Hartsock, MA, RN, AOCN
Associate Professor
Trinity College of Nursing
Moline, Illinois

Pam Harvey, MA, RN
College of Osteopathic Medicine and
    Surgery
University of Osteopathic Medicine and
    Health Sciences
Des Moines, Iowa

Marna Jacobi, MS, RN
Instructor
Marycrest International University
Davenport, Iowa

Shayna J. Johnson, MS, RN
Clinical Nurse Specialist
Mayo Medical Center
Rochester, Minnesota

Julie K. Katseres, MSN, ARNP
Program Associate
HIV Clinical Trials
The University of Iowa
Iowa City, Iowa

Gail Keenan, PhD, RN
Postdoctoral Fellow
College of Nursing
The University of Iowa
Iowa City, Iowa

Cathy Konrad, MA, RNC
Associate Professor
Trinity College of Nursing
Moline, Illinois

Vicki Kraus, MS, ARNP, CDE
Advanced Practice Nurse
Department of Nursing
The University of Iowa Hospitals and
    Clinics;
PhD Candidate
College of Nursing
The University of Iowa
Iowa City, Iowa

Jan Levsen, MA, RN
Staff, Cardiac Rehabilitation
Genesis Medical Center, East
Davenport, Iowa

Tom Martz, MSN, RNC-CNA
Patient Care Coordinator
VA Medical Center
Iowa City, Iowa

Becki Maxson, MS, RN
Assistant Professor
Black Hawk College
Associate Degree Nursing Program
Moline, Illinois

Heidi Nobiling, MA, MBA, RN
Manager, Internal Medicine Clinics
The University of Iowa Hospitals and
    Clinics;
Doctoral Student, College of Nursing
The University of Iowa
Iowa City, Iowa

Lisa Payden, MSN, RN
Trauma Coordinator
Trinity Medical Center
Moline, Illinois

Shelley-Rae Pehler, MSN, RN
Faculty
Scott Community College
Bettendorf, Iowa

Bev Soukup-Platz, MA, RNC
Psychiatric Nurse Clinician
VA Medical Center
Iowa City, Iowa

Cheryl Ramler, PhD, RN
Graduate Student in Nurse Anesthesia
College of Nursing
The University of Iowa
Iowa City, Iowa

Katie Brady-Schluttner, MS, RN
Nursing Education Specialist
Mayo Medical Center
Rochester, Minnesota

Sharron Schneider, BSN, RN
Staff Nurse, Methodist Hospital;
Graduate Student in Physiology
Mayo Medical Center
Rochester, Minnesota

Janet Specht, PhD, RN
Program Assistant, Family Involvement in
    Care Research Grant
College of Nursing
The University of Iowa
Iowa City, Iowa

Janice L. Stone, MS, RN
Clinical Nurse Specialist
Mayo Medical Center
Rochester, Minnesota

Dianne Wasson, MSN, RN, CDE
Assistant Professor
Trinity College of Nursing
Moline, Illinois

STUDENT MEMBERS

Kristine Bonnett, BSN, RN
Master's Student
College of Nursing
The University of Iowa
Iowa City, Iowa

Diane Davidson, MA, RN
Master's Student
College of Nursing
The University of Iowa
Iowa City, Iowa

Kerri Doeden, BA, RN
Master's Student
College of Nursing
The University of Iowa
Iowa City, Iowa

Linda Garand, MS, RN, CS
Doctoral Student
College of Nursing
The University of Iowa
Iowa City, Iowa

Yaseen Ahmed Hayajneh, MS, RN
Doctoral Student
College of Nursing
The University of Iowa
Iowa City, Iowa

Barbara J. Head, MSN, RN
PhD Candidate
College of Nursing
The University of Iowa
Iowa City, Iowa

Mary Ann Hovda, BSN, RN
Master's Student
College of Nursing
The University of Iowa
Iowa City, Iowa

Edith Lassegard, MS
Doctoral Student
Cornell University
Ithaca, New York

Melissa Lehan, BSN, RN
Staff Nurse
The University of Iowa Hospitals and Clinics
Medical Psychiatric Unit
Iowa City, Iowa

Linda McCabe, BSN, RN, PNP, ARNP
Pediatric Nurse Practitioner
Burlington Pediatric Association, PC;
Master's Student
College of Nursing
The University of Iowa
Iowa City, Iowa

Cindy A. Scherb, MS, RN
Doctoral Student
College of Nursing
The University of Iowa
Iowa City, Iowa

Sonia Van De Kieft
BSN Student
College of Nursing
The University of Iowa
Iowa City, Iowa

ADVISORY BOARD

Sheila Haas, PhD, RN
Professor and Chairperson, Community,
Mental Health and Administrative Nursing
Loyola University
Lake Shore Campus
Chicago, Illinois

Ada Jacox, PhD, RN, FAAN
Associate Dean for Research
Wayne State University
Detroit, Michigan

Kathleen A. McCormick, PhD, RN, FAAN
Senior Science Adviser
Office of Science and Data Development
Agency for Health Care Policy and
   Research
Rockville, Maryland

Polly Ryan, PhD, RN
Nurse Researcher
St. Joseph Hospital;
Clinical Assistant Professor
Marquette University
Milwaukee, Wisconsin

Joyce Verran, PhD, RN, FAAN
Professor
College of Nursing
University of Arizona
Tucson, Arizona

STAFF

Donna Laube
BSN Student
College of Nursing
The University of Iowa
Iowa City, Iowa

Lori J. Penaluna, BS
Program Associate
College of Nursing
The University of Iowa
Iowa City, Iowa

Donna Valiga, BS
Secretary
College of Nursing
The University of Iowa
Iowa City, Iowa

CONSULTANTS

Gloria Bulechek, PhD, RN, FAAN
Professor
College of Nursing
The University of Iowa
Iowa City, Iowa

Connie Delaney, PhD, RN
Associate Professor
College of Nursing
The University of Iowa
Iowa City, Iowa

Joanne McCloskey, PhD, RN, FAAN
Distinguished Professor
College of Nursing
The University of Iowa
Iowa City, Iowa

Toni Tripp-Reimer, PhD, RN, FAAN
Professor
Director, Office for Nursing Research
College of Nursing
The University of Iowa
Iowa City, Iowa

PREVIOUS MEMBERS

Rojann Alper, PhD, RN
Assistant Professor
Arizona State University
Tempe, Arizona

Anne Bodensteiner, MA, RN
Deceased

Lisa James, BSN, RN
Nurse Manager
University of Iowa Hospitals and Clinics
Iowa City, Iowa

Jeanette Miller-Criswell, MS, RN
Chief Nurse Executive
VA Medical Center
Wichita, Kansas

CONTRIBUTORS

Mary Kathleen Clark, PhD, ARNP, FNP
Assistant Professor
College of Nursing
The University of Iowa
Iowa City, Iowa

Perle Slavik Cowen, PhD, RN
Assistant Professor
College of Nursing
The University of Iowa
Iowa City, Iowa

Michele Eliason, PhD, RN
Assistant Professor
College of Nursing
The University of Iowa
Iowa City, Iowa

Sue Gettman, MSN, RN
Master's Student
College of Nursing
The University of Iowa
Iowa City, Iowa

Judy Maupin, MSN, RN
Nursing Education Manager
Columbus Regional Hospital
Columbus, Indiana

Patricia S. Moore, MSN, RN, CDE
Coordinator, Diabetes Education and
    Resource Center
Columbus Regional Hospital
Columbus, Indiana

Deborah Rapp, MSN, RN
Pulmonary Clinical Nurse Specialist
Columbus Regional Hospital
Columbus, Indiana

Jo Ann Wedig, MA, RN
Associate Professor
Trinity College of Nursing
Moline, Illinois

Since the initial draft of the book, the research team has been saddened by the death of two active members: Kathleen Kelly, co-investigator, and Rose Gebhart, team member.

Preface

This first edition of the *Nursing Outcomes Classification (NOC)* presents the first comprehensive standardized language used to describe the patient outcomes that are responsive to nursing intervention. The text contains 190 outcomes with more specific indicators that nurses can use to assess the effects of interventions. In addition, initial measurement scales have been developed to quantify the outcomes and indicators, which will aid nurses in evaluating and monitoring patient progress and in determining the effectiveness of interventions. Although the reliability and validity of the scales have not yet been estimated, the use of the outcome measures in computerized clinical information systems will make it possible to psychometrically evaluate the measures in the future.

The initial classification contains outcomes for individual patients and family caregivers. Future work will add more patient outcomes to the list as they are identified and developed. Outcomes for patient aggregates, families, organizations, and communities are recognized as important and their development is planned in future work.

Each outcome includes a label name, a definition, a set of indicators, a Likert-type measurement scale, and selected references. The format used to present each outcome is similar to the format used by the *Nursing Interventions Classification (NIC)*. The standardized language is the label name and definition. The NOC team expects that the indicators will be selected based on the particular circumstances for a patient population or individual. Although the scales are not yet fully tested, the team anticipates that the scales also will be standardized after more rigorous psychometric evaluation in future work.

The team currently is developing the taxonomic structure of the NOC. This aspect of the research was not completed in time for inclusion in the current text. When the taxonomic structure is completed and validated by nurse experts, the structure will be coded for uses such as clinical information systems. The taxonomic structure and codes will help nurses more easily locate and choose an outcome and will aid in the design and implementation of curricula and clinical nursing information systems.

Linkages between the North American Nursing Diagnosis Association (NANDA) diagnoses and the NOC are included in the text to help nurses more easily use the NOC. It is important to note that these linkages are not prescriptive and have not been validated with clinical data. They are provided as suggested linkages to assist nurses with identifying outcomes when a diagnosis is made. However, the nurse's clinical judgment remains the most important factor in selecting individual patient outcomes.

It is important that nurses provide the research team with feedback on the NOC. To encourage nurses to provide suggestions for revisions and to submit new outcomes, a form and procedure are included (see Appendix D). The expansion and refinement of the NOC is planned and will depend on the submission of useful feedback from nurse users.

There has never been a more important time for nursing to define the patient outcomes that are responsive to nursing interventions. The current emphasis on outcomes effectiveness in health policy decision making will continue as managed competition in health care evolves. The focus on the provision of care at the least cost will bring concerns about quality of care to the fore. Nursing plays a key role in the delivery of cost-effective care in every health care setting; therefore, it is imperative that nursing data be included in the evaluation of health care effectiveness. The NOC completes the nursing process elements of the Nursing Minimum Data Set. Standardized nursing languages, including standardized outcomes that are responsive to nursing interventions, are required if nursing data are to be included in computerized data bases that are analyzed and used in health policy decisions.

The NOC is a companion to the NIC and is comprehensive, as are NANDA diagnoses and the NIC. The study and teaching of diagnostic reasoning are facilitated by the standardized languages, as are the development of nursing theory and the testing of linkages between nursing diagnoses, interventions, and outcomes. Thus, standardized patient outcomes that are responsive to nursing intervention are important for the development of nursing knowledge.

Marion Johnson
Meridean Maas

Strengths of the Nursing-sensitive Outcomes Classification

Comprehensive. The NOC contains outcomes for individual patients and family caregivers that are representative for all settings and clinical specialties. Although all outcomes may not yet be developed, there are outcomes that are useful for the entire scope of nursing practice, and plans are to develop others as they are identified. At present the NOC does not include outcomes for patient aggregates, organizations, or communities, but there is a plan to develop these outcomes during a later phase of the research. Because each is comprehensive, the NANDA, NIC, and NOC provide standardized languages for the nursing process elements of the Nursing Minimum Data Set.[2]

Research-based. The research, conducted by a large team of University of Iowa College of Nursing faculty and students and clinicians from a variety of settings, began in 1991. Both qualitative and quantitative strategies were used. Methods included content analysis, focus group conduction of concept analysis, survey of experts, similarity analysis, hierarchical clustering analysis, multidimensional scaling, and clinical field site testing.

Developed inductively and deductively. Sources of data for initial development of the outcomes and indicators were nursing textbooks, care plan guides, nursing clinical information systems, standards of practice, and research instruments. Research team focus groups reviewed outcomes in eight broad categories that were drawn from the Medical Outcomes Study and nursing literature. Based on a review of literature, outcomes subsumed by the broad categories were identified and refined through concept analysis.

Grounded in clinical practice and research. Developed initially from nursing texts, care plan guides, and clinical information systems, the outcomes were reviewed by expert clinicians and are being tested in clinical field sites. Feedback from clinicians is solicited through a defined feedback process.

Uses clear, clinically useful language. Throughout the development of the NOC, clarity and usefulness of the language has been emphasized. Care has been taken to ensure that the language distinguishes NOC outcomes from nursing interventions and diagnoses.

Outcomes can be shared by all disciplines. Although the NOC emphasizes outcomes that are most responsive to nursing interventions, the outcomes describe patient states at a conceptual level. Thus the NOC provides a classification of patient outcomes that are potentially influenced by all disciplines. The NOC contains indicators for the outcomes that are expected to be most responsive to nursing intervention. Use of the outcomes by all members of the interdisciplinary team will provide needed standardization, yet allow the selection of indicators that are most responsive to each discipline.

Optimizes information for the evaluation of effectiveness. The outcomes and indicators are variable concepts. This allows measurement of the outcome states at any point on a continuum from most negative to most positive at different points in time. Rather than the limited information provided by the measurement of whether a goal is met, NOC outcomes can be used to monitor the extent of progress, or lack of progress, throughout an episode of care and across different care settings.

Funded by extramural grants. To date, the NOC research has received 5 years of peer-reviewed grant funding: 1 year from Sigma Theta Tau International and 4 years from the National Institute of Nursing Research (NINR).

Tested in clinical field sites. Testing of the NOC is planned in a variety of clinical field sites, including tertiary care hospitals, intermediate care hospitals, a nursing home, and a home health care setting. The field tests will provide important information about the clinical usefulness of the outcomes and indicators; linkages between nursing diagnoses, interventions, and outcomes; and the process of implementing the NOC in clinical nursing information systems.

Dissemination emphasized. This book describes the NOC research and the initial alphabetical classification of outcomes and indicators. In addition, a growing number of journal articles and book chapters are being published describing the NOC work. The NOC research is described on a University of Iowa College of Nursing World Wide Web home page (http://www.nursing.uiowa.edu/noc/), and *a listserv* is maintained to share information about the NOC and for dialogue with interested users. The NOC work has been disseminated in a number of national and international presentations and that will continue.

Linked to NANDA nursing diagnoses and NIC interventions. Initial linkages have been developed by the NIC and NOC research teams to assist nurses with the use of the classifications and to facilitate use in clinical information systems. NANDA-NOC linkages are presented in this volume. NANDA-NIC linkages have been published by the NIC team.[1] NIC-NOC linkages currently are under development by the NIC team and are available from the NIC research office at the College of Nursing, University of Iowa, Iowa City.

Developed as companion to the NIC. Experience with the NIC at Iowa has aided the NOC research. Both classifications are comprehensive, research-based, and reflect current clinical nursing practice.

References

1. Iowa Intervention Project. (1996). *Nursing Interventions Classification (NIC).* (2nd ed.). St. Louis: Mosby.
2. Werley, H.H. & Lang, N.M. (1988). (Eds.), *Identification of the Nursing Minimum Data Set.* New York: Springer.

Acknowledgments

Development of the Nursing-sensitive Outcomes Classification (NOC) and this publication would not have been possible without the work and support of numerous individuals and organizations that we would like to acknowledge:

1. Sigma Theta Tau International for a 1-year grant (1992-1993) and the Office of Nursing Research, University of Iowa, for a seed grant (1992-1993). These grants funded the pilot work and beginning development of the NOC.
2. The National Institute of Nursing Research, National Institutes of Health, for a 4-year grant (1993-1997) to develop the classification, construct the taxonomy, and field test the outcomes.
3. The investigators and clinicians who have devoted hours of work in addition to their regular jobs to develop the outcomes and associated indicators that appear in the NOC.
4. Gloria Bulechek and Joanne McCloskey, co-Principal Investigators of the intervention project, who have assisted and occasionally prodded us in the development of the NOC.
5. The American Nurses' Association for supporting the validation surveys and recognizing the work as a classification in development.
6. The field test sites and their staff who have worked diligently to include the NOC in their clinical information systems.
7. Nurses from a variety of nursing specialty organizations who served as expert respondents in the validation surveys. The samples were selected from the following organizations:

> Academy of Medical Surgical Nurses
> American Academy of Ambulatory Care Nursing
> American Association of Critical Care Nurses
> American Association of Neuroscience Nurses
> American Holistic Nurses Association
> American Psychiatric Nurses Association
> American Society for Parenteral & Enteral Nutrition
> ANA-Community Public Health
> ANA-General Practice
> ANA-Gerontology
> ANA-Medical Surgical
> ANA-Pediatrics
> ANA-Psychiatric/Mental Health
> ANCC-Clinical Specialist in Medical Surgical Nursing
> ANCC-Community Health Nurse
> ANCC-Family Nurse Practitioner
> Association of Nurses in AIDS Care
> Association of Rehabilitation Nurses
> Association of Women's Health, Obstetric and Neonatal Nurses
> Drug & Alcohol Nursing Association

National Association of Orthopedic Nurses
National Association of Pediatric Nurse Associates and Practitioners
National Association of School Nurses, Inc.
National Gerontological Nursing Association
North American Nursing Diagnosis Association
Oncology Nursing Society
Respiratory Nursing Society
Wound Ostomy and Continence Nurses Society

Although this is the first edition of the NOC, the team has received numerous requests for the classification from health care agencies, software companies, and educators who have become familiar with the work through presentations at conferences. The interest and support you have shown for this work has helped to make this edition possible.

Contents

PART ONE
Construction of the Outcomes Classification, *1*

Chapter One Outcome Development and Significance, *3*

Chapter Two Overview of the Nursing-sensitive Patient Outcomes Research, 18

Chapter Three Methods Used to Develop the Outcomes and Indicators, 32

Chapter Four The Current and Future Classification, 41

PART TWO
The Outcomes, *65*

PART THREE
Appendices, *313*

Appendix A: NANDA-NOC Linkages, *315*
Appendix B: Care Plans, *377*
Appendix C: Case Study, *387*
Appendix D: Nursing-sensitive Outcomes Classification Review Form, *397*

Detailed Contents

PART ONE
Construction of the Outcomes Classification, *1*

Chapter One Outcome Development and Significance, *3*

Outcome development in health care, *3*
  Outcome development in nursing, *4*
  Current outcome evaluation, *6*
Reasons for standardized outcomes for nursing, *8*
  Creation of a common nursing language, *8*
  Computerized nursing information systems, *9*
  Uniform nursing data sets, *9*
  National data sets, *10*
  Evaluation of nursing care quality, *10*
  Evaluation of nursing innovations, *12*
  Contribution to knowledge development, *12*
Summary, *14*

Chapter Two Overview of the Nursing-sensitive Patient Outcomes Research, *18*

Purposes and significance of the research, *18*
Preliminary work related to NOC, *19*
  Pilot studies of patient satisfaction outcomes, *19*
Development of the NOC research team, *20*
Resolution of issues and development of the initial list of outcomes, *20*
  Identification and resolution of conceptual and methodologic issues, *20*
    Who is the patient?, *20*
    What do patient outcomes describe?, *21*
    At what levels of abstraction should outcomes be developed?, *21*
    How should the outcomes be stated?, *23*
    What are nursing-sensitive patient outcomes?, *23*
    Are nursing-sensitive patient outcomes the resolution of nursing diagnoses?, *24*
    When should patient outcomes be measured?, *24*
  Methodologic issues and strategies, *25*
    What strategies were used?, *25*
    What sources were used to sample outcome statements?, *25*
    What criteria were used to select the sources from which outcome statements were extracted?, *25*
    How are nursing-sensitive outcomes and indicators validated?, *25*
    What methods will be used to develop the classification structure?, *27*
Development of the initial list of nursing-sensitive patient outcomes and indicators, *29*
Validation, field testing, and classification of the initial list of outcomes, *29*
  Refinement of the initial list of nursing-sensitive outcomes and indicators, *29*
  Field testing and classification of the list of outcomes and indicators, *30*
Validation of the NOC and testing of measurement procedures, *30*

Chapter Three Methods Used to Develop the Outcomes and Indicators, *32*

    Generation of the initial list of outcome labels, *32*
    Process for rating data sources, *32*
    Sources reviewed and extraction of outcome statements, *33*
    Grouping of outcome statements to develop nursing-sensitive outcome labels, *33*
    Data base management, *34*
    Placing the outcomes in broad categories for the assessment of content validity and refinement, *35*
    Focus group concept analyses, *35*
    Content validation by nurse experts, *37*
    Results of the surveys of nurse experts, *39*
    Field testing the nursing-sensitive outcomes and indicators, *39*

Chapter Four The Current and Future Classification, *41*

    The classification, *41*
    The classification—what it is, *41*
    The classification—what it is not, *44*
    The classification and its uses, *46*
    Uses in practice, *46*
    Outcome goals for individual patients, *46*
    Outcome goals for patient groups, *46*
    Outcome measures, *47*
    Use in research, policy formulation, and education, *48*
    Implementing the classification in practice, *48*
    Implementing the outcome, *48*
    Implementing the outcome indicators, *49*
    Implementing the measurement scales, *50*
    Commonly asked questions about the NOC, *51*
    The classification—ongoing and future work, *63*
    Request for feedback, *64*
    Summary, *64*

PART TWO
The Outcomes, *65*

Abuse Cessation, *67*
Abuse Protection, *68*
Abuse Recovery: Emotional, *69*
Abuse Recovery: Financial, *70*
Abuse Recovery: Physical, *71*
Abuse Recovery: Sexual, *72*
Abusive Behavior Self-Control, *73*
Acceptance: Health Status, *75*
Adherence Behavior, *76*
Aggression Control, *78*
Ambulation: Walking, *80*
Ambulation: Wheelchair, *81*
Anxiety Control, *82*
Balance, *84*
Blood Transfusion Reaction Control, *85*
Body Image, *86*
Body Positioning: Self-Initiated, *87*
Bone Healing, *88*
Bowel Continence, *89*

Bowel Elimination, *90*
Breastfeeding Establishment: Infant, *92*
Breastfeeding Establishment: Maternal, *93*
Breastfeeding Maintenance, *95*
Breastfeeding Weaning, *96*
Cardiac Pump Effectiveness, *98*
Caregiver Adaptation to Patient Institutionalization, *100*
Caregiver Emotional Health, *102*
Caregiver Home Care Readiness, *103*
Caregiver Lifestyle Disruption, *104*
Caregiver-Patient Relationship, *105*
Caregiver Performance: Direct Care, *106*
Caregiver Performance: Indirect Care, *107*
Caregiver Physical Health, *108*
Caregiver Stressors, *109*
Caregiver Well-Being, *110*
Caregiving Endurance Potential, *111*
Child Adaptation to Hospitalization, *112*

Child Development: 2 Months, *113*
Child Development: 4 Months, *114*
Child Development: 6 Months, *115*
Child Development: 12 Months, *116*
Child Development: 2 Years, *117*
Child Development: 3 Years, *118*
Child Development: 4 Years, *119*
Child Development: 5 Years, *120*
Child Development: Middle Childhood
  (6-11 Years), *121*
Child Development: Adolescence (12-17
  Years), *122*
Circulation Status, *123*
Cognitive Ability, *125*
Cognitive Orientation, *127*
Comfort Level, *128*
Communication Ability, *129*
Communication: Expressive Ability, *130*
Communication: Receptive Ability, *131*
Compliance Behavior, *132*
Concentration, *134*
Coping, *136*
Decision Making, *138*
Dignified Dying, *139*
Distorted Thought Control, *141*
Electrolyte & Acid/Base Balance, *143*
Endurance, *145*
Energy Conservation, *146*
Fear Control, *147*
Fluid Balance, *148*
Grief Resolution, *150*
Growth, *152*
Health Beliefs, *153*
Health Beliefs: Perceived Ability to
  Perform, *154*
Health Beliefs: Perceived Control, *155*
Health Beliefs: Perceived Resources, *156*
Health Beliefs: Perceived Threat, *157*
Health Orientation, *158*
Health Promoting Behavior, *159*
Health Seeking Behavior, *160*
Hope, *162*
Hydration, *163*
Identity, *164*
Immobility Consequences: Physiological,
  166
Immobility Consequences: Psycho-
  Cognitive, *167*
Immune Hypersensitivity Control, *168*
Immune Status, *170*
Immunization Behavior, *172*
Impulse Control, *174*
Infection Status, *176*
Information Processing, *178*
Joint Movement: Active, *179*
Joint Movement: Passive, *180*

Knowledge: Breastfeeding, *181*
Knowledge: Child Safety, *183*
Knowledge: Diet, *184*
Knowledge: Disease Process, *186*
Knowledge: Energy Conservation, *187*
Knowledge: Health Behaviors, *188*
Knowledge: Health Resources, *189*
Knowledge: Infection Control, *190*
Knowledge: Medication, *191*
Knowledge: Personal Safety, *193*
Knowledge: Prescribed Activity, *194*
Knowledge: Substance Use Control, *195*
Knowledge: Treatment Procedure(s), *196*
Knowledge: Treatment Regimen, *197*
Leisure Participation, *199*
Loneliness, *200*
Memory, *202*
Mobility Level, *203*
Mood Equilibrium, *204*
Muscle Function, *206*
Neglect Recovery, *207*
Neurological Status, *209*
Neurological Status: Autonomic, *211*
Neurological Status: Central Motor Control,
  213
Neurological Status: Consciousness, *214*
Neurological Status: Cranial Sensory/
  Motor Function, *215*
Neurological Status: Spinal Sensory/Motor
  Function, *216*
Nutritional Status, *217*
Nutritional Status: Biochemical Measures,
  218
Nutritional Status: Body Mass, *219*
Nutritional Status: Energy, *220*
Nutritional Status: Food & Fluid Intake,
  221
Nutritional Status: Nutrient Intake, *222*
Oral Health, *223*
Pain Control Behavior, *224*
Pain: Disruptive Effects, *225*
Pain Level, *226*
Parent-Infant Attachment, *227*
Parenting, *229*
Parenting: Social Safety, *231*
Participation: Health Care Decisions, *232*
Physical Aging Status, *234*
Physical Maturation: Female, *235*
Physical Maturation: Male, *236*
Play Participation, *237*
Psychosocial Adjustment: Life Change, *238*
Quality of Life, *239*
Respiratory Status: Gas Exchange, *240*
Respiratory Status: Ventilation, *241*
Rest, *243*
Risk Control, *244*

Risk Control: Alcohol Use, 246
Risk Control: Drug Use, 248
Risk Control: Sexually Transmitted
  Diseases (STD), 250
Risk Control: Tobacco Use, 252
Risk Control: Unintended Pregnancy, 254
Risk Detection, 256
Role Performance, 257
Safety Behavior: Fall Prevention, 258
Safety Behavior: Home Physical
  Environment, 259
Safety Behavior: Personal, 260
Safety Status: Falls Occurrence, 261
Safety Status: Physical Injury, 262
Self-Care: Activities of Daily Living (ADL),
  263
Self-Care: Bathing, 264
Self-Care: Dressing, 265
Self-Care: Eating, 266
Self-Care: Grooming, 267
Self-Care: Hygiene, 268
Self-Care: Instrumental Activities of Daily
  Living (IADL), 269
Self-Care: Non-Parenteral Medication, 271
Self-Care: Oral Hygiene, 272
Self-Care: Parenteral Medication, 273
Self-Care: Toileting, 274
Self-Esteem, 275

Self-Mutilation Restraint, 277
Sleep, 278
Social Interaction Skills, 279
Social Involvement, 280
Social Support, 281
Spiritual Well-Being, 282
Substance Addiction Consequences, 284
Suicide Self-Restraint, 285
Symptom Control Behavior, 287
Symptom Severity, 288
Thermoregulation, 289
Thermoregulation: Neonate, 291
Tissue Integrity: Skin & Mucous
  Membranes, 292
Tissue Perfusion: Abdominal Organs, 293
Tissue Perfusion: Cardiac, 295
Tissue Perfusion: Cerebral, 296
Tissue Perfusion: Peripheral, 297
Tissue Perfusion: Pulmonary, 298
Transfer Performance, 299
Treatment Behavior: Illness or Injury, 300
Urinary Continence, 302
Urinary Elimination, 304
Vital Signs Status, 306
Well-Being, 307
Will to Live, 308
Wound Healing: Primary Intention, 309
Wound Healing: Secondary Intention, 310

PART THREE
Appendices, 313

Appendix A: NANDA-NOC Linkages, 315
Gail Keenan

Appendix B: Care Plans, 377

Appendix C: Case Study, 387
Cindy A. Scherb

Appendix D: Nursing-sensitive Outcomes Classification Review Form, 397

Nursing Outcomes Classification (NOC)

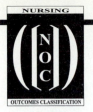

PART ONE

CONSTRUCTION OF THE OUTCOMES CLASSIFICATION

CHAPTER ONE

Outcome Development and Significance

T he restructuring of the U.S. health care system to increase economic efficiency has resulted in an emphasis on health care costs and patient outcomes as measures of system effectiveness. As health care costs have begun to stabilize, consumers and insurers have turned their attention to patient satisfaction and patient outcomes as criteria for selecting health care providers. The result has been the creation of a variety of evaluation tools designed to measure the outcomes of health care delivery systems. Although these measures have the potential to improve care delivery and to provide information about physician practice and organizational outcomes, the interventions and outcomes of nursing care are not readily apparent in most evaluation systems. As the nursing profession struggles to retain its identity in a health care system being restructured for greater efficiency, the need for nursing to define its interventions and outcomes has never been greater.

This book documents the development of standardized outcomes for the evaluation of nursing care. Part One provides background information for the standardized outcomes, which appear in Part Two. In Chapter One, outcome development in health care with an emphasis on nursing is described, and the need for a standardized outcome language for nursing is discussed. The research process used to develop the outcomes and the testing and implementation of the outcomes are described in the remaining chapters of Part One.

OUTCOME DEVELOPMENT IN HEALTH CARE

The systematic use of patient outcomes to evaluate health care began when Florence Nightingale recorded and analyzed health care conditions and patient outcomes during the Crimean War.[42,68] Since that time, attempts to identify, measure, and use patient outcomes in the evaluation of health care delivery have been sporadic, often discipline-specific, and commonly focused on physician practice.[33] Efforts to evaluate physician practice began in the early 1900s, when Codman, a Boston surgeon, proposed the use of outcome-based measures as indicators of medical care quality.[67] His work is considered the precursor of modern outcomes research. However, it wasn't until the mid-1960s that a model for assessing quality of physician practice was proposed by Donabedian.[12] This model, which emphasized structure, process, and outcome, was adopted by other health care disciplines and gained wide use as the preferred method of evaluating health care services. However, the complexity of problems inherent in identifying and measuring patient outcomes resulted in measures of structure and process developing more rapidly than measures of patient outcomes. Until the 1980s mortality, morbidity, and clinical signs served as traditional outcome measures,[43] and it wasn't until the emphasis on effectiveness in the mid-

1980s, fueled by political pressure and the availability of large data sets resulting from computerization, that attention again turned to measures of patient outcomes to evaluate physician practice. A recent, extensive study of physician practice, the Medical Outcomes Study (MOS), used a conceptual framework based on structure, process, and outcome to evaluate medical care effectiveness.[73] Outcome measures in the MOS were defined in the following four broad categories: *clinical end points,* which included signs and symptoms, laboratory values, and death; *functional status,* which included physical, mental, social, and role statuses; *general well-being,* which included health perceptions, energy/fatigue, pain, and life satisfaction, and *satisfaction with care,* which included access, convenience, financial coverage, quality, and general satisfaction. The study is significant for nursing because it was one of the first large national studies in which patient outcomes attributed to physician practice moved beyond the realm of disease-specific clinical outcomes to dimensions such as functional status, general well-being, and satisfaction. The study also has significance for health care in general because shortened versions of it, such as the Medical Outcomes Study Short Form-36 questions (MOS-SF-36),[76] used to evaluate physician practice have gained wide acceptance as general measures of health care delivery effectiveness.

Outcome Development in Nursing

The use of patient outcomes to evaluate nursing care quality began in the mid-1960s, when Aydelotte[3] used changes in behavioral and physical characteristics of patients to evaluate the effectiveness of nursing-care delivery systems. Since that time, additional patient outcome measures have been developed and tested for nursing[20] and a variety of patient outcomes have been used to evaluate the quality of nursing care and the effects of nursing interventions.[41,58,72]

In addition to the development and testing of outcome measures, nurses have expended considerable effort to categorize outcomes and define cardinal outcome measures. Early work to classify nursing-sensitive patient outcomes took place in the late 1970s. Hover and Zimmer[25] identified the following five general outcome criteria based on a review of patient outcomes used by nurses at that time:

- The patient's knowledge of illness and its treatments
- The patient's knowledge of medications
- The patient's self-care skills
- The patient's adaptive behaviors
- The patient's health status

Horn and Swain[24] conducted a major research effort to identify outcome measures useful for nursing research and categorized more than 300 indicators in the broad categories of universal demands and health deviation.

In the 1980s two outcome categorizations based on extensive reviews of outcomes used in nursing research were formulated. Lang and Clinton[41] identified the following six outcome categories:

- Physical health status
- Mental health status
- Social and physical functioning
- Health attitudes, knowledge, and behavior
- Use of professional health resources
- Patient perceptions of the quality of nursing care

Marek[47] identified the following 15 categories:

- Physiologic measures
- Psychosocial measures
- Functional status

- Client behaviors
- Client knowledge
- Symptom control
- Home maintenance
- Well-being
- Goal attainment
- Patient satisfaction
- Safety
- Frequency of service
- Cost
- Rehospitalization
- Resolution of nursing diagnoses

The increased importance placed on outcomes in the political arena in the 1990s resulted in a renewed emphasis on outcome development in nursing. McCormick[51] proposed a list of measurable outcomes that included process and patient outcomes as a method of evaluating nursing effectiveness. Patient outcomes identified as salient for nursing were normal fluid hydration, continence, mobility, and the absence of decubitus and mucosal membrane ulcers. A framework generated for use in hospital settings suggested the measurement of outcomes that evaluate patient/family education, facilitation of self-care, symptom distress management, provisions for patient safety, and enhancement of patient satisfaction.[17] Brown[6] proposed a conceptual framework for quality evaluation that included physiologic condition, psychologic status, health knowledge, and satisfaction. Naylor and associates[58] have suggested functional status, mental status, stress level, satisfaction with care, burden of care, and cost of care as appropriate outcomes for the evaluation of nursing care effectiveness.

Patient outcomes also have been developed for use in community and rehabilitative nursing practice. Daubert[9] proposed the following five categories to measure rehabilitation potential: (1) recovery, (2) self-care, (3) rehabilitation, (4) maintenance, and (5) terminal. Lalonde[40] developed and tested the following measures for home health evaluation: taking prescribed medications as instructed, general symptom distress, discharge status, caregiver status, functional status, knowledge of major health problems and diagnosis, and physiologic indicators. The Omaha Visiting Nurse Association has used the concepts of patient knowledge, patient behavior, and patient status to delineate specific outcomes for identified client problems.[49]

Most of the work done by the nursing profession in relation to outcome identification and categorization and the development of cardinal measures has been derived from literature reviews and practical experience rather than research or conceptual frameworks. A comparison of the outcomes developed for nurses and those for physicians demonstrates differences in the focuses of the two disciplines. Nursing outcomes have not emphasized laboratory values, death, access, and convenience. On the other hand, the nursing profession has included client knowledge and behaviors, safety, use of resources, home maintenance, and caregiver status—categories that may be influenced more by nursing care than by physician care and that seldom appear in current outcome evaluation tools.

Patient outcomes currently used to evaluate nursing practice are at three levels of abstraction. A number of broad outcome categories without specific measures (e.g., in the work of Marek) have been identified. At the other extreme, a multitude of specific outcome measures, or evaluation instruments, are used in clinical practice and clinical studies to evaluate patient outcomes related to specific nursing diagnoses and interventions. There also are an increasing number of outcomes at a middle level of abstraction in nursing care plans, critical paths, quality assurance programs, and nursing information systems. In general, specific outcome measures and intermediate level outcomes have not been used in a conceptual framework nor have they been placed in any of the current categorizations. An exception is the ongoing development of the Omaha Visiting Nurse Association system, in which their three broad categories of outcomes are being used to develop more specific measures of health status. Thus, there is a pressing need to (1) identify, label, define, and classify nursing-sensitive patient outcomes and indicators; (2) reconcile the classification with more general classifications of patient outcomes used in the health care sector; and (3) define specific measurement activities for the nursing-sensitive patient outcomes and indicators.[31]

Current Outcome Evaluation

Political interest in patient outcomes and health care costs initiated a revolution in health care in the late 1980s that has been labeled the "era of assessment and accountability."[27,65] This has put pressure on health care providers to justify their practice and its effects on patients and national health and has created a distinct area of study that Wennberg labeled "clinical evaluation science."[5,10] Basic questions being raised are: Is the care provided by one organization or agency worth the cost relative to the care provided by other organizations or agencies? What are the benefits patients receive from health care? What is the quality, and is it adequate in light of what is being paid?[69] What are the benefits to the health of the general population and individuals?[27] What outcomes can be expected, given various patient characteristics and states of health? If outcomes are not adequate, what changes are needed for improvement? If outcomes are adequate, can improvements still be achieved?[7] A variety of outcome measures have been developed in the last decade to answer these questions. Current outcome measures meet a number of needs, as illustrated in Fig. 1-1.

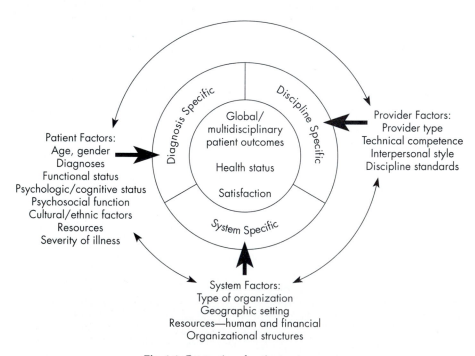

Fig. 1-1 Categories of patient outcomes.

Global, multidisciplinary patient outcomes tend to measure patient satisfaction with care and general health status, which often includes functional status, mental status, and role performance. In general, these measures were developed to evaluate the effectiveness of managed care systems or organizations and to provide information useful to insurers when selecting health care providers. Examples are HEDIS (Health Plan Employer Data and Information Set)[56,57] and the MOS-SF-36.[76] Although these global measures provide useful information, they often are not specific enough to determine accountability for changes necessary to improve outcomes. The inability to specify accountability occurs when responsibility for outcomes cannot be assigned to a health care provider or discipline. The fact that many of the widely used health status surveys are not suitable for monitoring the health and treatment status of individual patients, particularly those with chronic diseases,[53] contributes to the difficulty of identifying changes necessary to improve patient outcomes.

Diagnosis- or condition-specific outcomes, system-specific outcomes, and discipline-specific outcomes provide information about outcomes related to a specific diagnosis, organization, or discipline and may include measures that evaluate the effect on client knowledge, attitudes, and behaviors.[8] The outcomes in each of these areas are often intermediate outcomes that must be realized to achieve the more global, long-term outcomes related to health status and satisfaction with care.

Diagnosis-specific outcomes commonly are found in critical paths developed for use in an organization. A critical path may reflect current practices in a particular setting as well as practices identified through literature review. Outcomes commonly are stated as expected goals or end points. Standardized evaluation instruments, such as those developed by the Health Outcomes Institute,[19] assess treatment results for specific conditions but may focus primarily on physician-initiated treatments. Disease-specific outcomes normally are multidisciplinary- or physician-focused.

System-specific outcomes may include patient outcomes and structural or process outcomes that are used to evaluate the efficiency and effectiveness of a particular organization or managed care system. Global outcomes are used to evaluate patient status, and productivity measures, system costs, and system efficiencies may be used to evaluate the structure and process of the organization. These measures commonly are found in benchmarking or total-quality management systems put in place to evaluate organizational effectiveness and generally have a multidisciplinary focus.

System-specific measures that emphasize multidisciplinary outcomes provide valuable information about the effects of care, but make it difficult to determine accountability for outcomes.

Discipline-specific patient outcomes reflect the practice and standards of a health care discipline and are important for evaluating the performance and quality of that practice. To date, the focus of effectiveness research[64] using discipline-specific outcomes primarily has been on physician practices or process of care. Discipline-specific patient outcomes must be identified in each health care discipline so that each discipline can foster the development of knowledge and ensure that standards of care evolve as knowledge increases.

Attributes such as age, gender, functional status, and severity of illness are included in patient factors (see Fig. 1-1) because they can influence outcome achievement. These attributes are risk adjustment factors that must be considered when making outcome comparisons across settings or populations. Risk adjustment factors have been specified for a number of multidisciplinary or physician evaluation systems, but minimal work has been directed at the identification or risk adjustment factors for the evaluation of nursing practice.

REASONS FOR STANDARDIZED OUTCOMES FOR NURSING

For the nursing profession to become a full participant in clinical evaluation, it is essential that patient outcomes influenced by nursing care be identified and measured.[32,44,47] While it is recognized that the majority of patient outcomes, including those traditionally used to evaluate physician practice, are not influenced by any one discipline alone, it is essential for each discipline to identify the patient outcomes influenced by its practice to ensure that they are included in the evaluation of health care effectiveness. If nursing relies on physician-centered information only, "the impact of nursing care will remain largely unmeasured and therefore invisible."[46] For nurses to work effectively with managed care organizations to improve quality and reduce costs, nurses must be able to measure and document patient outcomes influenced by nursing care.[63] For example, the costs of decubitus ulcers are well-documented, and prevention is largely a function of nursing[52]; however, information about tissue integrity is not readily available in most clinical evaluation systems. The challenge facing the nursing profession is to create a common language that can be used to organize the phenomena of nursing practice without depersonalizing the patient.[39]

Creation of a Common Nursing Language

Creation of a common language for the nursing profession requires the identification, testing, and application of common terms and measures for nursing diagnoses, nursing interventions, nursing-care delivery structures and processes, and patient outcomes. Standardized nursing diagnoses have been under development since 1973, when the first invitational meeting of the National Conference Group for Classification of Nursing Diagnoses was convened in St. Louis.[77] Development of nursing diagnoses was formalized by the North American Nursing Diagnosis Association (NANDA) in 1982.[11] A comprehensive classification of nursing interventions has been developed by a research team at the University of Iowa.[30] This classification is coded for use in nursing information systems. Standard terminology for nursing diagnoses/patient problems, interventions/patient-care activities, and expected patient outcomes has been developed by Ozbolt and associates.[61] Work to standardize administrative data, including information about nursing-care delivery systems, currently is being conducted under the auspices of a team at the University of Iowa and the American Organization of Nurse Executives.[16]

In addition to the outcome work for nursing practice that was discussed earlier, there have been recent efforts to identify nursing-sensitive patient outcomes. The American Nurses' Association[2] has developed a Nursing Care Report Card for Acute Care. The report card identifies a core set of nursing quality indicators that includes structure, process, and outcome indicators. Outcome indicators include mortality rate, length of stay, adverse incidents, complications such as nosocomial infections and decubitus ulcers, and patient satisfaction with nursing care. A core set of outcomes has been identified and tested for home care.[69,70] The set consists of 12 global outcome measures applicable to all patients in home care and 13 outcome measures pertinent to patients with specified conditions[70] and has the added advantage of incorporating risk adjustment methods.

The outcomes presented in this text represent the work of a research team at the University of Iowa to identify outcomes and related measures at the individual patient level that can be used to evaluate nursing care across the patient care continuum. Although these measures are at the individual patient level, the outcome data can be aggregated in a number of ways to assess nursing care effectiveness within an organization and across various settings. This work differs from that previously mentioned because it is not specific to a condition or setting, although some outcomes and/or related measures will be used most frequently in a particular setting or with a particular patient population.

Computerized Nursing Information Systems

The growth of computerized nursing information systems creates a compelling need for a standardized language for nursing that includes, but is not limited to, patient outcomes influenced by nursing care. Nursing information systems have the potential for improving nursing performance, increasing nursing knowledge, and providing data and information necessary for nursing to participate in the formulation of health care policy.[26] Realizing the potential of such information systems, however, requires turning currently invisible nursing data into visible, productive data[71] that is standardized and can be aggregated and used to answer the pressing questions faced by the nursing profession. Unfortunately, few attempts have been made to standardize nursing data in clinical information systems, but rather current terminology and documentation have been automated.[29,51] As a consequence, software companies have tended to develop shells that can be individualized for each organization rather than producing software that creates comparable data across organizations. In 1984, Zielstorff noted that the lack of standard terminology for the nursing profession has been a major impediment to the development of nursing information systems,[80] and unfortunately the situation remains much the same today.

Outcomes in current nursing information systems appear in a variety of forms and normally are developed for use in one organization. Outcomes commonly appear as goal statements designed for use with either specific patient populations or multiple patient populations. Because they serve different purposes, goal statements vary in their degree of specificity. Statements may be quite specific and designed to reflect a discrete patient status or population (e.g., walks 10 feet without assistance, lists three expected effects of digitalis, and systolic blood pressure is between 100 and 150). Goal statements also may be more generic, applicable to a wide range of patients, and require a nursing judgment to determine whether a goal has been met (e.g., anxiety level is decreased, understands activity limitations, and blood pressure is in desired range).

One problem created by goal statements is that if the goal is not met, the health care professional has no way of knowing how close or how far the patient was from achieving the goal. Another problem is that information about patient status may be lost since patients may move from one health care setting to another over time. However, the major deficit is that goal statements developed at the organizational level create nonstandardized data that cannot be easily aggregated with those from other settings and populations. The use of a nationally standardized language and classification system with accepted coding would allow for the aggregation of data internally for organization reports and externally to add more comprehensive data to community and national data bases.[14]

Uniform Nursing Data Sets

A uniform data set "defines the central core of data needed on a routine basis by the majority of decision-makers about a given facet or dimension of the health care delivery system, and it establishes standard measurements, definitions, and classifications for this core."[55] Data-base development requires a common language and a standard way to organize data.[32] The essential first step in organizing and standardizing nursing information is to develop meaningful categories of data and establish uniform terminology.

A core set of data, referred to as the Nursing Minimum Data Set (NMDS), was identified in the 1980s under the leadership of Harriet Werley.[78] Consensus was reached on 16 core elements, which were grouped under the categories of nursing care, patient demographics, and service characteristics. Patient demographics and service characteristics are not unique to nursing and can be obtained from other health care data bases. The four elements in the nursing-care category—nursing diagnosis, nursing intervention, nursing outcome, and intensity of nursing care—are not available in a standardized data set because of the lack of a standardized language for each nursing care element.[11,48]

The National Association for Home Care has developed a uniform data set for home care and hospice. The data set is structured around organizational- and individual-level data items.[62] Items at the organizational level include service type and use and financial and personnel resources. Items at the individual level include patient demographics, medical diagnoses, surgical procedures, and patient use of services. The data set does not contain nursing diagnoses, interventions, or outcomes because these are areas without national consensus[62] and, thus, represent items that need to be developed.

Data sets facilitate the linkage of information in one data set to other data sets. This allows data in clinical information systems to be linked with administrative and other data sets for analysis. The use of logically linked data sets also decreases documentation work by reducing the need for repetitive documentation of information used for multiple purposes in an organization.[79]

National Data Sets

Physicians, health care organizations, and policy makers are extracting and analyzing data from national data sets to compare effectiveness and costs of care by provider and geographic area. "Results of such analyses increasingly form the basis of institutional, regulatory, and reimbursement policy decisions."[61] However, the majority of these data sets contain no information that reflects nursing practice, resulting in a lack of data supporting the effectiveness of nursing practice and its contributions to patient outcomes. The absence of nursing data is not the result of discrimination, but rather the result of the profession's failure to agree on and offer a set of clearly defined, valid, reliable, and standardized data elements for inclusion in national data sets.[60] Therefore the establishment of a set of standardized nursing data elements would allow data collected at the individual patient level to be coded and included in national data sets. This requires agreement on the data elements that are important and relevant for nursing, the measures or indicators to be used, a uniform coding system, and a cost-effective way to gather the data and input it into a computerized system.[59] The ideal solution for data input is the computerized clinical record that allows for data input at the point of service. The outcomes presented in Part Two will be coded for data input in the near future and can be input at the point of service.

In the current health care climate, nurses do not have the luxury of waiting for the future, because it is here. The nursing profession must be able to analyze the effectiveness of its interventions and practice and provide information about its role in patient welfare to influence health care policy.

Evaluation of Nursing Care Quality

The need for information about patient outcomes influenced by nursing has increased as organizations restructure to obtain greater efficiencies. Without this data, organizations have little information on which to base decisions about adjusting staff mix, determining the cost-effectiveness of various structural or process changes in the nursing-care delivery system, or providing information about the quality of nursing care available in the organization. Such information will be vital for organizations if

Congress passes the Patient Safety Act[22] or similar legislation requiring information about staffing and patient care quality.

Although quality of care can be examined from the perspectives of structure, process, and outcome, outcomes are essential components of any quality assurance or quality improvement program. "Outcomes are the changes, either favorable or adverse, in the actual or potential health status of persons, groups, or communities that can be attributed to prior or concurrent care."[13] Outcomes are the trigger for quality assurance programs since they answer the question, "Did the patient benefit or not benefit from the care provided?"[69] To facilitate continual quality improvement, information about patient outcomes should identify not only inadequate outcomes but also those that are marginal, adequate, and superior. Given that nursing care represents a majority of the hours of care provided in all settings except possibly physician offices and clinics,[1,15] it is essential that health care organizations and nursing practice settings be able to evaluate the quality of care provided by nursing staff. To do so, the identification and documentation of patient outcomes influenced by nursing practice is necessary, as well as the application of outcomes influenced by multiple health care providers. However, the Institute of Medicine[28] found in a review of nurse staffing and quality of care that existing work in outcome measurement typically has not focused on isolating the contribution of nursing to overall hospital quality.

The Nursing-sensitive Outcomes Classification described in this book is the first comprehensive list of standardized outcomes, definitions, and measures to describe patient outcomes influenced by nursing practice. The outcomes are presented as neutral concepts that reflect patient states (e.g., mobility, hydration, coping) that can be measured on a continuum rather than as discrete goals that are met or not met. This neutrality of concepts will facilitate the identification and analysis of outcomes currently achieved for specific patient populations and also facilitate the identification of realistic standards of care for specific populations.[45] For example, patients can be aggregated in a number of ways, such as by nursing or medical diagnoses, by service unit, or by severity of illness; and differences in outcome achievement can be analyzed by patient characteristics, such as age, gender, or functional status. This type of information can assist nurses in developing realistic standards that reflect currently achieved outcomes if the outcomes are satisfactory or can reflect desired, higher standards of achievement.[45] Such standards reflect variations in outcomes that occur within a patient population because of patient characteristics that cannot be changed. This is quite different from the usual practice of setting one standard or selecting one goal for all patients, regardless of individual patient characteristics that may constitute considerable risk in relation to outcome achievement. "From a quality improvement perspective, it is important to be able to identify a realistic outcome to be achieved. Unrealistic outcome expectations are inefficient in that resources may be expended to no good effect."[54] For comparison of quality across organizations it is necessary to ensure that the effects of structure and process on patient outcomes are being measured and not the effects of patient characteristics.[75]

Quality patient care requires the collaboration of all health care providers and is measured at the organizational level using outcomes that reflect a multidisciplinary approach to patient care. Illness-related measures have been the traditional measures of quality but are now being expanded to include wellness-related measures and patient satisfaction. The addition of nursing-sensitive patient outcomes related to wellness and satisfaction can contribute to organizational data used to evaluate health care quality. Additionally, knowledge of intermediate outcomes that may be influenced primarily by one discipline is necessary to identify and change structures and processes that inhibit the achievement of quality patient care. For example, functional status may be hindered by decubitus ulcers or inadequate patient knowledge—intermediate outcomes of concern primarily to nurses that will not be available for outcome analysis if not measured by nurses.

Evaluation of Nursing Innovations

Innovations are new ideas or techniques used to solve a problem.[36] They are necessary for the development and refinement of basic and applied knowledge. Nursing innovations can consist of new interventions, revised interventions, or the use of interventions in a new way to solve clinical problems. They also can be strategies, structures, or processes used to solve management problems.[50] In each instance, patient outcomes are desirable criteria for evaluating innovation effectiveness. In the case of clinical innovations, improved patient outcomes may be the only evaluation criterion. In the case of management innovations, patient outcomes need to be evaluated in conjunction with other outcomes, such as cost reduction or staff mix, to ensure the management innovation did not adversely affect patient outcomes.

Clinical innovations initially are evaluated through controlled clinical studies, with attention given to the measurement of desired or expected outcomes. Many clinical studies in nursing are conducted in one or a few sites and with relatively small samples. Generalizability of such studies can be increased using metaanalysis if study variables are similar. The use of standardized patient outcomes as one of the study variables would increase the ease with which findings can be compared across settings.

Management innovations may be initiated without an evaluation plan, and when such a plan is used, it may not include patient outcomes. The result is a paucity of empirical data about the relationships between structural measures, such as nurse staffing ratios, and quality of care in terms of patient outcomes[28] and the relationship between processes, such as the type of nursing delivery system, and quality of care. This is particularly bothersome in an era of restructuring and rapid change in health care organizations. Although managers may be forced to make decisions about structural and process changes without empirical data, potential problems can be alleviated if adequate outcome data, including patient outcome data, are identified and collected. The use of standardized outcomes will allow for the comparison of patient outcomes across sites and increase understanding of the effects of structural and process changes on patient outcomes and quality of care.

Contribution to Knowledge Development

The development of nursing knowledge requires the use of patient outcome measures. The effectiveness of a nursing intervention and the appropriateness of the decision-making process in selecting an intervention for a patient are determined by the resulting patient outcomes. Expanding this knowledge beyond the individual patient to patient populations requires massive amounts of clinical data that allow linkages to be drawn between and among diagnoses, patient characteristics, interventions, and outcomes.[29] Standardized data bases using a common language are the most feasible method of obtaining information necessary to analyze these linkages. Large data bases can provide information to a discipline about the effectiveness of current practices and assist in the development of performance goals and practice parameters. Practice parameters, such as the guidelines developed by the Agency for Health Care Policy and Research, provide strategies for patient management and assist clinicians in clinical decision making.[23]

Classifications of nursing diagnoses, nursing interventions, and nursing outcomes provide lexical elements for the development of middle-range theories that delineate the substantive structure or the aspects of health care that nurses address,[74] as illustrated in Fig. 1-2. Classifications that define the pattern of nursing diagnoses, interventions, and outcomes provide the vertical shafts for the development of middle-range theories used to build the substantive structure of nursing.[74] Using these classifications allows middle-range theory development to build on elements unique to nursing, as well as the "borrowed knowledge" and theories from other disciplines.[66,74] The usefulness of each classification relies on research that links the processes of care to outcomes and the development of explanatory theory.[4,37] Lexical and taxonomic development that provides standardized terms in a constructed classification fosters inductive theory formulation and the empirical testing of deductive theories. Although these classifications provide elements important for the development of substantive nursing theory, they will be expanded or complemented with other knowledge and theories as nursing knowledge develops.

A classification of nursing-sensitive patient outcomes may be the first, but not the only, step for the use of outcomes in the study of nursing practice. Issues related to outcome measurement have been well-documented in the literature,[4,18,21,35,38,43] but some of these issues will be best resolved with the use of standardized languages and data bases that can be used to study relationships between outcomes, between outcomes and patient characteristics, and between outcomes and nursing interventions.

For example, attributing a change in health status to nursing practice requires an understanding of factors that influence patient outcomes and the appropriate timing for data collection. The identification of patient characteristics or risk factors that influence outcome achievement has been used in the study of physician outcomes, but its use has been rare in nursing research. Identification of such factors is a prerequisite in the study of nursing-care effectiveness when the controls used in efficacy research

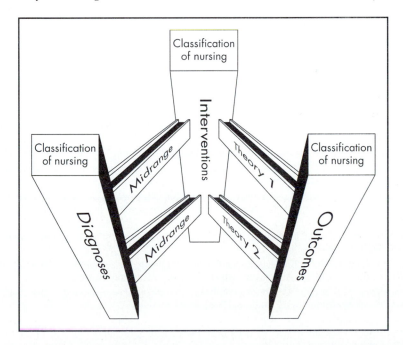

Fig. 1-2 Relationships of nursing diagnoses, interventions, and outcomes of midrange theories. (From Tripp-Reimer, T., Woodworth, G., McCloskey, J., Bulecheck, G.M. [1996]. The dimensional structure of nursing interventions. *Nursing Research,* 45[1].)

are not in place. Identification of risk factors also is necessary when comparing outcomes across settings. The anticipated change in patient health status may not occur immediately following a nursing intervention; however, the ideal time for evaluation of clinical outcomes, that is when treatment outcomes are sufficiently robust to be significant,[34] often is not known. These are only two examples of the questions that must be addressed for nursing to participate fully in outcomes research that focuses on the effectiveness, rather than the efficacy, of health care processes.

SUMMARY

There is a need for standardized language and data-base development in nursing if nursing is to become a full participant in health care restructuring. Policy decisions will not be responsive to a discipline that cannot provide data supporting its effectiveness. Nursing-sensitive patient outcomes provide one of the data elements for the Nursing Minimum Data Set. Development and use of such a data set will provide nurses the information needed for the determination of nursing practice effectiveness.

References

1. Aiken, L.A., Smith, H.L., & Lake, E.T. (1994). Lower Medicare mortality among a set of hospitals known for good nursing care. *Medical Care, 32*, 771-787.

2. American Nurses' Association. (1995). *Nursing Care Report Card for Acute Care.* Washington, DC: Author.

3. Aydelotte, M. (1962). The use of patient welfare as a criterion measure, *Nursing Research, 11*, 10-14.

4. Bond, S. & Thomas, L.H. (1991). Issues in measuring outcomes of nursing. *Journal of Advanced Nursing, 16*, 1492-1502.

5. Brook, H.L. (1989). Practice guidelines and practicing: Are they compatible? *Journal of the American Medical Association, 262*, 3027-3030.

6. Brown, D.S. (1992). A conceptual framework for the evaluation of service quality. *Journal of Nursing Care Quality, 6*, 66-74.

7. Carey, R.G. & Lloyd, R.C. (1995). *Measuring Quality Improvement in Healthcare: A Guide to Statistical Process Control Applications.* New York: Quality Resources, a Division of the Kraus Organization Limited.

8. Centers for Disease Control and Prevention (1992). *The Planned Approach to Community Health: A Guide for the Local PATCH Coordinator.* Atlanta: U.S. Department of Health and Human Services, Public Health Service.

9. Daubert, E.A. (1979). Patient classification and outcome criteria. *Nursing Outlook, 27*, 450-454.

10. DeFriese, G.H. (1990). Measuring the effectiveness of medical interventions: New expectations of health services research. *Health Services Research, 25*, 697-708.

11. Delaney, C., Mehmert, P.A., Prophet, C,. Bellinger, S.L., Huber, D.H., & Ellerbe, S. (1992). Standardized nursing language for healthcare information systems. *Journal of Medical Systems, 16*(4), 145-159.

12. Donabedian, A. (1966). Evaluating the quality of medical care. *Milbank Memorial Fund Quarterly, 44*(3), 166-206.

13. Donabedian, A. (1985). *The Methods and Findings of Quality Assessment and Monitoring: An Illustrated Analysis,* Vol. 3. Ann Arbor, MI: Health Administration Press.

14. Donaldson, M.S. & Lohr, K.N. (Eds.). (1994). *Health Data in the Information Age: Use, Disclosure, and Privacy.* Washington, DC: National Academy Press.

15. Flarey, D.L. & Blancett, S.S. (1995). Management and organizational restructuring: Reforming the corporate system. In S. S. Blancett & D. Flarey (Eds.), *Reengineering Nursing and Health Care.* Gaithersburg, MD: Aspen.

16. Gardner, D.L., Delaney, C., Crossley, J., Mehmert, P., & Ellerbe, S. (1992). A nursing management minimum data set: Significance and development. *Journal of Nursing Administration, 22*, 7.

17. Gillette, B., & Jenko, M. (1991). Major clinical functions: A unifying framework for measuring outcomes. *Journal of Nursing Care Quality, 6,* 20-24.

18. Harris, M.R. & Warren, J.J. (1995). Patient outcomes: Assessment issues for the CNS. *Clinical Nurse Specialist, 9*(2), 82-86.

19. Health Outcomes Institute. (1993). *Condition-specific Type Specifications.* Bloomington, MN: Author.

20. Heater, B.S., Becker, A.M. & Olson, R.K. (1988). Nursing interventions and patient outcomes: A meta-analysis of studies. *Nursing Research, 37,* 303-307.

21. Hegyvary, S. (1991). Issues in outcomes research. *Journal of Nursing Quality Assurance, 5*(2), 1-6.

22. Helmlinger, C.S. (1996). ANA's landmark patient safety legislation debuts on Capitol Hill. *The American Nurse, 28*(4), 1 & 10.

23. Hirshfeld, E.B. (1994). Practice parameters versus outcome measurements: How will prospective and retrospective approaches to quality management fit together? *Nutrition in Clinical Practice, 9*(6), 207-215.

24. Horn, B.J. & Swain, M.A. (1978). *Criterion Measures of Nursing Care.* (DHEW Pub. No. PHS 78-3187). Hyattsville, MD: National Center for Health Services Research.

25. Hover, J, & Zimmer, M. (1978). Nursing quality assurance: The Wisconsin system. *Nursing Outlook, 26,* 242-248.

26. Huber, D. & Delaney, C. (1996). Unpublished manuscript. Iowa City, IA: The University of Iowa.

27. Iezzoni, L.I. (1994). Risk and outcomes. In L.I. Iezzoni (Ed.), *Risk Adjustment for Measuring Health Care Outcomes* (pp. 1-28). Ann Arbor, MI: Health Administration Press.

28. Institute of Medicine. Wunderlich, G.S., Sloan, F.A., & Davis, C.K. (Eds.) (1996). *Nursing Staff in Hospitals and Nursing Homes: Is It Adequate?* Washington, DC: National Academy Press.

29. Iowa Intervention Project. (1992). *Nursing Interventions Classification (NIC).* St. Louis: Mosby.

30. Iowa Intervention Project. (1996). *Nursing Interventions Classification (NIC)* (2nd ed.). St. Louis: Mosby.

31. Jenkins, C.D. (1992). Assessment of outcomes of health interventions. *Social Science Medicine, 35*(4), 367-375.

32. Jennings, B.M. (1991). Patient outcomes research: Seizing the opportunity. *Advances in Nursing Science, 14*(2), 59-72.

33. Johnson, M. & Maas, M. (1994). Nursing-focused patient outcomes: Challenge for the nineties. In J. McCloskey & H. Grace (Eds.), *Current Issues in Nursing* (pp. 643-649) (4th ed.). St. Louis: Mosby.

34. Johnston, M.V. & Granger, C.V. (1994). Outcomes research in medical rehabilitation. *American Journal of Physical Medicine & Rehabilitation, 73*(4), 296-303.

35. Jones, K.R. (1993). Outcomes analysis: Methods and issues. *Nursing Economics, 11,* 145-152.

36. Kanter, R.M. (1983). *The Change Masters: Innovation for Productivity in the American Corporation.* New York: Simon & Schuster.

37. Keith, R.A. (1995). Conceptual basis of outcome measures. *American Journal of Physical Medicine & Rehabilitation, 74*(1), 73-80.

38. Kelsey, A. (1995). Outcome measures: Problems and opportunities for public health nursing. *Journal of Nursing Management, 3,* 183-187.

39. Kritek, P.V. (1989). An introduction to the science and art of taxonomy. In American Nurses Association (Ed.), *Classification Systems for Describing Nursing Practice: Working Papers* (pp. 6-12). Kansas City, KS: American Nurses' Association.

40. Lalonde, B. (1988). Assuring the quality of home care via the assessment of client outcomes. *Caring, 12*(1), 20-24.

41. Lang, N.M. & Clinton, J.F. (1984). Assessment of quality of nursing care. *Annual Review of Nursing Research 2,* 135-163.

42. Lang, N.M. & Marek, K.D. (1990). The classification of patient outcomes. *Journal of Professional Nursing, 6,* 153-163.

43. Lohr, K.N. (1988). Outcome measurement: Concepts and questions. *Inquiry, 25*(1), 37-50.

44. Lower, M.S. & Burton, S. (1989). Measuring the impact of nursing interventions on patient outcomes: The challenge of the 1990s. *Journal of Nursing Quality Assurance,* 4(1), 27-34.

45. Maas, M.L., Johnson, M.R., & Kraus, V.L. (1996). In K. Kelly (Ed.), *Outcomes of Effective Management Practice, SONA 8* (pp. 20-35). Thousand Oaks, CA: Sage.

46. Mallison, M.B. (1990). Editorial: Access to invisible expressways. *American Journal of Nursing,* 90(9), 7.

47. Marek, K.D. (1989). Outcomes measurement in nursing. *Journal of Nursing Quality Assurance,* 4(1), 1-9.

48. Mark, B.A. & Burleson, D.L. (1995). Measurement of patient outcomes: Data availability and consistency across hospitals. *Journal of Nursing Administration,* 25(4), 52-59.

49. Martin, K.S. & Scheet, N.J. (1992). *The Omaha System: Applications for Community Health Nursing.* Philadelphia: W.B. Saunders.

50. McCloskey, J.C., Maas, M.L., Huber, D.G., Kasparek, A., Specht, J.P., Ramler, C.L., Watson, C., Blegen, M., Delaney, C., Ellerbe, S., Etscheidt, C., Gongaware, C., Johnson, M.R., Kelly, K.C., Mehmert, P., & Clougherty, J. (1996). Nursing management innovations: A need for systematic evaluation. In K. Kelly (Ed.), *Outcomes of Effective Management Practice, SONA 8.* Thousand Oaks, CA: Sage.

51. McCormick, K. (1991). Future data needs for quality care monitoring, DRG considerations, reimbursement and outcome measurement. *Image,* 23(1), 29-32.

52. McFarland, G.K. & McFarlane, E.A. (1993). *Nursing Diagnosis and Intervention: A Model for Clinical Practice.* St. Louis: Mosby.

53. McHorney, C.A. & Tarlov, A.R. (1995). Individual-patient monitoring in clinical practice: Are available health status surveys adequate? *Quality of Life Research,* 4, 293-307.

54. Mills, W.C. (1994). Tacking through troubled waters: Toward desired outcomes. In R.M. Carroll-Johnson & M. Paquette (Eds.), *Classification of Nursing Diagnosis: Proceedings of the Tenth Conference* (pp. 126-130). Philadelphia: J.B. Lippincott.

55. Murnaghan, H. (1978). Uniform basic data sets for health statistical systems. *International Journal of Epidemiology,* 7, 263-269.

56. National Committee for Quality Assurance. (1993). *Health Plan Employer Data and Information Set 2.0 (HEDIS 2.0).* Washington, DC: Author.

57. National Committee for Quality Assurance. (1995). *Health Plan Employer Data and Information Set 2.1 (HEDIS 2.1).* Washington, DC: Author.

58. Naylor, M.D., Munro, B.H., & Brooten, D.A. (1991). Measuring the effectiveness of nursing practice. *Clinical Nurse Specialist,* 5, 210-215.

59. Niemeyer, L.O. & Foto, M. (1995). Using outcomes data. *REHAB Management,* April/May, 105-106.

60. Ozbolt, J. (1991). Strategies for building nursing databases for effectiveness research. Invited paper presented to National Center for Nursing Research, September 11-13, Rockville, MD.

61. Ozbolt, J.G., Fruchtnight, J.N., & Hayden, J.R. (1994). Toward data standards for clinical nursing information. *Journal of the American Medical Informatics Association,* 1(2), 175-185.

62. Pace, K.B. (1995). Data sets for home care organizations. *Caring,* 14:3, 38-42.

63. Phoon, J., Corder, K., & Barter, M. (1996). Managed care and total quality management: A necessary integration. *Journal of Nursing Care Quality,* 10(2), 25-32.

64. Prescott, P.A. (1993). Nursing: An important component of hospital survival under a reformed health care system. *Nursing Economics,* 11, 192-199.

65. Relman, A.S. (1988). Assessment and accountability: The third revolution in medical care. *New England Journal of Medicine,* 319, 1220-1222.

66. Retsas, A. (1995). Knowledge and practice development: Toward an ontology of nursing. *The Australian Journal of Advanced Nursing,* 12(2), 20-25.

67. Reverby, S. (1981). Stealing the golden eggs: Ernest Amory Codman and the science and management of medicine. *Bulletin of the History of Medicine,* 55, 156-171.

68. Salive, M.E., Mayfield, J.A. & Weissman, N.W. (1990). Patient outcomes research teams and the Agency for Health Care Policy and Research. *Health Services Research,* 25, 697-708.

69. Shaughnessy, P.W. & Crisler, K.S. (1995). *Outcome-based Quality Improvement: A Manual for Home Care Agencies on How to Use Outcomes.* Washington, DC: National Association for Home Care.

70. Shaughnessy, P.W., Crisler, K.S., Schlenker, R.E., & Arnold, A.G. (1995). Outcome-based quality improvement in home care. *Caring,* 14:2, 44-49.

71. Simpson, R. (1991). Adopting a nursing minimum data set. *Nursing Management,* 22(2), 20-21.

72. Sovie, M.D. (1989). Clinical nursing practices and patient outcomes: Evaluation, evolution, and revolution. *Nursing Economics, 7,* 79-85.

73. Tarlov, A.R., Ware, J.E., Greenfield, S., Nelson, E.C., Perrin, E, & Zubkoff, M. (1989). The Medical Outcomes Study: An application of methods for monitoring the results of medical care. *Journal of the American Medical Association,* 262, 925-930.

74. Tripp-Reimer, T., Woodworth, G., McCloskey, J.C., & Bulechek, G.M. (1996). The dimensional structure of nursing interventions. *Nursing Research,* 45, 10-17.

75. United States General Accounting Office. (1994). *Health Care Reform "Report Cards" are Useful but Significant Issues Need to Be Addressed* (Pub. No. GAO/HEHS 94-219). Gaithersburg, MD: Author.

76. Ware, J.E. & Sherbourne, C.D. (1992). The MOS 36-item short-form health survey (SF-36). I. Conceptual framework and item selection. *Medical Care,* 30, 473-481.

77. Warren, J.J. & Hoskins, L.M. (1991). The development of NANDA's nursing diagnosis taxonomy. *Nursing Diagnosis,* 1, 162-168.

78. Werley, H. & Lang, N. (1988). *Identification of the Nursing Minimum Data Set.* New York: Springer.

79. Westra, B. & Raup, G. (1995). Computerized charting: An essential tool for survival. *Caring,* 14:8, 57-61.

80. Zielstorff, R.D. (1984). Why aren't there more significant automated nursing information systems? *Journal of Nursing Administration,* 14(1), 7-10.

CHAPTER TWO

Overview of the Nursing-sensitive Patient Outcomes Research

T his chapter is an overview of the research conducted thus far to develop and test the Nursing-sensitive Outcomes Classification (NOC). Preliminary work to classify nursing interventions laid the foundation for the NOC research, specifically the conceptualization of outcomes responsive to nursing interventions and the qualitative and quantitative methods used to develop the outcomes and to assess the content validity of the outcomes and indicators. In Phase I of the research, conceptual and methodologic issues were identified and resolved, and outcome statements used by nurses were gathered, organized in clusters, and given conceptual outcome labels. Phase II included the refinement and content validation of each outcome through concept analysis and surveys of nurse experts. Field testing of the nursing-sensitive patient outcomes is ongoing in Phase II, and the outcomes and indicators are being organized in a classification structure, with defined rules and principles that determine the structure; at present the outcomes are classified in an alphabetical list. Plans for Phase III of the research focus on testing measurement scales and procedures, including risk adjustments, for the outcomes and indicators. Plans also call for the validation of the classification structure and further field testing to describe the use of the outcomes and linkages between diagnoses, interventions, and outcomes in specific patient populations and health care settings.

PURPOSES AND SIGNIFICANCE OF THE RESEARCH

The purpose of the NOC research is threefold: (1) to identify, label, validate, and classify nursing-sensitive patient outcomes and indicators; (2) to field test and validate the classification; and (3) to define and test measurement procedures for the outcomes and indicators.

The NOC is complementary to taxonomies of the North American Nursing Diagnosis Association (NANDA)[15,17] and the Nursing Interventions Classification (NIC).[9] The NOC provides the language for the evaluation step of the nursing process and the content for the outcomes element in the Nursing Minimum Data Set. The documentation of the outcomes has been encouraged by NANDA's work to develop a taxonomy of nursing diagnoses; the advancement of the Nursing Minimum Data Set[22,23]; the work to classify nursing interventions[7,9,18]; the development of computerized information systems in health care and the associated large uniform data bases; and the emphasis on demonstrating medical effectiveness. However, the definition and classification of clinically useful nursing-sensitive patient outcomes had not been accomplished before the NOC. Further, there are few conceptual frameworks of nursing-sensitive patient outcomes, and existing ones tend to describe broad categories of outcomes and are not validated. The NOC is especially significant because standardized languages for nursing diagnoses, interventions, and outcomes that can be computerized are needed for the study of linkages between diagnoses, interventions, and outcomes discovered through the documentation and study of actual patient care.

PRELIMINARY WORK RELATED TO NOC

Related work at the University of Iowa College of Nursing laid the foundations for the NOC research. The research to classify nursing interventions[9] provided the impetus for the NOC research by creating a heightened awareness of the need to classify nursing phenomena, including nursing-sensitive outcomes, and by providing some methods and experiences that were adapted for the classification of outcomes and indicators. Nursing Service Administration faculty at the university developed a conceptual framework, the Iowa Model of Nursing Administration, that depicts the relationships between individual, organizational, and environmental provider and outcome variables.[6,10] Several members of the NOC research team also were members of the Nursing Administration Research Team (NART) at the University of Iowa. The NART team designed a portfolio of methods and instruments to be used by nursing and other health care managers to evaluate the outcomes of innovations in health services organizations.[13]

Pilot Studies of Patient Satisfaction Outcomes

Two pilot studies were conducted to test the methodology of validating nursing-sensitive patient outcomes and indicators. The Fehring method was used to assess content validity. Patient satisfaction with nursing outcomes and related indicators also were included in these studies. The identified outcomes based on a review of literature included satisfaction with the following:
- Physical environment
- Availability and access to care
- Provision for patient rights
- Caring
- Technical aspects of care
- Meeting physical needs
- Continuity of care
- Functional status
- Teaching/counseling
- Communication
- Symptom control
- Costs and finances
- Safety

The pilot studies were conducted by two students in the master's program to meet thesis requirements. Study results supported the methodology used to validate the NOC outcomes and supported the need for further work.

The master's program students used an adaptation of the Fehring technique[4,5] to validate patient satisfaction with nursing outcomes among a sample of inpatients and their nurses in an acute hospital medical/surgical setting and among a sampling of outpatients and nurses in a medical ambulatory–care setting. Patients had no difficulty responding to how important particular indicator items are to patient satisfaction; however, they had great difficulty identifying nursing's contribution to the outcomes and indicators. Nurses, on the other hand, were able to identify both the importance of the indicator items and the contribution of nursing. Based on the findings, the following changes were made in the surveys for content validation of the remaining nursing-sensitive patient outcomes and indicators. First, the number of indicators were kept to a minimum and did not exceed 20 for each identified outcome. Second, patients were not asked to validate outcomes and indicators. Although the team continues to believe data from patients are important and had originally hoped to have a sampling of patients respond to what they perceive as nursing's contribution to each outcome, the use of patient ratings or interviews is planned for a later phase of the research. Overall, the results of content validation of patient satisfaction with nursing outcomes using an adaptation of the Fehring method[4,5] indicated that the method was a useful approach. In addition, most patient satisfaction outcomes and indicators identified through the literature review were rated as content valid and nursing responsive.

DEVELOPMENT OF THE NOC RESEARCH TEAM

The NOC research team was formed in August 1991 at the University of Iowa. Its purpose was to conceptualize, label, and classify nursing-sensitive patient outcomes. The team consists of 17 investigators, including a biostatistician, seven graduate students (four doctoral students), two postdoctoral students, and four consultants. Initially, work began to identify and resolve conceptual and methodologic issues and to generate an initial list of nursing-sensitive patient outcome labels and indicators. As the work progressed, more than 20 master's-degreed clinicians from surrounding hospitals and nursing and community health practice sites joined the research team to assist with the development and refinement of the outcomes and indicators.

RESOLUTION OF ISSUES AND DEVELOPMENT OF THE INITIAL LIST OF OUTCOMES
Identification and Resolution of Conceptual and Methodologic Issues

To prepare for the identification and resolution of conceptual and methodologic issues, the team reviewed the literature on patient outcomes, information systems, the science of taxonomic classification, and relevant qualitative and quantitative methods. Team members reviewed multiple sources of patient outcomes used by nurses (textbooks, nursing information systems, critical pathways and care plans, outcome studies, standards of practice), conceptual frameworks, and outcome classifications.

The following seven questions that provided the conceptual approach for the Nursing-sensitive Outcomes Classification (NOC) were identified and resolved:
1. Who is the patient?
2. What do patient outcomes describe?
3. At what levels of abstraction should outcomes be developed?
4. How should the outcomes be stated?
5. What are nursing-sensitive patient outcomes?
6. Are nursing-sensitive patient outcomes the resolution of nursing diagnoses?
7. When should patient outcomes be measured?

These issues were resolved as follows, although in research of this type, issues continue to arise that the team must address.

1. **Who is the patient?** Patient outcomes focus on the recipient of care; however, the traditional use of the term *patient* is too limiting for evaluation of all nursing practice purposes. *Patient* traditionally has been defined as an individual recipient of care; however, because family caregivers and significant others often are integrally involved with patients and their care, they also are recipients of nursing care. The term *patient* is used regardless of the care setting, even though the team recognizes that the care recipient may be called "client" or "resident" in some settings.

Data ordinarily are collected on individuals and aggregated to characterize other units of analysis (e.g., patient groups, organizations, communities), but some outcomes may require data to be collected at a group level.[8] Because of the need to limit the scope of the research and to address outcomes of priority importance, the research team decided to use individuals as the focal unit for the development of the NOC, with family caregivers included to assess the full impact of nursing on individuals. Outcomes for other units, such as family, community, and organization will be developed in a later phase of the research.

2. **What do patient outcomes describe?** Like nursing diagnoses, the phenomena of concern with nursing-sensitive patient outcomes are individual patient or family caregiver states or behaviors, including perceptions or subjective states.[3] These phenomena are in contrast to nursing interventions, in which the phenomena of concern are nurse behaviors.[9] The phenomena of concern with nursing-sensitive patient outcomes also are in contrast to nursing diagnoses, in which the phenomena of concern are patient states identified for improvement. Patient states that are assessed but do not follow an intervention are not outcomes. *Outcomes* describe patient states that follow and are expected to be influenced by an intervention. For the team's research, a *nursing-sensitive patient outcome* is defined as a variable patient or family caregiver state, behavior, or perception that is responsive to a nursing intervention and conceptualized at middle levels of abstraction (e.g., mobility level, nutritional status, health beliefs). *Nursing-sensitive outcome indicators* are defined as variable patient or family caregiver states, behaviors, or perceptions at a low level of abstraction that are responsive to nursing intervention and used for determining a patient outcome (e.g., for the outcome Mobility Level, indicators include "joint movement," "transfer performance," and "ambulation: walking"). The definitions and indicators acknowledge that nurses, family caregivers, and patients supply outcomes data and that both the patient and family caregiver are the focus of outcomes. Definitions of terms used in the research are listed in Box 2-1.

In contrast to the Joint Commission on Accreditation of Healthcare Organizations' use of the term *indicator* as a quantitative measure,[14,16] the team uses the term *nursing-sensitive outcome indicator* to describe the specific patient states that are most sensitive to nursing interventions and for which measurement procedures can be defined. To facilitate measurement of change, outcomes are conceptualized as nonevaluative, variable patient states influenced by nursing intervention. Thus, patient outcomes represent patient states that vary and can be measured and compared with a baseline over time. As Bond and Thomas[1] note, the requirement of predetermined outcomes that require a specific change is unnecessary. Unintended consequences of nursing interventions and maintenance of steady states also are valid and may be desirable outcomes.[1] Therefore nursing-sensitive patient outcomes are **not** viewed as goals, although the outcomes and indicators can be used to set goals for specific patients with baseline status and change in status assessed over time.

3. **At what levels of abstraction should outcomes be developed?** When complete, the NOC is expected to contain patient outcomes and indicators at four levels of abstraction, with measurement procedures at the empirical level (Fig. 2-1). At the highest levels of abstraction, outcome categories and classes will be derived from the results of hierarchic clustering, which is a statistical procedure, and qualitative strategies used in the research. These results will be compared with outcome cate-

---

BOX 2-1
Definition of Terms

Classification of Nursing-sensitive Patient/Family Outcomes*

The ordering, or arranging, of nursing-sensitive patient outcomes and indicators into groups or sets on the basis of their relationships and the assigning of labels and definitions to these groups.

Nursing-sensitive Patient Outcome

A measurable patient or family caregiver state, behavior, or perception that is conceptualized as a variable and is largely influenced by and sensitive to nursing interventions. A nursing-sensitive patient outcome is at the conceptual level. To be measured, an outcome requires identification of a series of more specific indicators. Nursing-sensitive patient outcomes define the general patient state, behavior, or perception resulting from nursing interventions.

Nursing-sensitive Patient Outcome Indicator

A specific variable referent of a nursing-sensitive patient outcome that is sensitive to nursing interventions. An indicator is an observable patient state, behavior, or self-reported perception or evaluation. Nursing-sensitive patient outcome indicators characterize a patient state at the concrete level. Examples of indicators are: "describes reasons why medication must be taken according to prescribed dose and schedule;" "notifies caregiver when needs to urinate."

Nursing-sensitive Outcome Measures

The operations or activities that describe precisely what outcome indicator is to be measured, how it is to be measured, and how it will be quantified. Quantification will reflect a continuum, such as 1 = toilets self independently; 2 = requires some assistance with clothing for toileting; 3 = requires assistance with transfer for toileting; and 4 = requires total assistance for toileting.

---

*When reference is made to nursing-sensitive outcomes the term *patient* also includes family caregiver.

Most abstract	Nursing-sensitive outcome categories
High-middle level abstraction	Nursing-sensitive outcome classes
Middle level abstraction	Nursing-sensitive outcome labels
Low level abstraction	Nursing-sensitive outcome indicators
Empirical level	Measurement activities for outcomes

Fig. 2-1 Levels of outcomes in the taxonomy.

gories promulgated by the Medical Outcomes Study (MOS)[20] and with current nursing outcome categories.[11,12] The least abstract level will contain indicator statements for each outcome label. Outcome labels are at middle levels of abstraction; and in some instances indicators for more abstract, global outcomes also are developed as more specific, less abstract outcomes. For example, an indicator for the outcome Mobility Level is "joint movement," whereas neck is an indicator for the

---

BOX 2-2

Rules for Standardization of Nursing-sensitive Outcomes

An outcome label is concise; stated in five or fewer words.

An outcome label is stated in nonevaluative terms rather than as a decreased, increased, or improved state.

An outcome label does **not** describe a nurse behavior or intervention.

An outcome label is **not** stated as a nursing diagnosis.

An outcome label describes a patient state, behavior, or perception that is inherently variable and can be measured and quantified.

An outcome label is conceptualized and stated at a middle level of abstraction.

Colons are used to make broader concept labels more specific; however, the broader label is stated first, with the colon and more specific label following (e.g., Nutritional Status: Intake or Nutritional Status: Energy Level).

---

outcome Joint Movement: Active. The empirical level will include measurement activities for each outcome and its indicators.

It is important that all outcome measures are quantifiable and psychometrically sound for the development of manageable computerized data bases that are optimally useful for assessing the efficacy and effectiveness of nursing interventions. Activities to develop and test the measurement procedures for each outcome are planned for a later phase of the research.

4. **How should the outcomes be stated?** Because the outcomes and indicators are conceptualized as variable patient or family caregiver states, behaviors, or perceptions, they are given labels representing concepts that can be measured along a continuum as negative or positive states. Whenever possible the team avoided labels that describe an undesirable state. However, because of the common use of some labels or difficulty identifying an antonym, some outcome labels do describe an undesirable state (e.g., the outcomes Infection Status and Pain Level).

Conceptualization of the outcomes as variable patient states allows for the description of negative or positive changes or a lack of change resulting from nursing interventions.[3] The research team defined a set of rules (Box 2-2) to guide the conceptualizion of the outcomes and the writing of nursing-sensitive outcome labels.

5. **What are nursing-sensitive patient outcomes?** To be useful for assessing the effectiveness of nursing, outcomes and indicators that are influenced by nursing and comprehensive enough to assess all aspects of nursing practice must be identified. The team recognized that the majority of patient outcomes, including those traditionally used to evaluate physician care, are not influenced by any one discipline alone. Even so, for nursing to monitor and improve its practice, it is important that outcomes influenced by nursing care be identified.

The more abstract and global the outcome, the more likely its achievement will be the result of interventions from several health care disciplines. Specific disciplines will have more influence on certain intermediate outcomes than others. For example, at different times, nursing, medicine, and physical therapy each have the most impact on the outcome Joint Movement: Active, and, overall, each influences the outcome. Specific indicators of outcomes are more likely to be sensitive to the interventions of a single discipline; therefore, it is essential to identify the indicators most sensitive to nursing interventions so that nurses can document the effects of their interventions and be held individually and collectively accountable for care delivered to patients. To develop and refine the list of nursing-sensitive outcomes and indicators, the team defined a set of criteria for evaluating evidence of nursing sensitivity or responsiveness to nursing intervention. These criteria are listed in Box 2-3.

6. **Are nursing-sensitive patient outcomes the resolution of nursing diagnoses?** The majority of nursing-sensitive patient outcomes represent the resolution of nursing diagnoses, although some outcomes are more generic and not necessarily related to specific diagnoses. Clearly, patient satisfaction and the financial charges to patients resulting from nursing care are not diagnosis specific and cannot be conceived as the resolution of a diagnosis. At this time, it appears that the more general (abstract) the outcome, such as Quality of Life, the less likely it will be diagnosis specific, and conversely, the less abstract the outcome concept, such as Self Care: Hygiene, the more likely it will be nursing-diagnosis–specific.

7. **When should patient outcomes be measured?** The appropriate time to measure patient outcomes will vary. Some outcomes respond very quickly to intervention and others respond over a longer period. The outcomes of health promotion interventions, for example, are likely to occur over a considerable time period, while the response to interventions to improve nutritional intake could be immediate. There also are outcomes such as Transfer Performance in which the full response may take several weeks. The difficulty is selecting a time for measuring an outcome close enough to the intervention for the nurse to be confident that change resulted from the intervention, but far enough removed from the intervention to be able to measure a change. This is why medicine has begun to place more emphasis on intermediate outcomes. Thus, it is important that the measurement of nursing-sensitive outcomes be repeated over time, but the timing and intervals of measurement are critical and must be determined for specific conditions, interventions, and expected outcomes. This aspect of measurement will be an important consideration in the later phase of the research in which measurement procedures will be defined and tested.

BOX 2-3
Criteria for Evaluating Nursing Sensitivity

Evidence a nursing intervention produced a positive outcome
Evidence a nursing intervention influenced a positive outcome
Evidence a nursing intervention is carried out with the intent to produce or influence the outcome
Evidence a nursing intervention produced improvement or maintenance of the outcome or prevented deterioration or occurrence of a negative outcome
Evidence the nursing intervention occurred before observation of the outcome
Evidence a failure to provide nursing intervention resulted in failure to achieve a positive outcome or to prevent a negative outcome
Evidence the interventions that produced or influenced the outcome are within nursing's scope of practice

METHODOLOGIC ISSUES AND STRATEGIES

The NOC team identified and resolved the following five methodologic issues to develop and validate the initial list of nursing-sensitive patient outcomes:

1. What strategies are used (inductive or deductive, qualitative or quantitative)?
2. What sources were used to sample outcome statements?
3. What criteria were used to select the sources from which outcome statements were extracted?
4. How are nursing-sensitive outcomes and indicators validated?
5. What methods will be used to develop the classification structure?

What Strategies Were Used?

Combinations of inductive and deductive and qualitative and quantitative strategies were required for the development of the classification of nursing-sensitive patient outcomes.[3] Inductive and deductive approaches[19] also are used in taxonomy development, in which concept development is intertwined with conceptual framework development. The classification methods used for the NIC project were adapted for the NOC research.[2,9]

What Sources Were Used to Sample Outcome Statements?

Nurses have written about outcomes and have included them in plans of care for many years. Although typically stated as goals, these statements have been readily available in textbooks, care planning guides, clinical information systems, and standards of care. Just as in the NIC work, the NOC team decided to inductively identify nursing-sensitive outcome concepts by sampling a variety of nursing sources. To ensure the representativeness and comprehensiveness of the outcome statements, a sampling plan was developed. The plan detailed clinical emphases, settings, and patient age groups to be represented in the sources. The sources were selected to represent medical/surgical, critical care, maternal and child, rehabilitation, and mental health clinical practices; acute care, nursing home, community, and ambulatory settings; and elderly, adult, child, and infant populations. Health promotion and illness management perspectives also were incorporated. The sampling scheme depicted in Table 2-1 shows the clinical areas, settings, and patient age groups represented by the sources selected.

What Criteria Were Used to Select the Sources From Which Outcome Statements Were Extracted?

Literature sources were selected according to the following predetermined criteria (Box 2-4) that the source:

1. Presented clear statements that described specific states or behaviors of patients/family members
2. Included a comprehensive list of outcome statements
3. Presented outcome statements that were measurable
4. Presented outcome statements that were designed to evaluate nursing interventions
5. Added outcome statements that were needed according to the sampling plan

A source rating form (Fig. 2-2) was developed to evaluate the acceptability of each source. The sources selected are listed in Table 2-2.

How Are Nursing-sensitive Outcomes and Indicators Validated?

Three methods were selected to validate the outcome indicators as representative of the outcome definition and as nursing sensitive. First, concept analysis and re-

TABLE 2-1
Sampling Scheme for Data Sources

Clinical emphasis	Age group	Setting		
		Acute hospital	Nursing home	Community
Medical/Surgical	Elderly	X	X	X
	Adult	X	X	X
Critical Care	Elderly	X	NA	NA
	Adult	X	NA	NA
	Child	X	NA	NA
	Infant	X	NA	NA
Maternal/Child	Adult	X	NA	X
	Child	X	X	X
	Infant	X	NA	X
Rehabilitation	Elderly	X	X	X
	Adult	X	X	X
	Child	X	X	X
Mental Health	Elderly	X	X	X
	Adult	X	X	X
	Child	X	X	X

BOX 2-4
Criteria for Selection of Sources

1. Presents clear statements that describe specific states or behaviors of patients/families
2. Includes a comprehensive list of outcome statements
3. Presents outcome statements that are measurable
4. Presents outcome statements that are specifically designed to evaluate nursing interventions
5. Adds outcome statements that are needed according to the sampling plan

---

view of the literature provided evidence of the indicator content and responsiveness to nursing interventions. Second, surveys of master's-degreed nurses representing cross sections of clinical specialties, settings, and client age groups were used to rate which indicators are most important to determine each outcome and to rate which indicators are most sensitive to nursing intervention. Third, a field test of the initial list of outcomes and indicators is planned in the following five practice settings: two tertiary-care hospitals, an acute-care community hospital, a long-term–care facility, and a community health agency. Evidence of the indicators' usefulness and sensitivity to nursing interventions in these settings will be indicated by frequency of use and linkages to specific nursing interventions.

Date: _____

Specific Topic/Content: _____

Citation: _____

Description: _____

Location of Copies:

Rating:

1. Setting for which designed: _____

2. Patient population for which designed: _____

3. Refers to current practice? _____ Yes _____ No

4. Has an empirical base? _____ Yes _____ No

5. Indicator statements:

Criteria:

Measurability:	Not measurable	Measurable	Measurable with revision
Specificity:	Not specific to nursing	Specific to intervention	Specific to nursing
Clarity:	Not clear	Clear to nurses in specific setting	Clear to nurses

6. Framework for presenting outcome indicators (e.g., nursing dx, care standards of book/ article/database

_____

7. Adopt as source of indicators? _____ Yes _____ No

8. Reviewer Name _____

Adapted from the Source Rating Form, Iowa Intervention Project: NIC (1992)
1-30-92

Fig. 2-2 Nursing-sensitive patient outcomes classification (NOC) research rating form.

The research team, which includes faculty content experts and clinical nurse experts, will review the logic of conceptual links between each outcome and indicator, NIC interventions, and NANDA diagnoses. They also will review to what extent these linkages are empirically validated according to reported research and will review evidence obtained from the field tests. Finally, evidence from each validation method will be used to refine the outcome concepts, definitions, and indicators. Fig. 2-3 illustrates the process of refinement over time.

What Methods Will Be Used to Develop the Classification Structure?

Similarity-dissimilarity analysis, using hierarchic clustering procedures, will be conducted to develop the nursing-sensitive outcomes classification structure. The classification structure will: (1) relate outcomes and indicators in terms of levels of abstraction and (2) group outcomes and indicators according to rules that define commonalities in the groups. As stated, the classification is expected to have four increasingly general levels of outcomes (see Fig. 2-1).

TABLE 2-2

Outcome Sources Accepted

Source	Setting
American Association of Critical Care Nurses. (1990). *Outcome Standards for Nursing Care of the Critically Ill.* Laguna Niguel, CA: Author.	Hospital Critical care
Bedrosian, C.A. (1989). *Home Health Nursing: Nursing Diagnoses & Care Plans.* East Norwalk, CT: Appleton & Lange.	Home care Long-term/Chronic
Carpenito, L.J. (1992). *Nursing Diagnosis: Application to Clinical Practice* (4th ed.). Philadelphia: J.B. Lippincott.	Multiple settings Acute/Chronic
Doenges, M.E., Moorhouse, M.F., & Geissler, A.C. (1989). *Nursing Care Plans: Guidelines for Planning Patient Care.* Philadelphia: F.A. Davis.	Hospital Acute
Gulanick, M., Klopp, A. & Galanes, S. (1980). *Nursing Care Plans: Nursing Diagnosis and Interventions.* St. Louis: Mosby.	Hospital Maternal health
Holloway, N. (1988). *Medical Surgical Care Plans.* Springhouse, PA: Springhouse.	Hospital/Community Medical/Surgical
Horn, B.J. & Swain, M.A. (1978). *Criterion Measures of Nursing Care* (DHEW Pub. No. PHS 78-3187). Hyattsville, MD: National Center for Health Services Research.	Multiple settings Acute/Chronic
Jaffee, M.S. & Skidmore-Roth, L. (1988). *Home Health Nursing Care Plans.* St. Louis: Mosby.	Community Acute/Chronic
Johanson, B.C., Dungaca, C.U., Hoffmeister, D., & Wells, S.J. (1985). *Standards for Critical Care* (2nd ed.). St. Louis: Mosby.	Hospital Critical care
March, C.S. (1992). *The Complete Care Plan Manual for Long Term Care.* Chicago: American Hospital Association.	Multiple settings Long-term/Adults
McFarland, G.K. & McFarlane, E.A. (1993). *Nursing Diagnoses & Intervention: Planning for Patient Care* (2nd ed.). St. Louis: Mosby.	Multiple settings Acute/Chronic
Nursing staff: Iowa City VA Medical Center. (1989). *Guidelines for Patient Care.* Iowa City, IA: Author.	Hospital Acute/Chronic
Patrick, M., Woods, S., Cravens, R., Rokosky, J., & Bruno, P. (1991). *Medical Surgical Nursing.* Philadelphia: J.B. Lippincott.	Multiple settings Acute/Chronic
Potter, P.A. & Perry, A.P. (1989). *Fundamentals of Nursing: Concepts, Process, and Practice* (2nd ed.). St. Louis: Mosby.	Multiple settings Acute/Chronic
Schriger-Krebs, M.J. & Larson, K. (1988). *Applied Psychiatric-Mental Health Nursing Standards in Clinical Practice.* New York: John Wiley & Sons.	Hospital/Ambulatory care Mental health
Soenges, M., Kenby, J., & Moorhouse, M. (1988). *Maternal-New-born Careplans: Guidelines for Client Care.* Philadelphia: F.A. Davis.	Hospital/Community Maternal/Newborn
Townsend, M.C. (1988). *Nursing Diagnosis in Psychiatric Nursing: A Pocket Guide for Care Plan Construction.* Philadelphia: F.A. Davis.	Multiple settings Mental health
Wong, D.L. (1993). *Whaley & Wong's Essentials of Pediatric Nursing* (4th ed.). St. Louis: Mosby.	Hospital/Community Pediatrics
Schirger-Krebs, M.J. & Larson, K. (1988). *Applied Psychiatric-Mental Health Nursing Standards in Clinical Practice.* New York: John Wiley & Sons.	Ambulatory

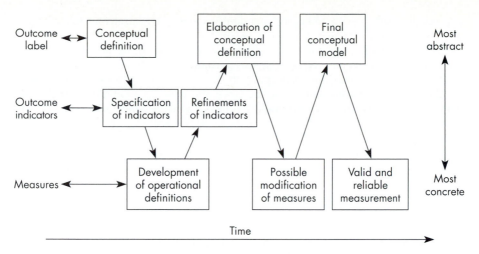

Fig. 2-3 Explication and synthesis of outcomes and indicators. (Adapted from Walizer M.H., Wiener P.L. [1978]. *Research methods and analysis: searching for relationships* [p. 37]. New York: Harper & Row.)

DEVELOPMENT OF THE INITIAL LIST OF NURSING-SENSITIVE PATIENT OUTCOMES AND INDICATORS

The outcome indicator statements that describe patient states or behaviors nurses currently use to evaluate nursing interventions were the initial data used in the research. The nursing literature contains broad patient outcome concepts and classifications, and nursing textbooks, critical paths, instruments, care plans, and research studies contain many concrete patient outcome statements that are proposed as the desired results of nursing interventions. Although there is considerable similarity in the several broad categorizations of outcomes from these sources, none are the same. In addition the specific goals listed for the same nursing diagnoses and patient characteristics or the same interventions usually are not stated in the same way. In many settings, nurses state their own goals, or if a list of goals is available, it is not apt to be the same as a list provided in another setting. For example, goals for a patient with the diagnosis Impaired Mobility in one setting may be very different from the desired outcomes or goal statements for a similar patient with the same nursing diagnosis in another setting. Differences also are found when comparing nursing textbooks and care planning manuals. Thus to develop a classification that contains a useful number of outcomes, the team decided to use the abundant concrete goal statements as the data to group for inductive formation of the outcomes. Goal statements were extracted from sources purposively selected to represent all areas of nursing practice. Outcome labels were given to groups of similar goal statements to form the initial list of outcomes and indicators.

VALIDATION, FIELD TESTING, AND CLASSIFICATION OF THE INITIAL LIST OF OUTCOMES
Refinement of the Initial List of Nursing-sensitive Outcomes and Indicators

Each outcome label and associated goal statements on the initial list was assigned to a focus group composed of research team members. To facilitate this process, broad outcome categories were derived from the MOS and broad nursing outcome categories.[11,12] To group the outcome labels in the broad categories the team used a Delphi process (i.e., each team member independently assigned each outcome to a category and then the team, through discussion, reached a consensus on the placement of the outcomes). The outcomes and their indicators assigned to one of the categories were distributed to one of eight focus groups, each chaired by an NOC investigator with a doctorate degree. A modified concept analysis was performed for each outcome to validate the indicator content, refine the label, and develop a definition for the outcome label. Surveys of advanced practice nurses also were conducted to validate indicators for each outcome and to validate the nursing sensitivity of each outcome and its indicators. Data from the surveys were reviewed by the principal investigators and approved by the research team. The refined initial list of outcomes and indicators was then approved for field testing and construction of the classification structure.

Field Testing and Classification of the List of Outcomes and Indicators

Five-point Likert-type scales were developed for each outcome (see outcomes in Part Two) and its indicators to prepare for field testing. The outcomes are being used in a clinical information system for community settings, and the research team currently is working on arranging the outcome list in an initial taxonomic structure.

VALIDATION OF THE NOC AND TESTING OF MEASUREMENT PROCEDURES

The next phase of the research will be devoted to field testing and validation of the classification structure and to the development and psychometric evaluation of measurement procedures for each nursing-sensitive outcome. Funding from Sigma Theta Tau International and the National Institute for Nursing Research was obtained to complete Phases I and II of the research, and a second grant proposal seeking funding for Phase III research will be submitted. Initial plans for the Phase III proposal include surveys of nurses expert in theory development who will be asked to assess the clarity of the NOC language, and the homogeneity, inclusiveness, mutual exclusiveness, and theory neutrality of outcomes in each class of the taxonomic structure. Field tests will be used to evaluate the adequacy of the classification structure in the development and use of the outcomes in clinical nursing information systems. Field test data also will be used to evaluate the reliability and validity of measurement procedures. In the next chapter, the methods used to develop the NOC are described in detail.

References

1. Bond, S. & Thomas, L.H. (1991). Issues in measuring outcomes on nursing. *Journal of Advanced Nursing,* 16, 1492-1502.

2. Cohen, M., Kruckeberg, T., McCloskey, J., Bulechek, G., Craft, M., Crossley, J., Denehy, J., Glick, O., Maas, M., Prophet, C., Tripp-Reimer, T., Carlson, D., Wyman, M., & Titler, M. (1991). A taxonomy of nursing interventions: Inductive methodology with a research team and a large data set. *Nursing Outlook,* 39(4), 162-165.

3. Erben, R., Franzkowiak, P., & Wenzel, E. (1992). Assessment of the outcomes of health interventions. *Social Science Medicine,* 35(4), 359-365.

4. Fehring, R.J. (1986). Validating diagnostic labels: Standardized methodology. In M.E. Hurley (Ed.), *Classification of Nursing Diagnoses: Proceedings of the Sixth Conference.* St. Louis: Mosby.

5. Fehring, R.J. (1987). Methods to validate nursing diagnoses. *Heart & Lung,* 16(6), 625-629.

6. Gardner, D., Kelly, K., Johnson, M., McCloskey, J., & Maas, M. (1991). Nursing administration model for administrative practice. *Journal of Nursing Administration,* 21(3), 37-41.

7. Grobe, S.J. (1990). Nursing intervention lexicon and taxonomy study: Language and classification methods. *Advances in Nursing Science,* 13(2), 22-33.

8. Hegyvary, S.T. (1991). Issues in outcomes research. *Journal of Nursing Quality Assurance,* 5(2), 1-6.

9. Iowa Intervention Project. (1996). *Nursing Interventions Classification (NIC)* (2nd ed.). St. Louis: Mosby.

10. Johnson, M., Gardner, D., Kelly, K., Maas, M., & McCloskey, J. (1991). The Iowa Model: A proposed model for nursing administration. *Nursing Economics,* 9(4), 255-262.

11. Lang, N.M., & Clinton, J.F. (1984). Assessment of quality of nursing care. In H.H. Werley & J.J. Fitzpatrick (Eds.), *Annual Review of Nursing Research, Vol. 2* (pp. 135-163). New York: Springer.

12. Marek, K.D. (1989). Outcome measurement in nursing. *Journal of Nursing Quality Assurance,* 4(1), 1-9.

13. McCloskey, J.C., Maas, M.L., Huber, D.G., Kasparek, A., Specht, J.P., Ramler, C.L., Watson, C., Blegen, M., Delaney, C., Ellerbe, S., Etscheidt, C., Gongaware, C., Johnson, M.R., Kelly, K.C., Mehmert, P., & Clougherty, J. (1994). Nursing management innovations: A need for systematic evaluation. *Nursing Economics,* 12(1), 35-44.

14. Nadzam, D.M. (1991). The agenda for change: Update on indicator development and possible implications for the nursing profession. *Journal of Nursing Quality Assurance,* 5(2), 18-22.

15. North American Nursing Diagnosis Association (NANDA). (1994). *Nursing Diagnoses: Definitions & Classification, 1995/1996.* Philadelphia: Author.

16. Podgorny, K.L. (1991). Developing nursing-focused quality indicators: A professional challenge. *Journal of Nursing Care Quality,* 6(1), 47-52.

17. Rantz, M.J. & LeMone, P. (Eds). (1995). Classification of nursing diagnoses: Proceedings of the eleventh conference of the North American Nursing Diagnosis Association. Glendale, CA: CINAHL Information Systems.

18. Saba, V.K. (1992). The classification of home health care nursing diagnoses and interventions. *Caring,* 11(3), 50-57.

19. Suppe, F. & Jacox, A. (1985). Philosophy of science and the development of nursing theory. In H.H. Werley & J. Fitzpatrick (Eds.), *Annual Review of Nursing Research, Vol. 3,* (pp. 241-267). New York: Springer.

20. Tarlov, A.R., Ware, J.E., Greenfield, S., Nelson, E.C., Perrin, E., & Zubkoff, M. (1989). The Medical Outcomes Study: An application of methods for monitoring the results of medical care. *Journal of the American Medical Association,* 262, 925-930.

21. Walizer, M.H. & Wienir, P.L. (1978). *Research Methods and Analysis: Searching for Relationships.* New York: Harper & Row, p. 37.

22. Werley, H.H., & Lang, N.M. (Eds.). (1988). *Identification of the Nursing Minimum Data Set.* New York: Springer.

23. Werley, H.H. & Devine, E.C. (1987). The Nursing Minimum Data Set: Status and implications (pp. 540-551). In K.J. Hanna, et al. (Eds.), *Clinical Judgment and Decision Making: The Future of Nursing Diagnosis.* New York: John Wiley & Sons.

CHAPTER THREE

Methods Used to Develop the Outcomes and Indicators

GENERATION OF THE INITIAL LIST OF OUTCOME LABELS

The research team began generating the initial list of outcomes in August 1991. Abstract patient outcome concepts and classifications were in the literature. Further, there were many concrete patient outcome statements proposed as the desired results of nursing interventions in nursing textbooks, critical paths, instruments, care plans, and research studies. Both inductive and deductive approaches were needed to classify and develop nursing-sensitive patient outcomes and indicators at middle levels of abstraction. The difficulty was collecting the more specific, less abstract indicators and, using an inductive approach, to group and label them at a more abstract level. Another difficulty was using existing broad, abstract categories to explicate less abstract nursing-sensitive outcomes and indicators. Thus an inductive approach was required to identify and develop nursing-sensitive outcomes by synthesizing indicators, whereas a deductive approach was used to ensure that a comprehensive list of nursing-sensitive outcomes had been identified. Further, existing abstract outcome categories provided a framework for patient outcomes that have become generally accepted by health care disciplines and by health care policy makers.[14] The most critical task was to identify and standardize nursing-sensitive patient outcomes and indicators that are clinically useful and sensitive to nursing intervention. This work was necessary for the assessment of nursing's influence and effectiveness in achieving expected patient outcomes, the advancement of the development of nursing knowledge, and the enhancement of clients' and policy makers' understanding about nursing's contribution to health care.

Process for Rating Data Sources

The process for rating each data source (adapted from the process used by the Iowa Intervention Project: NIC[6]) was as follows:

1. A potential data source was identified and obtained.
2. The team member most familiar with the source or specialty area identified representative sections of the source (including title/author page, preface/overview, table of contents, and two to three chapters/sections) and gave them to all team members for review.
3. Each team member read the material and came prepared to a team meeting to discuss it.
4. The team member who had reviewed the entire source and identified representative sections for distribution led the discussion.

5. Each team member completed the NOC Source Rating Form (see Fig. 2-2) after discussing the material and came to a consensus on each criterion.
6. An overall score (1 = poor to 5 = excellent) based on the consensus of the team was determined for each source.

Sources Reviewed and Extraction of Outcome Statements

Thirty sources were reviewed for the extraction of concrete outcome statements (e.g., goals used by clinicians). The sources were representative of setting, clinical emphasis, and type (e.g., textbook, information system, research study). A minority of sources contained research-based outcome statements, and if the basis of the research was indicated, it was noted on the NOC Source Rating Form. Of the 30 sources (mostly books) that were reviewed, 19 were accepted as actual data sources (see Table 2-2).

Team members reviewed information system data bases including one each from a tertiary-care hospital and from an intermediate-care hospital in Iowa. An extensive file of research instruments that measure outcomes was available in The College of Nursing Service Administration (NSA) Laboratory. Critical paths developed in a number of settings across the nation also were available in the NSA laboratory.[2] The team decided that the NSA laboratory sources added a much-needed practice dimension to the textbook sources, which were written chiefly by theorists and educators. The sampling of sources continued until all areas included in the sampling scheme (see Table 2-1) were represented and very few new indicators were obtained.

More than 4,500 outcome statements were extracted from the sources, and an initial list of 282 nursing-sensitive patient outcome labels was developed. The outcome statements were at varied levels of abstraction and usually were stated as goals or standards (e.g., from broad statements, such as prevention of complications and maintenance of optimal activity level; to midlevel statements, such as knowledge of proper dressing care; to very specific statements, such as cardiac index 2.5 to 4 liters per minute). About 150 to 200 outcome indicator statements were selected from each source; if the source contained more than 200 indicators, 150-200 statements were randomly selected from the source.

In summary, the selection of data sources for the generation of the initial list of outcomes was accomplished by a purposive, systematic sampling of nursing textbooks, critical paths, measurement instruments, standards of practice, nursing information systems, and nursing-diagnoses and care-planning books that contain specific nursing outcome statements. The team selected sources that reflected nursing practice in hospital, nursing home, community, and ambulatory settings with varied clinical emphases and patient age groups. No list of nursing-sensitive outcomes can be complete, and new outcomes and indicators will always need to be added as the profession matures. However, the methodology developed by the team has provided a means of identifying the most common nursing-sensitive patient outcomes that are most commonly taught and used in practice and research.

Grouping of Outcome Statements to Develop Nursing-sensitive Outcome Labels

The nursing-sensitive outcome statements extracted from sources were analyzed, grouped, and labeled as follows: (1) the 150 to 200 outcome statements selected from each source were entered into a computer file; (2) each statement was printed on a separate piece of paper and copies of the statements were distributed in a series of exercises to all research team members; and (3) each team member independently grouped the statements and gave each grouping an outcome label.

Team members generated labels based on their knowledge and experience, and used approximately 175 outcome statements in each exercise because team members felt this was a manageable number.

Anywhere from 3 to 25 outcome statements were grouped under each of the outcome labels and were used as the basis for the development of indicators for each outcome label. Twenty exercises were determined sufficient because of the large number of outcome statements identified in the sampling scheme. The labels and associated outcome statements from each exercise and team member were entered into a computer data base. As the list of outcome labels grew, team members reviewed the labels to eliminate redundancy and to standardize semantics and grammar according to the rules in Box 2-2. Table 3-1 contains examples of outcome labels and associated outcome statements developed in the initial content analysis exercises that were subsequently revised to form the initial list of outcomes and indicators. The content analysis exercises were very labor intensive, each requiring 4 to 6 hours per researcher, as well as the many more hours required to enter the outcome statements and the results of the exercises into the computer. Each of the nursing-sensitive outcome statements was coded to correlate with its associated outcome label.

Data Base Management

A computer program was designed to assist with the coding, manipulation, categorization, and retrieval of the initial outcome labels and associated indicators. Tom Kruckeberg, College of Nursing Systems programmer and investigator for the research team, designed the program by using the Paradox data base.[6,7] The program was patterned after the program initially designed for the NIC project and assisted the biostatistician, a consultant for the NOC research team, with the analysis of data, principally in the areas of refining the outcomes and indicators. The team also anticipates its usefulness for the analyses required to develop the taxonomic structure and for coding the outcomes in the structure.

In summary, team members completed 20 grouping exercises to generate the initial list of 282 nursing-sensitive outcome labels and associated indicators. When only a few new outcome labels were produced through the exercises and when the indicators were completely redundant of earlier ones, the team determined that an initial list of nursing-sensitive patient outcomes and indicators had been generated and decided to move to the next step of the research—validation and refinement of the outcomes and indicators.

TABLE 3-1

Examples of Outcome Labels and Associated Outcome Statements
on Initial List Before Refinement

Outcome labels	Outcome statements
Mobility Level: Ambulation	Progressive moderate exercising and ambulation Increased ambulation daily
Nutritional Status	Decreased appetite improved Patient consumes most of food on meal tray
Pain Level	Verbalizes relief and/or absence of pain Absence of associated pain

PLACING THE OUTCOMES IN BROAD CATEGORIES FOR THE ASSESSMENT OF CONTENT VALIDITY AND REFINEMENT

The redundancy among the outcome statements existed because many were listed in more than one source and because some identical ones were grouped under more than one outcome label. To facilitate the validation and refinement process, the nursing-sensitive outcome labels initially were placed in the Medical Outcomes Study (MOS) and other broad nursing-outcome categories.

The research team considered how their list of outcomes and indicators fit in the MOS outcome categories[14] and other categories such as those offered by Lang & Clinton[8] and Marek.[9] Because the MOS classification is generally accepted and used by health services researchers, the team revised the MOS framework to include other broad outcome categories that are in the nursing literature. The team's initial list of nursing-sensitive outcome labels and indicators were grouped in these generally accepted broad outcome categories to facilitate the focus groups' concept analyses of each of the outcome labels.

Focus Group Concept Analyses

The research team was divided into eight focus groups of three to four members each, with as many different practice settings and areas of clinical expertise as possible represented in each group. A doctorate-degreed faculty investigator and a part-time research assistant were assigned to each group, and expert clinicians were added to each group to assist with the work. The clinicians were extremely valuable and spent long hours working as volunteers on the outcomes. The use of focus groups was demonstrated as a very effective means to refine intervention concept labels and activities, identify supporting literature, and develop definitions.[6]

To refine the outcome labels and statements and to identify any nursing-sensitive outcomes and indicators not included in the initial list, the outcome labels were placed in the following eight broad categories based on the MOS[14] and nursing literature[8,9]:

- Physiological status
- Psychological and cognitive status
- Social and role status
- Physical functional status
- Safety status
- Family caregiver status
- Health attitudes, knowledge, and behavior
- Perceived well-being

As previously mentioned, a Delphi process was used to group the outcome labels in the broader categories. First, the team determined what revisions were needed in the MOS framework, based on their judgment and the current nursing outcomes literature. Next, each team member grouped the outcome labels within the revised framework, and then these groupings were analyzed. Outcome labels that were grouped in the same category by at least 75% of the team members were placed in that category. The results were shared with team members, and the outcome labels that did not meet the criterion were distributed to each team member and again grouped in broad categories. The team discussed outcome labels that did not meet the criterion after the second grouping and assigned, by consensus, those labels to a broad category. Each of the broad categories was then assigned to one of the eight focus work groups.

For each outcome label, the focus group reviewed nursing and allied research, instruments measuring the outcome concepts, and other pertinent literature for concept analysis; refined the outcome labels and indicators; and reviewed the initial validation of nursing sensitivity.

Each focus group reviewed the outcome labels in its category, combined similar labels, as appropriate, and added new labels as needed. Each label was reviewed according to the rules listed in Box 2-2, and each outcome statement in the initial list was refined to reflect the indicators for the label. Additional indicators based on the literature review and concept analysis were added and others deleted, and a definition for the label, based on the concept analysis, was developed.

The concept analysis of each outcome was conducted according to a procedure adapted from Rodgers[10] and Waltz, Strickland, & Lenz.[16] The purposes of the analyses were to (1) evaluate the completeness of the outcome concepts subsumed in a category and develop labels for any missing concepts, (2) develop a definition of the outcome label, and (3) evaluate and refine the indicators generated in Phase I, based on the literature review and expertise of the focus group members. The following steps were used for the concept analysis:

1. Identification of literature related to the concept, including instruments that measure the concept.
2. Review of each source for definitions, indicators, linkages to nursing interventions, and patient populations.
3. Comparison of indicators derived from the literature with indicators generated in Phase I of the research.
4. Development of an outcome label, a proposed definition for the outcome label, and a list of indicators that reflect all dimensions of the outcome using information from the literature review and indicator lists generated in Phase I of the research. Rules for development of outcomes definitions and indicators are listed in Boxes 3-1 and 3-2. Rules for stating outcome labels are in Box 2-2.

BOX 3-1
Rules for Development of Outcome Definitions

The definition describes the complete meaning of the outcome concept
The definition as a whole is synonymous with the outcome concept
The definition is clear and simple
The definition refers to all indicators included with the concept; describes all dimensions of the outcome

---

BOX 3-2
Rules for Development of Indicator Definitions

Terms are explicit, specific, and precise
The meaning is adequate if there is congruence between the outcome and the indicators
Terms are used in a consistent manner
All dimensions of the outcome are represented by indicators; indicators are inclusive
The indicators are measurable; empirical measures can be developed for all indicators
The indicators have utility; all are sensitive and useful for nursing

5. Determination of the appropriateness of the outcome label and presentation to the focus group and the NOC team for their review and approval. The final product included an outcome label, a conceptual definition, a list of indicators, and a list of selected references used for the concept analysis.

Focus groups presented a summary of the concept analysis of each outcome and the outcome label, definition, and indicators to the research team for review. The research team reviewed the final product for compatibility with the rules of standardization and consistency and for overlap with other outcomes and indicators. Then, five-point Likert-type scales were added to each outcome and indicator for field testing. Following adoption, the outcomes and indicators were ready for content validation surveys and field testing.

Content Validation by Nurse Experts

Surveys of master's-degreed nurses representing cross sections of clinical specialties, settings, and client age groups were used to rate which indicators are most important to determine each outcome and to rate which indicators were most sensitive to nursing intervention. A revision of Fehring's methodology[3,4] for assessing content validity of nursing diagnoses was used to estimate the outcomes' and indicators' content validity and sensitivity to nursing interventions.

Fehring's methodology[3,4] for determining content validity for nursing diagnoses was adapted and tested in the preliminary work to validate the content of the nursing-sensitive patient outcomes by using satisfaction with nursing outcomes. A variant of this method also was used by the Iowa Intervention Project: NIC[6] to establish the content validity of nursing interventions and the NIC.[1] McCloskey and Bulechek[6] argue that the adaptation of Fehring's method is consistent with recommendations of ways to construct taxonomies.[5] The successful use of Fehring's method to validate nursing interventions and the team's pilot work with patient satisfaction of outcomes supported the use of the method to assess the content validity of the outcomes.

The adaptation of Fehring's methodology for validating the nursing-sensitive patient outcomes is as follows:

1. The nursing-sensitive outcome indicators refined by the focus groups were listed beneath the outcome label and definition. Some (two to three) indicators that were not retained by the focus groups and were considered not important for assessing the outcome also were included.
2. The nurse experts rated the indicators for each nursing-sensitive outcome for sensitivity to nursing intervention and for importance for evaluating the outcome concept. The experts also were asked to suggest any indicators they believe were omitted.
3. Weighted ratios were calculated for each indicator statement (for importance and sensitivity ratings). The ratios were obtained by adding the weights assigned to each response and then dividing the sum by the total number of responses. The weights suggested by Fehring were used: $5 = 1, 4 = .75, 3 = .50, 2 = .25$ and $1 = 0$.
4. Nursing-sensitive outcome indicators with importance and sensitivity ratios greater than .80 were declared major sensitive indicators, and those with importance and sensitivity ratios equal to or less than .60 were discarded. Indicators were determined to be supporting factors in determining patient status in relation to the outcome if the mean was between .61 and .79.[11] Sparks and Lien-Gieschen raised the lower bound coefficient for minor characteristics to .60 to achieve a manageable number of defining characteristics for a nursing diagnosis. The NOC team adopted and altered the revised criterion to retain a minimum set of indicators with high content validity estimates.

5. Outcome content validity and outcome score sensitivity values were formed for each outcome by summing and averaging the indicator importance and sensitivity ratings.

Master's-degreed nurse experts were selected to rate the indicators because of their clinical expertise and their greater familiarity with concept development, research techniques, the need for nursing nomenclatures and classifications, and clinical practice theory. The names and addresses of the expert nurses were obtained from the following specialty organizations:

Academy of Medical Surgical Nurses
American Academy of Ambulatory Care Nursing
American Association of Critical Care Nurses
American Association of Neuroscience Nurses
American Holistic Nurses Association
American Psychiatric Nurses Association
American Society for Parenteral & Enteral Nutrition
ANA*-Community Public Health
ANA-General Practice
ANA-Gerontology
ANA-Medical Surgical
ANA-Pediatrics
ANA-Psychiatric/Mental Health
ANCC*-Clinical Specialist in Medical Surgical Nursing
ANCC-Community Health Nurse
ANCC-Family Nurse Practitioner
Association of Nurses in Aids Care
Association of Rehabilitation Nurses
Association of Women's Health, Obstetric and Neonatal Nurses
Drug & Alcohol Nursing Association
National Association of Orthopedic Nurses
National Association of Pediatric Nurse Associates and Practitioners
National Association of School Nurses, Inc.
National Gerontological Nursing Association
North American Nursing Diagnosis Association
Oncology Nursing Society
Respiratory Nursing Society
Wound Ostomy and Continence Nurses Society

The lists obtained were reviewed, and duplicate names were removed. A random sampling of nurse experts was drawn from the appropriate lists for each survey and stratified by practice setting, clinical emphasis, and patient age group served. The samples were mostly female and represented the distribution of other minorities in the nation's population of master's-degreed nurses who belong to these organizations.

Each survey was mailed to 175 or more randomly selected nurse experts who were asked to return the completed questionnaire within 2 weeks of receiving it. The team expected a return rate of about 50%, but rates between 30% and 44% were achieved. Stamped, addressed envelopes were mailed with the survey questionnaires and one follow-up postcard reminder was sent 3 weeks after the first mailing. Each survey contained 8-10 outcome concepts and from 6-15 nursing-sensitive indicators. The nurse experts were asked to rate each indicator as to: (1) the extent each is influenced by nursing interventions (sensitivity) (1 = no contribution; 5 = contribution is mainly nursing), and (2) the importance to the outcome concept (1 = never important; 5 = always important).

---

*ANA = American Nurses' Association; ANCC = American Nurses Credentialing Center.

Results of the Surveys of Nurse Experts

Only a few minor changes in relation to the definitions were suggested on the surveys returned, and in each case the outcome label and definition were reevaluated and a change made, if indicated. In general, the majority of indicators were rated at .60 or more, and many met the .80 criterion. Respondents suggested a few additional indicators, and after review by the research team investigators and clinicians, a few new indicators were added. The results of the surveys indicated that important indicators of the outcomes were not missing and that nurses believe that nursing's contribution to most outcomes and indicators is substantial. The survey findings provided evidence that the selection, development, and refinement of nursing-sensitive outcomes and indicators, based on the qualitative and concept analyses, were valid.

In summary, the initial nursing-sensitive patient outcomes the team generated were placed in the MOS and broad nursing-outcome categories and refined and validated using concept analysis and surveys of nurse experts. Thus both concept synthesis and concept analysis strategies were used to develop and validate nursing-sensitive patient outcomes and indicators.[15] The outcomes and indicators were then prepared for field testing in a variety of practice settings.

FIELD TESTING THE NURSING-SENSITIVE OUTCOMES AND INDICATORS

As previously mentioned, field tests of the refined list of outcomes and indicators are being conducted in five practice settings—two tertiary care hospitals, an acute-care community hospital, a long-term–care facility, and a community health agency. Evidence of the outcomes' and indicators' sensitivity to nursing interventions as perceived by nurses practicing in the different types of settings will be demonstrated by frequency of use and linkage to nursing diagnoses and interventions. Although the ultimate validation of nursing's influence on specific outcomes must await systematic, controlled research, this type of research will be facilitated by the use of standardized nursing languages. Standardized nursing-sensitive outcomes (NOC) for which there is some evidence of responsiveness to nursing interventions will be especially important for nursing research to assess effectiveness and to influence health policy.[12,13] Field testing before publication of a second edition of the NOC will facilitate the classification's development and use in clinical settings across the United States.

When the NOC taxonomic structure is completed, its content, at all levels, will be coded to aid its implementation in nursing clinical information systems. Implementing the NOC in clinical test site information systems to assess the clinical usefulness and comprehensiveness of the classification structure, outcomes, and indicators will provide critically important information for future refinement and for testing measurement procedures.

Data being collected from the information systems include the following: patient age, medical diagnoses, nursing diagnoses, nursing interventions, and nursing-sensitive outcomes and indicators. The outcomes and indicators chosen for different age groups, medical diagnoses, nursing diagnoses, and interventions will be described. The clinical usefulness and comprehensiveness of the nursing-sensitive outcomes will be evaluated by the following:

1. The number of times each outcome and indicator is used by nurses
2. The use of each outcome and indicator to evaluate specific nursing interventions for different patient groups defined by age, medical diagnoses, and nursing diagnoses
3. Identification of outcomes that are not on the NOC list but are chosen by practicing nurses

4. Discussion of the use or lack of use of the outcomes and indicators by staff nurses in each of the settings and documentation of reasons for use or nonuse

The research team focus groups, composed of faculty content experts and clinical nurse experts, will review the logic of conceptual links between each outcome and indicator, NIC interventions, and NANDA diagnoses; the extent these linkages are empirically validated according to reported research; and the evidence obtained from the study. Finally, evidence from the field tests will be used to refine the outcome concepts, definitions, indicators, and measures.

The results of the field testing will prepare the team to continue the work into the measurement phase. The electronic capability provided by clinical information systems will make it possible to download clinical nursing data for analysis at the University of Iowa College of Nursing's computer center and to gather the outcomes measures as they are developed for psychometric evaluation. The team also will be able to examine the association between diagnoses, interventions, and outcomes for teaching methods and for conducting nursing effectiveness research.

References

1. Bulechek, G. & McCloskey, J. (1992). Nursing interventions. *Nursing Clinics of North America,* 27:289-598.

2. Clougherty, J., McCloskey, J., Johnson, M., Gardner, D., Kelly, K., & Maas, M. (1991). Software evaluation and usage in nursing service administration laboratory and classes. *Computers in Nursing,* (March/April), 69-74.

3. Fehring, R.J. (1986). Validating diagnostic labels: Standardized methodology. In M.E. Hurley (Ed.), *Classification of Nursing Diagnoses: Proceedings of the Sixth Conference.* St. Louis: Mosby.

4. Fehring, R.J. (1987). Methods to validate nursing diagnoses. *Heart & Lung,* 16(6), 625-629.

5. Fleishman, E.A. & Quaintance, M.K. (1984). *Taxonomies of Human Performance: A Description of Human Tasks.* Orlando, FL: Academic Press.

6. Iowa Intervention Project. (1992). *Nursing Interventions Classification (NIC).* St. Louis: Mosby.

7. Iowa Intervention Project. (1996). *Nursing Interventions Classification (NIC)* (2nd ed.). St. Louis: Mosby.

8. Lang, N.M. & Clinton, J.F. (1984). Assessment of quality of nursing care. In H.H. Werley & J.J. Fitzpatrick (Eds.), *Annual Review of Nursing Research,* Vol. 2, 135-163, New York: Springer.

9. Marek, K.D. (1989). Outcome measurement in nursing. *Journal of Nursing Quality Assurance,* 4(1), 1-9.

10. Rodgers, B.L. (1989). Concepts, analysis and the development of nursing knowledge: the evolutionary cycle. *Journal of Advanced Nursing,* 14(4):330-335.

11. Sparks, S.M. & Lien-Gieschen, T. (1994). Modification of the diagnostic content validity model. *Nursing Diagnosis,* 5(1):31-35.

12. Stewart, B.J. & Archbold, P.G. (1992). Nursing intervention studies require outcome measures that are sensitive to change. Part I. *Research in Nursing and Health,* 15, 477-481.

13. Stewart, B.J. & Archbold, P.G. (1993). Nursing intervention studies require outcome measures that are sensitive to change. Part II. *Research in Nursing and Health,* 16, 77-81.

14. Tarlov, A.R., Ware, J.E., Greenfield, S., Nelson, E.C., Perrin, E., & Zubkoff, M. (1989). The Medical Outcomes Study: An application of methods for monitoring the results of medical care. *Journal of the American Medical Association,* 262, 925-930.

15. Walker, L.O. & Avant, K.C. (1988). *Strategies for Theory Construction in Nursing* (pp. 51-61) (2nd ed.). Norwalk, CT: Appleton & Lange.

16. Waltz, C.G., Strickland, O.L., & Lenz, E.R. (1991). *Measurement in Nursing Research.* Philadelphia: F.A. Davis.

CHAPTER FOUR

The Current and Future Classification

I dentifying outcomes responsive to nursing, rather than depending on the use of interdisciplinary outcomes developed mostly for physician practice, is important for the control of quality patient care and the development of nursing knowledge. Agreement on standardized nursing-sensitive patient outcomes will allow nurses to study the effects of nursing interventions along a continuum of patient care and across care settings. Standardized outcomes will provide data to elucidate nursing knowledge and advance nursing theory development, and will provide information about nursing effectiveness for health care policy formulation. Nurses have been documenting the outcomes of their interventions for decades, but the lack of a common language and associated measures for outcomes has impeded data aggregation, analysis, and the synthesis of information about the effects of nursing interventions and nursing practice. Outcome evaluation in health care has expanded to include not only the efficacy of health care interventions, but also the effectiveness of interventions. In efficacy research, the outcomes of interventions are studied under controlled conditions,[4] whereas in effectiveness research, outcomes are studied in an uncontrolled practice situation. In a sense, efficacy research illustrates what outcomes are possible, given ideal conditions and without consideration for cost, and effectiveness research demonstrates what outcomes are achieved in practice and at what cost. An important result of the emphasis put on the evaluation of health care effectiveness has been the recognition that all initiatives to evaluate effectiveness require the identification, standardization, and valid measurement of patient outcomes.[5]

THE CLASSIFICATION

This book presents one way to standardize terminology for nursing-sensitive patient outcomes. Each outcome presented in Part Two represents a concept that can be used to assess the state, behavior, or perception of a patient or family caregiver to evaluate the effects of nursing interventions. Each outcome has a definition, a measurement scale, and associated indicators and measures. At this stage of development, the list of outcomes is presented alphabetically. Work to group common outcomes and create a taxonomy of nursing-sensitive patient outcomes is under way and when complete will facilitate the ease with which outcomes can be located. An alphabetical listing of the outcomes and their page numbers is provided in the Contents in the beginning of the text to make it easier to find an outcome.

The Classification—What It Is

The current classification is a list of 190 outcomes with definitions, indicators, and measurement scales. Outcomes in the classification are for use at the individual level—either for individual patients or for individual family caregivers in the home. The research team recognizes that outcomes for other units, be they families, communities, or organizations, are important outcomes for nursing, and the team anticipates the development of family- and community-centered outcomes as future steps necessary to complete the classification. Some of these outcomes may be aggregated measures of individual patient outcomes.

The term *patient* is used in the classification to denote an individual who is the recipient of nursing care. It is recognized that the term *client* is used in many community and health-maintenance settings and that *resident* is used in many long-term settings. For purposes of brevity, the term patient was selected since it is commonly used in nursing and health care literature. Likewise, the terms *caregiver* and *family* are used to denote a family member, a significant other, a friend, or another person who cares for or acts on behalf of the patient.

As noted earlier, the outcomes are variable concepts that can be measured along a continuum, which means the outcomes are stated as concepts that reflect a patient's actual condition rather than as expected goals. It also means that the outcomes are neutral, that is they don't specify the desired patient condition. This retains the variability of the outcome and allows measurement of the patient condition at any point in time. For example, the outcome Cognitive Ability is measured on a five-point scale from "extremely compromised" to "not compromised" and Caregiver Performance: Direct Care is measured on a five-point scale from "not adequate" to "totally adequate." This allows nurses to follow changes in or maintenance of patient or caregiver conditions as the patient is cared for over time or moves from one practice setting to another.

Outcomes in the classification are at a higher level of abstraction than goal statements typically are. In some instances, the use of a variable concept and a five-point measurement scale allows what may have been two or more outcomes to be represented as one outcome. For example, the scale used to measure self-care outcomes (e.g., Self-Care: Dressing, Self-Care: Hygiene) has the following anchors:
1. "Dependent, does not participate"
2. "Requires assistive person and device"
3. "Requires assistive person"
4. "Independent with assistive device"
5. "Completely independent"

Each of these levels, except "dependent, does not participate" might have represented a separate goal statement for each type of self-care. In other instances, the indicators used to determine patient condition in relation to an outcome represent the intermediate, specific outcomes often reflected in goal statements. For example, a few of the indicators used to determine the outcome Cognitive Ability are: "demonstrates immediate memory," "demonstrates remote memory," "communicates clearly and appropriately for age and ability," and "processes information." While these may serve as intermediate outcomes or indicators of cognitive ability, when used alone they do not measure the multidimensional aspects of the concept Cognitive Ability. The use of midlevel concepts facilitates the use of outcomes in computerized systems and the aggregation of data for effectiveness research and policy formulation, which tend to focus on patient conditions that influence functional and health status. The midlevel concept also may be useful in efficacy research. For example, a researcher evaluating an intervention to improve memory can use outcome indicators to determine the effects of the intervention not only on memory but on other factors that determine cognitive ability. Whereas the outcomes currently do not provide tested measures for assessing the effects of an intervention on memory, they do suggest other factors to consider and can be used in conjunction with tested measures to arrive at a determination of how improvement of memory influences cognitive ability. Further, if found to be psychometrically sound, there is potential for the use of outcomes to measure impact variables in efficacy research. Development and testing of outcome measures that have practical use in clinical settings and are valid for use in research have important implications for documenting the nursing profession's contributions to health care and providing data to influence health care policy.

The outcomes, while representative of broad, midlevel concepts, are at varied levels of specificity. For example, Risk Control is a broad outcome defined as "actions to eliminate or reduce actual, personal, and modifiable health threats" that can be used with any nursing intervention directed at assisting patients to identify and control risks. However, more specific outcomes for risks of common concern to nurses' area of care (e.g., Risk Control: Alcohol Use and Risk Control: Drug Use) are in the classification. As the taxonomic structure is developed, one of the criteria for categorization will be the level of abstraction, which will facilitate the ease with which the classification can be used.

The language used in the outcomes reflects the language used by nurses in nursing literature. Language used most consistently by nurses, rather than by those in other disciplines, was selected for the outcomes whenever possible. However, there are exceptions when terminology most familiar to nurses is too specific to reflect a broad patient state or is stated as a negative outcome. For example, decubiti, or skin breakdown, is a common term used by nurses, but the term used in the classification to describe the condition of the skin is Tissue Integrity: Skin & Mucous Membranes. The wording allows the outcome to be stated as a neutral term and as a midlevel concept that is addressed by nursing interventions. In some instances, undesirable or negative patient conditions are used as the outcome when the concept cannot be captured adequately with a neutral term. For example, the classification contains the outcomes Pain Level and Infection Status, both undesirable patient states that represent important outcomes that need to be monitored but cannot be adequately described by terms such as "comfort level" or "immune status." Undesirable patient conditions also are used as outcomes when the language is commonly accepted and used by both health care providers and policy makers. For example, the Agency for Health Care Policy and Research uses Pain Level in published guidelines, as do researchers and practitioners when evaluating the effects of interventions on pain.

The classification structure uses colons to separate broad outcome terms from terms that make the outcomes more specific. As much as possible, the first term in the outcome reflects the term that the practitioner might select when looking for the outcome. For example, recovery from abuse is found under the broad category abuse recovery but is further specified by Abuse Recovery: Emotional; Abuse Recovery: Financial; Abuse Recovery: Physical; and Abuse Recovery: Sexual.

Each concept represents a patient state, behavior, or perception sensitive in varying degrees to nursing interventions. Although the team assessed sensitivity to nursing interventions by (1) selecting the concepts from outcomes in nursing literature and clinical information systems, (2) determining that the outcomes have been used to measure the effects of nursing interventions, and (3) surveying expert nurses about the importance of the outcomes as measures of nursing care, it is recognized that the ultimate test of sensitivity will be the widespread selection and use of outcomes in practice and research. Because the outcomes have been developed for use in all settings where nurses provide care, some of the outcome indicators may be more applicable in one setting than another. For example, blood values and other diagnostic results used as indicators may be pertinent in an intensive- or acute-care setting, but may be less useful in a home- or nursing-home–care setting.

Many of the nursing-sensitive patient outcomes are not specific for nursing interventions only and thus could be used to evaluate the care provided by other health care disciplines. For example, physical therapists may highly influence certain patients' Mobility Level, which may be an appropriate outcome to assess the collaborative results of nursing care and physical therapy. While the outcomes may be used in other disciplines, the indicators used to assess patient condition in relation to the outcome may vary from discipline to discipline. For example, physical therapists may use indicators that measure progress with the use of equipment not routinely used by nursing. The classification also contains outcomes most often associated with nursing interventions (e.g., Breastfeeding Establishment: Infant; Bowel Elimination; Health Promoting Behavior; and Knowledge: Treatment Procedure[s]). As standardized outcomes are selected and used in practice, more information will be available to determine their frequency of use and conditions under which they are selected.

The Classification—What It Is Not

Although the classification of outcomes presented in this text contains outcomes frequently used by nurses, at this stage of development the text does not include all outcomes that might be important for nursing. As nurses review the outcomes and use them in practice and research, other outcomes will be identified and current outcomes may require modification. The project investigators anticipate that any classification of outcomes will undergo modification to reflect changes in nursing practice and health care delivery, and therefore, the classification will be continually evolving.

The current list of outcomes has not been placed in a taxonomy, but this work is in progress and will be published when complete. Coding the outcomes for their use in information systems will be done when the taxonomic work is complete. Coding outcomes is an important prerequisite for the aggregation and analysis of data since it will allow data to be collected using a code number rather than a more lengthy outcome statement.

As noted earlier, the current list of outcomes does not contain outcomes for client groups with which nurses intervene. However, this does not mean that the outcomes cannot be aggregated for patient populations (e.g., by a nursing or medical diagnosis, by a diagnostic related group [DRG], by the unit or geographic location in which care is provided, or by the nurse providing the care). It does mean that family, community, and population outcomes need to be developed to assess the effectiveness of nursing interventions aimed at these patient groups. It is possible that some of the outcomes can be modified for use with aggregates, and this type of feedback from users will be extremely helpful to the investigators. The outcome classification also does not contain outcomes of organizational performance or the cost of health care. These outcomes are important in effectiveness research, but do not reflect the effects of interventions on a patient.

The outcomes are not prescriptive. They are not goals for individual patients or patient populations, although they can be translated into goals by identifying the desired patient condition on the measurement scale. They are not prescribed for a particular nursing diagnosis or nursing intervention, but can be selected for a diagnosis or intervention based on the judgment of the nurse responsible for the care of an individual patient or based on the collective judgment of the health care providers responsible for developing a critical path for a patient population. Possible linkages to NANDA nursing diagnoses are suggested and can be found in Appendix A. These linkages are presented in this text to assist the user in the selection of outcomes and to stimulate study of the suggested linkages.

The outcomes are not nursing diagnoses, although many of them assess the same patient states, behaviors, or perceptions addressed by nursing diagnoses. A diagnosis identifies a patient condition that is altered, has the potential to be altered, or has the potential to be improved whereas an outcome assesses the actual patient condition at a given point in time using a five-point measurement scale. Table 4-1 illustrates some of the differences in diagnostic and outcome language using NANDA diagnoses and NOC outcomes.

The comparisons in Table 4-1 illustrate the difference between the language used to identify a patient condition for which a diagnosis is made and the patient condition that is measured as an outcome. They also illustrate that some outcomes are more specific than a related diagnosis (e.g., knowledge outcomes), while some diagnoses are more specific than the related outcome (e.g., diagnoses of bowel function). There also are some global outcomes for which similar language is not used in the NANDA diagnoses; however, these outcomes might be selected for a number of the diagnoses.

Outcomes are not patient assessments, although indicators may represent patient states, behaviors, or perceptions evaluated during a patient assessment. No outcome represents the total range of patient states, behaviors, or perceptions that comprise a comprehensive assessment. The patient assessment provides information needed to identify actual or potential patient problems and nursing diagnoses and to select nursing interventions and patient outcomes. Although the defining assessment data for a diagnosis should correspond with the outcome indicators that describe the same patient state, the validation of nursing diagnoses and nursing-sensitive patient outcomes needed to achieve correspondence or complete similarity has not yet been done. As discussed later in the chapter, when an outcome is selected, the patient's condition will need to be evaluated and rated on the measurement scale to provide a baseline measure for comparison with post-intervention measures.

The classification does not contain patient satisfaction outcomes. This is not because these outcomes are less important indicators of nursing care effectiveness, but because their development was delayed because of the extensive work being done in the area of patient satisfaction. Patient satisfaction with nursing care remains an important component of the classification for future development.

TABLE 4-1
Comparison of NANDA Diagnoses and NOC Outcomes

NANDA diagnosis	NOC outcome
Impaired Physical Mobility	Mobility Level
Hopelessness	Hope
Knowledge Deficit	Knowledge: Disease Process Knowledge: Medication Knowledge: Health Behaviors Knowledge: Treatment Regimen
Constipation Diarrhea	Bowel Elimination
Bowel Incontinence	Bowel Continence Symptom Control Well-being Will to Live

THE CLASSIFICATION AND ITS USES

The classification can be used in nursing practice, research, and education. It provides a framework for the evaluation of nursing practice, whether in the clinical setting or in research studies. It also can be used by students and novice nurses to develop clinical decision-making skills. Some of the uses, with an emphasis on its use in practice, are elaborated in the following pages.

Uses in Practice

The outcomes are adaptable for a variety of uses in practice. Although the outcomes are neutral concepts developed for use at the individual patient level, they can be used as expected outcomes or goals and will provide data that can be aggregated and analyzed in a number of ways. The following examples of possible use are not inclusive.

Outcome goals for individual patients. In addition to evaluating an individual patient's condition, outcomes can be used as desired outcomes, or goals. After completing a patient assessment, the nurse will rate the patient on the selected outcome scale and identify the desired rating to be achieved following the intervention. For example, the patient may enter the care situation with the outcome Cognitive Ability rated as "extremely compromised," and because the cause of the impaired cognition cannot be completely eliminated, the desired goal for this patient following treatment may be to achieve a rating of "moderately compromised." In some instances, this goal may not be achieved following a brief care episode but will need to be evaluated at a later time, either during a home or clinic visit. However, the patient may demonstrate improvement in some of the indicators during the brief care episode, which would indicate progress toward the long-term goal of "moderately compromised." Another patient may have "extremely compromised" Cognitive Ability because of a condition that can be eliminated or completely controlled, and the desired outcome status following even a brief episode of care may be "not compromised." Outcomes stated as variable concepts allow goal statements to be individualized for each patient while maintaining standardized outcome language and measures. They also give recognition to what all nurses know, that not all patients will be able to achieve the most desirable state despite the most intensive care. Variable outcomes measured along a continuum allow the nurse to evaluate the amount of progress or lack of progress for individual patients. This information is not available when outcomes represent only the most desirable patient state and the evaluation at the conclusion of a care episode represents a goal not met. However, if a desired outcome has been identified, the option always remains to record that the outcome goal was met or not met for a specific data base purpose.

Outcome goals for patient groups. The outcomes also can be used as goals in critical paths or in standardized care plans (see Appendix B for examples). In these situations, the outcome is stated with a specific desired measurement point on the scale. For example, the desired goal at the end of an acute-care episode for stroke patients with "extremely compromised" Cognitive Ability at the time of admission might be "substantially compromised" with a goal of "moderately compromised" or "mildly compromised" following rehabilitation. If the acute-care episode is extremely short, the goal may be to maintain the patient at the "extremely compromised" level with some improvement in specified indicators—the intermediate outcomes that indicate progress toward improvement in Cognitive Ability.

On the other hand, the desired goal for patients with hepatic encephalopathy and "extremely compromised" Cognitive Ability at the time of admission may be to have the patients progress to "moderately compromised" or "mildly compromised" Cognitive Ability after an acute-care episode. This group of patients also represents a population of patients for which follow-up monitoring of the outcome Cognitive Ability is important because deterioration in this outcome may be an early indication of disease progression. For patients with acute confusion and "substantially compromised" Cognitive Ability resulting from chemical imbalances, the desired goal after an acute-care episode may be Cognitive Ability, "not compromised." If the cause of the chemical imbalance stems from an acute rather than a chronic condition, indicators for Cognitive Ability likely would not be measured over time since the underlying pathologic factor would no longer exist and no changes in Cognitive Ability would be anticipated.

Outcome measures. The outcomes also can be adapted for data aggregation and analysis for populations of patients. For example, the outcome Pain Level can be used as an outcome measure with any patient population in which pain is a symptom and interventions to alleviate pain are initiated. Pain Level is defined as the "amount of reported or demonstrated pain." The pain measurement scale rates pain as: (1) severe, (2) substantial, (3) moderate, (4) slight, and (5) none. These ratings constitute the **numerator** of an outcome measure. The **denominator** is any patient population in which pain management is an intervention and the level of pain is an important outcome. In the following example the patient population is defined as patients with lung cancer.*

> The outcome measure, or ratio, can be defined as the percent of lung cancer patients with Pain Level ratings of either 1, 2, 3, 4, or 5. In this example, the equation to determine a measure, or ratio, of lung cancer patients with various levels of pain would be set up as follows:
>
> **NUMERATOR:** number of lung cancer patients with a rating of either 1, 2, 3, 4, or 5 on the Pain Level scale
> **DENOMINATOR:** number of lung cancer patients who have undergone surgery, nonsurgical therapy, or palliative care
>
> If five points in the **numerator** are too many, the ratings can be combined and the outcome measure defined as the percent of lung cancer patients with ratings of 1 and 2; 3; or 4 and 5, which will provide three numbers rather than five numbers in the numerator to determine the ratio. If desired, the **denominator** also can be more specific, and ratios can be determined separately for lung cancer patients who have had surgery, for those receiving nonsurgical therapy, and for those receiving palliative care. The nonsurgical therapy patients can be further specified as those receiving chemotherapy and those receiving radiation therapy. However the measure is set up, data about the pain levels achieved with treatment in a specified group of patients can be determined. If desired, mean pain levels for any patient group can be determined by weighting each pain level to reflect the number of patients with a rating of 1, 2, 3, 4, or 5.

Timing of the measurement of an outcome also needs to be defined. Possible times for data collection in the preceding example could be the day of admission, every 3 days, and the day of discharge. Timing of data collection might vary if the denominator is more specifically related to the type of therapy provided. One could also identify sug-

---

*This example was developed by G. Bulechek, B. Head, M. Johnson, J. McCloskey, and B. Wakefield, faculty and doctoral students at the University of Iowa.

gested nursing interventions for pain control; using NIC interventions, these might include, but not be limited to: biofeedback, medication administration, pain management, simple relaxation therapy, and simple guided imagery. If the sample size is sufficient, the mean pain level following any of these nursing interventions also could be calculated.

The advantage of collecting data that identify patients with a pain level of "slight" or "none" versus only those with "severe" or "substantial" pain following interventions designed to alleviate pain is that a health provider can review patient records to determine the factors that differ in the two populations. For example, is it a characteristic of the patient, the extent of the pathologic condition, or is there variation in the intervention used? This type of analysis is not possible when only the undesired outcome is aggregated—in this case patients with "severe" or "substantial" pain levels following interventions.

Use in Research, Policy Formulation, and Education

The classification, because it provides standardized outcomes, can be used to expand nursing knowledge through theory development and efficacy research. Implications for its use in these areas have been discussed in Chapter One and in previous sections of this chapter.

The classification also can be used to provide information for effectiveness research and policy development. Health service researchers use effectiveness, equity, and efficiency of health care delivery to assess the performance of the U.S. medical care system.[1] In this context "effectiveness concerns the benefits of medical care measured by improvements in health."[1] Although health service researchers tend to include the delivery of all health care under the term *medical care*, emphasis is placed on the benefits of physician care. To ensure that the benefits of nursing care that affect improvements in health are recognized and included in health services research, the nursing profession must develop standardized measures that enable data aggregation. Inclusion in health services research is important because this research provides basic, descriptive data about the performance of the U.S. health care system that is used in the formulation of health care policy.

The classification will be useful for teaching decision-making skills to student nurses and novice practitioners. Because the classification is not prescriptive, it forces the nurse to identify outcomes based on knowledge of the patient's nursing and medical diagnoses and the interventions available to the nurse. In addition, since the outcomes are not stated as goals, the nurse must determine individual outcomes based on knowledge of the individual patient's condition and resources. Formulation of outcomes for groups of patients requires knowledge of pertinent research describing the outcomes achieved with various interventions. If the learner is asked to develop a nursing care plan for the patient, this can be done using the outcome classification. An example of such a plan can be found in Appendix C.

IMPLEMENTING THE CLASSIFICATION IN PRACTICE

Possible uses of the classification in practice have been illustrated in the preceding section. This section discusses how the classification is applied in the practice setting for individual patients or groups of patients, with emphasis on the application of the various components of the outcome—the outcome label, the indicators, and the measurement scales.

Implementing the Outcome

The outcome label and the outcome definition are the standardized components of the outcome, meaning the terminology should not change. The scale also will be standardized when its reliability and validity have been tested. The times at which outcomes should be evaluated are not specified, but the minimum requirement is measuring an outcome when care is initiated (i.e., the baseline measure) and measuring an outcome when care is completed (i.e., the discharge measure). Since measurement times are not standardized, reporting the time at which measures were obtained is important for making comparisons between populations and across settings. These reports will help enable the eventual development of recommended intervals for outcome measurement.

As previously discussed, the outcome appropriate for an individual patient or patient group will be selected in much the same manner that an outcome goal is selected. That is, after assessing the patient and determining the pertinent nursing diagnoses and patient problems, the outcomes to evaluate care effectiveness will be identified. If the patient has a nursing diagnosis Breathing Pattern: Ineffective, possible outcomes would be Respiratory Status: Gas Exchange or Respiratory Status: Ventilation. Both outcomes might be selected or only one chosen, depending on the cause of the ineffective breathing pattern. After selecting the outcome(s), the nurse will rate the patient's condition on the provided outcome scale—in this case from "extremely compromised" to "not compromised." Then the practitioner may determine a point on the scale that is the desired outcome for the individual patient or patient group. The practitioner also may choose not to determine a desired outcome if knowledge about achievable outcomes is inadequate. In either case, the patient condition in relation to the outcome should be reevaluated at specified intervals and at the time of discharge. Changes in patient condition or lack of change will be immediately illustrated through the patient ratings. For example, a patient may be admitted with the outcome rating Respiratory Status: Ventilation "extremely compromised" and leave the care situation with the outcome rating Respiratory Status: Ventilation "moderately compromised." If the desired goal was to have the patient's condition "not compromised," the use of a rating scale would more likely result in an analysis of the care than if a goal of "respiratory status improved" was used since that goal would be met and further analysis of care would not be done.

Implementing the Outcome Indicators

The purpose of the outcome indicators is to help a nurse determine a patient rating for an outcome; they can be considered as more specific outcomes used to determine the patient rating on the outcome scale. Two abbreviations used in the indicators are IER, which means "in expected range," and WNL, which means "within normal limits." These abbreviations have been used in lieu of specifying ranges that may differ with disease pathology or with laboratory techniques used in a specific setting.

The language of the indicators should remain standardized as much as possible. However, practitioners may wish to add some indicators that are pertinent to a specialized area of practice or make the indicators more specific. For example, specific ranges for an individual patient or patient population may be substituted when the indicator states IER or WNL. Also, some of the indicators may be deleted if they are not pertinent to an individual patient or patient group.

Selecting the indicators important for the individual patient and rating the patient, either mentally or on paper for the selected indicators, will help determine the patient's rating on the outcome scale. As a nurse uses an outcome and becomes familiar with its associated indicators, it may be unnecessary to rate a patient on the indicator scales since the nurse will automatically assess the patient's condition for the indicators he or she is accustomed to using.

The source of data for the indicators will vary. Some data may be obtained from the patient record (e.g., information about chemical measures or vital signs). Some data will be obtained from observation or physical assessments (e.g., for the following indicators—"negotiates for care preferences," "nausea not present," or "auscultated breath sounds IER"). Other indicators may require soliciting information or perceptions from the patient (e.g., "describes strategies to maximize health," "perceived isolation," or "satisfaction with health status").

The indicators are less abstract than the outcome and may at times serve as intermediate outcomes in a critical-path or standardized-care plan. If an indicator is considered an important measure of patient progress, nurses may choose to aggregate data on a particular indicator as well as on the outcome. This may be particularly true for patients with short episodes of care in which progress in relation to the outcome will not be possible, but progress in relation to significant indicators may be achieved.

Implementing the Measurement Scales

The classification contains 16 measurement scales, which are illustrated in Table 4-2. Because the outcomes are variable concepts representing patient states, behaviors, and perceptions, a method of measuring the concepts is essential. Based on the advice of practitioners in the field sites and measurement experts, a five-point Likert-type scale was selected. The scale provides an adequate number of options to demonstrate variability in the patient state, behavior, or perception depicted in the outcome. The scale also limits the degree of precision required for a 10-point scale. Although the scales have been used in pilot studies and field testing, statistical analysis of the scales is necessary to ensure reliability and validity.

Each scale is constructed so the fifth, or end point, reflects the most desirable patient condition relative to the outcome. As previously indicated, the most desirable condition will not be achievable in all patients or patient groups, and the desired outcome for an intervention in a given situation may be less than the most desirable patient condition. As nursing knowledge increases and more effective interventions are developed, improvement in the outcomes achieved may be expected. The following scales are described briefly, with their ranges given:

- Scale 1, which ranges from "extremely compromised" to "not compromised," is used to measure physiologic and psychologic outcomes that do not have quantifiable or standardized ranges.
- Scale 2, which ranges from "extreme deviation from expected range" to "no deviation from expected range," is used with physiologic states with known ranges (see Table 4-2).
- Scale 3 measures the degree of dependency for functional status and self-care outcomes and ranges from "dependent, does not participate" to "completely independent."
- Scale 6 measures the level of adequacy for outcomes related to patient performance and safety and has a range from "not adequate" to "totally adequate."
- The extent of patient states, behaviors, and knowledge are measured using Scale 9, which ranges from "none" to "extensive."
- The anchors in Scale 9 are reversed in Scale 8 for the outcomes for Caregiver Stressors and Loneliness, in which the desired condition is "none."
- Scale 10 is adjusted for wound healing to depict "complete healing," a measurable state with wound healing but not necessarily the end point for patient outcomes for which a measure of "complete" is not possible.
- Scale 13, which ranges from "never demonstrated" to "consistently demonstrated," is used to measure outcomes for a number of patient behaviors in

which the consistency with which the behavior is used is an important outcome measure.

Other scales and their associated outcomes that are used less frequently also can be found in Table 4-2.

Scales to measure both the outcome and the outcome indicators are provided, and in all instances the same scale is used for both the outcome and its indicators, as illustrated in Table 4-3.

Although the indicator scales will assist in determining the patient's rating on the outcome scale, they currently are not weighted to provide a mean or summated rating. It is recommended that the practitioner use both the range and the frequency of patient ratings on the indicator scale as an aid in arriving at the outcome rating. In general, the lower ratings on the indicators should be used to determine the outcome rating since they indicate that the higher level has not been consistently achieved. For example, in the outcome illustrated in Table 4-3, a consistent rating of 3s and 4s on the indicators would suggest that Caregiver Emotional Health is "moderately compromised" since some of the indicators of emotional health are rated as moderate. However, if the indicator ratings range from "extremely compromised" for frustration to "mild" and "none" for the remainder of the indicators, the nurse will need to determine whether frustration was a preexisting caregiver trait exacerbated by the caregiving role. If so, the nurse will rate the overall emotional health as "mildly compromised," but if frustration is a direct result of caregiving, the nurse should consider the extreme degree of frustration created by caregiving, decrease the rating one step to "moderately compromised," and initiate interventions to relieve caregiver frustration.

Information about the importance of each indicator for determining the outcome is available from the surveys and will be used in the validation of the measurement scales. Also, feedback from users will assist in the psychometric evaluation of the current scales.

Commonly Asked Questions About the NOC

To summarize information provided in this and previous chapters and to encourage better understanding and thus greater use of the NOC, the most commonly asked questions about the classification are listed in the following paragraphs with brief responses.

1. **Why are the outcomes not stated as goals for the patient?** The research team developed the outcomes as variable concepts so that patient status in response to nursing interventions could be documented and monitored over time and across settings and yield more information than just whether a goal was met. For clinical and research purposes, either/or type data provide a very limited amount of information and will not allow nurses to adequately evaluate the effectiveness of their interventions. If goals are not met, it is important to know whether any progress was made or the extent that the patient's status deteriorated, if at all. It is important to note, however, that the NOC outcomes can be used to state a goal for the patient.

2. **How are the outcomes different from nursing diagnoses?** NOC outcomes describe a variable patient state, behavior, or perception. The outcome state for a particular patient at a particular time can be at any point on a negative to positive continuum. Nursing diagnoses, on the other hand, describe patient states that are in some way less positive than what is desired. Nursing diagnoses describe patient problems, actual or potential, that the nurse seeks to resolve through intervention.

Text continued on p. 60.

TABLE 4-2

Measurement Scales Used in NOC

Scale #		NOC scales	
1	Extremely compromised	Substantially compromised	Moderately compromised

		Outcomes
Mildly compromised	**Not compromised**	Bowel Elimination
		Cardiac Pump Effectiveness
		Caregiver Emotional Health
		Caregiver Physical Health
		Caregiver Well-Being
		Caregiver-Patient Relationship
		Circulation Status
		Cognitive Ability
		Communication
		Communication: Expressive Ability
		Communication: Receptive Ability
		Electrolyte & Acid/Base Balance
		Endurance
		Fluid Balance
		Hydration
		Immune Status
		Muscle Function
		Neurological Status
		Neurological Status: Autonomic
		Neurological Status: Central Motor Control
		Neurological Status: Consciousness
		Neurological Status: Cranial Sensory/Motor Function
		Neurological Status: Spinal Sensory/Motor Function
		Nutritional Status
		Nutritional Status: Energy
		Oral Health
		Quality of Life
		Respiratory Status: Gas Exchange
		Respiratory Status: Ventilation
		Rest
		Sleep
		Spiritual Well-Being
		Thermoregulation
		Thermoregulation: Neonate
		Tissue Integrity: Skin & Mucous Membranes
		Tissue Perfusion: Cardiac
		Tissue Perfusion: Cerebral
		Tissue Perfusion: Peripheral
		Tissue Perfusion: Pulmonary
		Tissue Perfusion: Abdominal Organs
		Urinary Elimination
		Well-Being
		Will to Live

Continued.

TABLE 4-2

Measurement Scales Used in NOC—cont'd

Scale #		NOC scales	
2	Extreme deviation from expected range	Substantial deviation from expected range	Moderate deviation from expected range
3	Dependent, does not participate	Requires assistive person & device	Requires assistive person
4	No motion	Limited motion	Moderate motion
5	Not at all	To a slight extent	To a moderate extent
6	Not adequate	Slightly adequate	Moderately adequate

		Outcomes
Mild deviation from expected range	**No deviation from expected range**	Growth Nutritional Status: Biochemical Measures Nutritional Status: Body Mass Physical Aging Status Physical Maturation: Female Physical Maturation: Male Vital Signs Status
Independent with assistive device	**Completely independent**	Ambulation: Walking Ambulation: Wheelchair Balance Body Positioning: Self-Initiated Mobility Level Self-Care: Activities of Daily Living (ADL) Self-Care: Bathing Self-Care: Dressing Self-Care: Eating Self-Care: Grooming Self-Care: Hygiene Self-Care: Instrumental Activities of Daily Living (IADL) Self-Care: Non-Parenteral Medication Self-Care: Oral Hygiene Self-Care: Parenteral Medication Self-Care: Toileting Transfer Performance
Substantial motion	**Full motion**	Joint Movement: Active Joint Movement: Passive
To a great extent	**To a very great extent**	Blood Transfusion Reaction Control Dignified Dying Energy Conservation Grief Resolution Immune Hypersensitivity Control
Substantially adequate	**Totally adequate**	Abuse Protection Breastfeeding Establishment: Infant Breastfeeding Establishment: Maternal Breastfeeding Maintenance Breastfeeding Weaning Caregiver Performance: Direct Care Caregiver Performance: Indirect Care Caregiving Endurance Potential Leisure Participation Nutritional Status: Food & Fluid Intake Nutritional Status: Nutrient Intake Parenting Parenting: Social Safety Play Participation

Continued.

TABLE 4-2
Measurement Scales Used in NOC—cont'd

Scale #		NOC scales	
6—cont'd			
7	Over 9	7-9	4-6
8	Extensive	Substantial	Moderate
9	None	Limited	Moderate
10	None	Slight	Moderate
11	Never positive	Rarely positive	Sometimes positive

		Outcomes
		Role Performance Safety Behavior: Fall Prevention Safety Behavior: Home Physical Environment Safety Behavior: Personal
1-3	**None**	Safety Status: Falls Occurrence
Limited	**None**	Caregiver Stressors Loneliness
Substantial	**Extensive**	Abuse Recovery: Emotional Abuse Recovery: Financial Abuse Recovery: Physical Abuse Recovery: Sexual Acceptance: Health Status Caregiver Adaptation to Patient Institutionalization Caregiver Home Care Readiness Child Adaptation to Hospitalization Comfort Level Hope Knowledge: Breastfeeding Knowledge: Child Safety Knowledge: Diet Knowledge: Disease Process Knowledge: Energy Conservation Knowledge: Health Behaviors Knowledge: Health Resources Knowledge: Infection Control Knowledge: Medication Knowledge: Personal Safety Knowledge: Prescribed Activity Knowledge: Substance Use Control Knowledge: Treatment Procedure(s) Knowledge: Treatment Regimen Psychosocial Adjustment: Life Change Social Interaction Skills Social Involvement Social Support
Substantial	**Complete**	Bone Healing Wound Healing: Primary Intention Wound Healing: Secondary Intention
Often Positive	**Consistently Positive**	Body Image Self-Esteem

Continued.

TABLE 4-2
Measurement Scales Used in NOC—cont'd

Scale #		NOC scales	
12	**Very Weak**	Weak	Moderate
13	**Never demonstrated**	**Rarely demonstrated**	Sometimes demonstrated

		Outcomes
Strong	**Very strong**	Health Beliefs Health Beliefs: Perceived Ability to Perform Health Beliefs: Perceived Control Health Beliefs: Perceived Resources Health Beliefs: Perceived Threat Health Orientation
Often demonstrated	**Consistently demonstrated**	Abusive Behavior Self-Control Adherence Behavior Aggression Control Anxiety Control Bowel Continence Cognitive Orientation Compliance Behavior Concentration Coping Decision Making Distorted Thought Control Fear Control Health Promoting Behavior Health Seeking Behavior Immunization Behavior Identity Impulse Control Information Processing Memory Mood Equilibrium Pain Control Behavior Parent-Infant Attachment Participation: Health Care Decisions Risk Control Risk Control: Alcohol Use Risk Control: Drug Use Risk Control: Immunization Risk Control: Sexually Transmitted Diseases (STD) Risk Control: Tobacco Use Risk Control: Unintended Pregnancy Risk Detection Self-Mutilation Restraint Suicide Self-Restraint Symptom Control Behavior Treatment Behavior: Illness or Injury Urinary Continence

Continued.

TABLE 4-2
Measurement Scales Used in NOC—cont'd

Scale #		NOC scales	
14	Severe	Substantial	Moderate
15	No evidence	Limited evidence	Moderate evidence
16	Extreme delay from expected range	Substantial delay from expected range	Moderate delay from expected range

3. **At what intervals should the outcomes be assessed and documented?** Research is needed to definitively answer this question. At present, the nurse will determine the intervals for measurement and documentation of the outcome based on clinical judgment as to when the effects of intervention need to be assessed. However, at minimum, the outcomes should be assessed and documented: (1) when a patient is admitted to a care setting or makes an initial visit to a nurse for care, and (2) when the patient is discharged, transferred, or referred to another setting or clinician for care.

4. **How are the outcomes used in critical paths?** NOC outcomes are very useful in clinical pathways because they allow quantification of the patient state, behavior, or perception that is expected to occur at specific points in time during an episode of care. Examples of use in critical paths are included in Appendix B of this edition. A major advantage of their use is the ability to monitor and compare the achievement of specific states across settings and providers. Use of the standardized outcomes will greatly facilitate the development of large data bases across settings and providers, rather than the more limited, unique setting or provider data bases that result when setting- or provider-specific outcomes are used in critical pathways.

5. **Why is it necessary for nurses to have their own list of outcomes?** NOC outcomes are patient outcomes that are responsive to nursing interventions. They are not in-

		Outcomes
Slight	**None**	Caregiver Lifestyle: Disruption Immobility Consequences: Physiological Immobility Consequences: Psycho-Cognitive Infection Status Pain Level Pain: Disruptive Effects Safety Status: Physical Injury Substance Addiction Consequences Symptom Severity
Substantial evidence	**Extensive evidence**	Abuse Cessation Neglect Cessation

Mild delay from expected range	**No delay from expected range**	Child Development: 2 Months
		Child Development: 4 Months
		Child Development: 6 Months
		Child Development: 12 Months
		Child Development: 2 Years
		Child Development: 3 Years
		Child Development: 4 Years
		Child Development: 5 Years
		Child Development: Middle Childhood
		   (6-11 Years)
		Child Development: Adolescence
		   (12-17 Years)

tended to be unique to nursing. Clearly most, if not all, patient outcomes are influenced by multiple health care providers. However, it is important for nurses to measure the effects of their interventions on patient outcomes. The NOC provides indicators for each outcome that are more sensitive to nursing interventions. Thus whereas the team expects all disciplines to use the majority of the outcomes, different indicators will be of most use to different health care disciplines. Without discipline-specific indicators for shared outcomes, it will be impossible to monitor the accountability of each discipline for its contribution to outcome improvement or deterioration.

6. **Why is it important to assess outcomes across care settings?** Continuity of care always has been an important value for the nursing profession. Yet, communication between settings and nurse providers has been constrained. A major obstacle has been the lack of standardized nomenclatures to describe the patient problems nurses treat, the interventions used, and the resulting patient outcomes. The inability to optimize continuity of care is costly to the patient and to the health care system. In the current resource-constrained environment, more emphasis is placed on continuity of care to reduce costs. Further, providers are developing networks that include providers and settings across the continuum of care to enhance continuity and reduce costs. There also is an emphasis on the demonstration of outcomes effectiveness. NOC outcomes provide a standardized language for outcomes that can be

---

TABLE 4-3

Caregiver Emotional Health

DEFINITION: Feelings, attitudes and emotions of a family care provider while caring for a family member or significant other over an extended period of time

CAREGIVER EMOTIONAL HEALTH	Extremely compromised 1	Substantially compromised 2	Moderately compromised 3	Mildly compromised 4	Not compromised 5
INDICATORS:					
Satisfaction with life	1	2	3	4	5
Sense of control	1	2	3	4	5
Self-esteem	1	2	3	4	5
Free of anger	1	2	3	4	5
Free of resentfulness	1	2	3	4	5
Free of guilt	1	2	3	4	5
Free of depression	1	2	3	4	5
Free of frustration	1	2	3	4	5
Free of ambivalence concerning situation	1	2	3	4	5
Certainty about future	1	2	3	4	5
Perceived social connectedness	1	2	3	4	5
Perceived spiritual well-being	1	2	3	4	5
Free of perceived burden	1	2	3	4	5
Perceived adequacy of resources	1	2	3	4	5
Use of psychotropic drugs	1	2	3	4	5
Other _____ Specify					

measured across the entire continuum of care, providing essential information that clinicians need to achieve continuity and to assess the cost-effectiveness of care.

7. **Why is it necessary to use the outcome labels when the indicators may be more useful?** Along with medicine, the nursing profession is a key member of the interdisciplinary health care team. The profession's contribution to interdisciplinary patient outcomes must be documented and the effectiveness of nursing interventions must be evaluated. Large, standardized data bases will contain NOC outcomes, but likely not discipline-specific indicators in all cases because of space limitations. Therefore, it is essential that the nursing profession use the standardized outcome labels that are included in large data bases so that the profession's influence on outcomes will be assessed to affect health policy.

8. **Why is the standardization of outcomes advocated when each patient is an individual?** Standardizing the language used to describe patient outcomes in no way interferes with assessing each patient as an individual. Rather, use of the NOC outcomes will enable nurses to measure each outcome state for each individual and will provide more information for monitoring the progress of each patient as an individual. Further, specific quantified goals can be set for each individual, and the extent that the goals are or are not met can be documented over time and across settings.

THE CLASSIFICATION—ONGOING AND FUTURE WORK

The current classification represents the completion of the beginning phases of research to develop a taxonomy of nursing-sensitive patient outcomes. Development of the taxonomy is in progress using similarity ratings and hierarchical clustering techniques. This will provide the broad domains in which similar outcomes will be clustered. After the taxonomy is completed, the outcomes will be coded for use in computerized systems. The taxonomy and coding will be developed to allow for additional outcomes. This work will be completed during the current phase of the research.

Identification and development of additional outcomes is ongoing. New outcomes are identified through feedback from nurses familiar with the classification and through comparisons of outcomes identified in nursing and related literature. Currently, 56 additional outcomes have been identified for development. Examples include:

- Accident Prevention
- Medication Effects
- Sensory Status
- Sexual Function
- Activity Tolerance
- Exercise Status
- Physical Fitness
- Motivation

While focus groups continue to do the majority of this work, graduate students have elected to develop outcomes related to their clinical specialities as part of their graduate work.

Psychometric testing of the outcomes will be the next phase of the research. Areas that need to be addressed as the reliability and validity of the scales are assessed include the following:

1. Are all of the indicators necessary? Should some be eliminated, should some be added, and should the indicators be weighted?
2. Should a five-point scale be used? Would a three-point or seven-point scale be more reliable?
3. How many scales should be used? Do anchors need to be more descriptive for each outcome, or can generic anchors be used?
4. Are the scales user-friendly? Can nurses use them with ease and without increasing the time used to identify and assess outcomes?

Two forms of reliability will be determined—interrater reliability and internal consistency reliability. Content validity has been assessed for the outcome indicators. If existing measures are available, criterion validity will be assessed. Construct validity also will be assessed.

Other questions related to outcome measurement also need to be addressed, especially the identification of risk-adjustment factors. Risk adjustment is a way to reduce the effects of confounding factors in effectiveness research, where cases are not randomly assigned to different treatments.[3] The key confounding factors are those aspects of health status that are causally related to the outcome under study.[2] Risk adjustment allows the evaluator to distinguish between the natural progression of a disease in various patient populations and the effects of the care provided.[6] Known risk factors for the outcomes in the classification will be identified through literature review.

Further field testing of the outcomes is needed to complete the evaluation of their usefulness and adaptability in clinical settings and to validate suggested linkages between nursing diagnoses, nursing interventions, and nursing-sensitive patient outcomes. This is planned for future research.

A taxonomy of nursing-sensitive patient outcomes will never be complete, but will be expanded and improved with further knowledge, development, and research. Therefore a means to keep the classification current is needed. In most disciplines, the classification work is done by a professional organization. The American Nurses' Association has not had the resources to do this work; therefore a Center for Nursing Classification has been established at the University of Iowa for the purpose of maintaining the NIC and NOC classifications. Although the center has received approval from the governing board of the institution, the center is not funded by the institution, and currently a fund-raising project for the center is ongoing.

Request for Feedback

Readers and users of the classification are encouraged to provide feedback to the research team. Identification of problems, issues, and outcomes for future development is encouraged. Appendix D contains a review form that can be completed and returned to the investigators.

SUMMARY

This chapter provided an overview of the current outcome classification and suggested uses in practice, research, and education. The components of the outcomes were described and suggestions for implementation in the practice setting were provided. Although implementation was described only in relation to practice, use of the outcomes is similar in research and education. Ongoing and future work includes continued development and psychometric evaluation of the classification.

References

1. Aday, L.A., Begley, C.E., Lairson, D.R., & Slater, C.H. (1993). *Evaluating the Medical Care System Effectiveness, Efficiency, and Equity.* Ann Arbor, MI: Health Administration Press.

2. Blumberg, M.S. (1993). Biased estimates of acute myocardial infarction mortality using Medis-Groups admission serverity groups. *Journal of the American Medical Association,* 265(22), 2965-2970.

3. Iezzoni, L.I. (1994). Risk and outcomes. In L.I. Iezzoni (Ed.), *Risk Adjustment for Measuring Health Care Outcomes* (pp. 1-28). Ann Arbor, MI: Health Administration Press.

4. Lohr, K.N. (1988). Outcome measurement: Concepts and questions. *Inquiry,* 25(1), 37-50.

5. McCloskey, J.C. & Bulechek, G.M. (1994). Standardizing the language for nursing treatments: An overview of the issues. *Nursing Outlook,* 42(2), 56-63.

6. Shaughnessy, P.W. & Crisler, K.S. (1995). *Outcome-based Quality Improvement: A Manual for Home Care Agencies on How to Use Outcomes.* Washington, DC: National Association for Home Care.

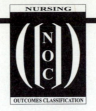

PART TWO

THE OUTCOMES

Abuse Cessation

DEFINITION: Evidence that the victim is no longer abused

ABUSE CESSATION	No evidence	Limited evidence	Moderate evidence	Substantial evidence	Extensive evidence
	1	**2**	**3**	**4**	**5**
INDICATORS:					
Cessation of abuse reported by victim	1	2	3	4	5
Physical abuse has ceased	1	2	3	4	5
Emotional abuse has ceased	1	2	3	4	5
Sexual abuse has ceased	1	2	3	4	5
Neglect has ceased	1	2	3	4	5
Financial exploitation has ceased	1	2	3	4	5
Other _____ Specify	1	2	3	4	5

BACKGROUND READINGS:

Amundson, M.J. (1989). Family crisis care: A home based intervention program for child abuse. *Issues in Mental Health Nursing, 10,* 285-296.

Cowen P. (1991). *The Iowa Crisis Nursery Project as a factor in the prevention of abuse.* Unpublished doctoral dissertation, University of Iowa, Iowa City.

Hunka, C.D., O'Toole, A.W., & O'Toole, R. (1985). Self-help therapy in Parents Anonymous. *Journal of Psychosocial Nursing, 23*(7), 24-32.

Olds, D.L., Henderson, C.R., Chamberlin, R., & Tatelbaum, R. (1986). Preventing child abuse and neglect: A randomized trial of nurse home visitation. *Pediatrics, 78*(1), 65-78.

Reuter, M.M. (1988). Parenting needs of abusing parents: Development of a tool for evaluation of parent education class. *Journal of Community Health Nursing, 5*(2), 129-140.

Abuse Protection

DEFINITION: Protection of self or dependent others from abuse

ABUSE PROTECTION	Not adequate 1	Slightly adequate 2	Moderately adequate 3	Substantially adequate 4	Totally adequate 5
INDICATORS:					
Plans for leaving situation	1	2	3	4	5
Safety of residence	1	2	3	4	5
Plans for avoiding abuse	1	2	3	4	5
Implementation of plan to avoid abuse	1	2	3	4	5
Safety of self	1	2	3	4	5
Safety of children	1	2	3	4	5
Obtaining restraining order as necessary	1	2	3	4	5
Self-advocacy	1	2	3	4	5
Facilitation of abuser obtaining counseling	1	2	3	4	5
Withdrawal when relationship is unsafe	1	2	3	4	5
Severance of relationship as needed	1	2	3	4	5
Other _____ Specify	1	2	3	4	5

BACKGROUND READINGS:

Brendtro, M., & Bowker, L.H. (1989). Battered women: How can nurses help? *Issues in Mental Health Nursing, 10*(2), 169-180.

Helton, A., McFarlane, J., & Anderson, E. (1987). Prevention of battering during pregnancy: Focus on nurse behavioral change. *Public Health Nursing, 4*(3), 166-174.

Hoff, L.A. (1992). Battered women—understanding, identification, and assessment: A psychosocial perspective, Part 1. *Journal of the American Academy of Nurse Practitioners, 4*, 148-155.

Hoff, L.A. (1993). Battered women—intervention and prevention: A psychosocial cultural perspective, Part 2. *Journal of the American Academy of Nurse Practitioners, 5*(1), 34-39.

Outcomes

Abuse Recovery: Emotional

Outcomes

DEFINITION: Healing of psychological injuries due to abuse

ABUSE RECOVERY: EMOTIONAL	None	Limited	Moderate	Substantial	Extensive
	1	2	3	4	5

INDICATORS:

Resolution of depression	1	2	3	4	5
Demonstration of confidence	1	2	3	4	5
Demonstration of self-esteem	1	2	3	4	5
Appropriate affect for situation	1	2	3	4	5
Decrease in suicide attempts	1	2	3	4	5
Resolution of trauma-induced psychoneurotic behaviors	1	2	3	4	5
Seeking of appropriate attention from others	1	2	3	4	5
Resolution of trauma-induced conduct disorders	1	2	3	4	5
Resolution of trauma-induced learning difficulties	1	2	3	4	5
Decrease in self-injurious behavior	1	2	3	4	5
Resolution of neurotic behaviors	1	2	3	4	5
Demonstration of impulse control	1	2	3	4	5
Self-advocacy	1	2	3	4	5
Expressions of feeling empowered	1	2	3	4	5
Recognition of abusive relationship(s)	1	2	3	4	5
Demonstration of comfort with caretaker or partner	1	2	3	4	5
Demonstration of comfort with returning home	1	2	3	4	5
Demonstration of insight into abusive relationship	1	2	3	4	5
Demonstration of adequate social interaction	1	2	3	4	5
Demonstration of positive interpersonal relation-ships	1	2	3	4	5
Demonstration of positive adjustment to change in living arrangement	1	2	3	4	5
Other _____ Specify	1	2	3	4	5

BACKGROUND READINGS:

Campbell J., McKenna, L.S., Torres, S., Sheridan, D., & Landenburger, K. (1993). Nursing care of abused women. In J. Campbell & J. Humphreys (Eds.), *Nursing care of survivors of family violence.* St. Louis: Mosby.

Campbell, J., & Fishwick, N. (1993). Abuse of female partners. In J. Campbell & J. Humphreys (Eds.), *Nursing care of survivors of family violence.* St. Louis: Mosby.

Abuse Recovery: Financial

DEFINITION: Regaining monetary and legal control or benefits following financial exploitation

ABUSE RECOVERY: FINANCIAL	None 1	Limited 2	Moderate 3	Substantial 4	Extensive 5
INDICATORS:					
Control of personal possessions	1	2	3	4	5
Access to Social Security and pension checks	1	2	3	4	5
Control of personal finances	1	2	3	4	5
Control of legal matters	1	2	3	4	5
Exercise of legal rights	1	2	3	4	5
Control of withdrawal of money from account(s)	1	2	3	4	5
Information about finances	1	2	3	4	5
Information about legal matters	1	2	3	4	5
Participation in financial security planning	1	2	3	4	5
Pursuit of vocation or occupation	1	2	3	4	5
Control of earned income	1	2	3	4	5
Protection of financial assets	1	2	3	4	5
Court-ordered benefits received	1	2	3	4	5
Other _____ Specify	1	2	3	4	5

BACKGROUND READINGS:

Anetzberger, G.J. (1987). *The etiology of elder abuse of adult offspring.* Springfield, IL: Charles C Thomas, Publisher.

Baumhover, L.A., Beall, S.C., & Pieroni, R.E. (1990). Elder abuse: An overview of social and medical indicators. *Journal of Health and Human Resources Administration, 12*(4), 414-443.

Hudson, M.F., & Johnson, T.F. (1986). Elder neglect and abuse: A review of the literature. *Annual Review of Nursing Research, 6*(3), 81-134.

Outcomes

Abuse Recovery: Physical

DEFINITION: Healing of physical injuries due to abuse

ABUSE RECOVERY: PHYSICAL	None 1	Limited 2	Moderate 3	Substantial 4	Extensive 5
INDICATORS:					
Healing of physical injuries	1	2	3	4	5
Evidence of regular bowel elimination	1	2	3	4	5
Evidence of timely treatment of injuries	1	2	3	4	5
Evidence that therapeutic health care obtained when needed	1	2	3	4	5
Evidence that preventive health care obtained when needed	1	2	3	4	5
Occurrence of expected response to treatment	1	2	3	4	5
Resolution of physical health problems	1	2	3	4	5
Evidence of adequate nutrition	1	2	3	4	5
Evidence of urinary continence	1	2	3	4	5
Other _____ Specify	1	2	3	4	5

BACKGROUND READINGS:

Campbell, J., McKenna, L.S., Torres, S., Sheridan, D., & Landenburger, K. (1993). Nursing care of abused women. In J. Campbell & J. Humphreys (Eds.), *Nursing care of survivors of family violence.* St. Louis: Mosby.

Campbell, J., & Fishwick, N. (1993). Abuse of female partners. In J. Campbell & J. Humphreys (Eds.), *Nursing care of survivors of family violence.* St. Louis: Mosby.

Outcomes

Abuse Recovery: Sexual

DEFINITION: Healing following sexual abuse or exploitation

ABUSE RECOVERY: SEXUAL	None	Limited	Moderate	Substantial	Extensive
	1	2	3	4	5

INDICATORS:

Verbalization of details of abuse	1	2	3	4	5
Acknowledgment of right to disclose abusive situation	1	2	3	4	5
Verbalization of feelings about the abuse	1	2	3	4	5
Verbalization of appropriate and inappropriate guilt	1	2	3	4	5
Expressions of right to have been protected from abuse	1	2	3	4	5
Verbalization that physical damage to body is absent or healed	1	2	3	4	5
Freedom from sleep disturbances	1	2	3	4	5
Resolution of depression	1	2	3	4	5
Expressions of anger in non-destructive ways	1	2	3	4	5
Self-advocacy	1	2	3	4	5
Expressions of feeling empowered	1	2	3	4	5
Expressions of hope	1	2	3	4	5
Consistency of behavior with social norms	1	2	3	4	5
Evidence of appropriate same-sex relationships	1	2	3	4	5
Evidence of appropriate opposite-sex relationships	1	2	3	4	5
Expressions of confidence with gender identity	1	2	3	4	5
Expressions of confidence with sexual orientation	1	2	3	4	5
Resolution of eating disorders	1	2	3	4	5
Resolution of self-mutilation	1	2	3	4	5
Decrease in suicide attempts	1	2	3	4	5
Verbalization of accurate information about sexual functioning	1	2	3	4	5
Other _____ Specify	1	2	3	4	5

BACKGROUND READINGS:

Bass, E., & Davis, L. (1988). *The courage to heal: A guide for women survivors of child sexual abuse.* New York: Harper & Row.

DePanfilis, D. (1986). *Literature review of sexual abuse* (DHHS Publication No. [OHDSA] 87-30530). Washington, DC: USDHHS, National Center on Child Abuse & Neglect.

Sgroi, S.M. (1982). *Handbook of clinical intervention in child sexual abuse.* Lexington, MA: Lexington Books.

Sgroi, S.M. (Ed). (1988). *Vulnerable populations: Evaluation and treatment of sexually abused children and adult survivors* (Vol. 1). Lexington, MA: Lexington Books.

Sgroi, S.M. (Ed). (1988). *Vulnerable populations: Sexual abuse treatment for children, adult survivors, offenders, and persons with mental retardation* (Vol. 2). Lexington, MA: Lexington Books.

Outcomes

Abusive Behavior Self-Control

DEFINITION: Management of own behaviors to avoid abuse and neglect of dependents or significant others

ABUSIVE BEHAVIOR SELF-CONTROL	Never demonstrated 1	Rarely demonstrated 2	Sometimes demonstrated 3	Often demonstrated 4	Consistently demonstrated 5
INDICATORS:					
Avoids physically abusive behavior	1	2	3	4	5
Avoids emotionally abusive behavior	1	2	3	4	5
Avoids sexually abusive behavior	1	2	3	4	5
Avoids neglect of dependent's basic needs	1	2	3	4	5
Uses alternative coping mechanisms for stress	1	2	3	4	5
Discusses the abusive behavior	1	2	3	4	5
Identifies factors contributing to abusive behavior	1	2	3	4	5
Expresses feelings about victim	1	2	3	4	5
Identifies available community resources for help	1	2	3	4	5
Expresses frustrations	1	2	3	4	5
Uses nurturing behavior toward victim	1	2	3	4	5
Demonstrates self-esteem	1	2	3	4	5
States expectations congruent with developmental level	1	2	3	4	5
Applies appropriate caregiving techniques	1	2	3	4	5
Uses support network	1	2	3	4	5
Expresses empathy for victim	1	2	3	4	5
Demonstrates impulse control	1	2	3	4	5
Demonstrates knowledge of correct role behaviors	1	2	3	4	5

Continued.

Outcomes

ABUSIVE BEHAVIOR SELF-CONTROL— cont'd	Never demonstrated 1	Rarely demonstrated 2	Sometimes demonstrated 3	Often demonstrated 4	Consistently demonstrated 5
Seeks treatment as needed	1	2	3	4	5
Participates in treatment as needed	1	2	3	4	5
Other _____ Specify	1	2	3	4	5

BACKGROUND READINGS:

Altemeier, W.A., O'Connor, S., Vietze, P., Sandler, H., & Sherrod, K. (1984). Prediction of child abuse: A prospective study of feasibility. *Child Abuse and Neglect, 8,* 393-400.

Amundson, M.J. (1989). Family crisis care: A home based intervention program for child abuse. *Issues in Mental Health Nursing, 10,* 285-296.

Anderson, C.L. (1987). Assessing parenting potential for child abuse risk. *Pediatric Nursing, 13*(5), 323-327.

Cowen P. (1991). *The Iowa Crisis Nursery Project as a factor in the prevention of child abuse.* Unpublished doctoral dissertation, University of Iowa, Iowa City.

Hunka, C.D., O'Toole, A.W., & O'Toole, R. (1985). Self-help therapy in Parents Anonymous. *Journal of Psychosocial Nursing, 23*(7), 24-32.

Olds, D.L., Henderson, C.R., Chamberlin, R., & Tatelbaum, R. (1986). Preventing child abuse and neglect: A randomized trial of nurse home visitation. *Pediatrics, 78*(1), 65-78.

Marshall, E., Buckner, E., & Powell, K. (1991). Evaluation of a teen parent program designed to reduce child abuse and neglect and to strengthen families. *Journal of Child and Adolescent Psychiatric and Mental Health Nursing, 4*(3), 96-100.

Reuter, M.M. (1988). Parenting needs of abusing parents: Development of a tool for evaluation of parent education class. *Journal of Community Health Nursing, 5*(2), 129-140.

Taylor, D.K., & Beauchamp, C. (1988). Hospital-based primary prevention strategy in child abuse: A multi-level needs assessment. *Child Abuse and Neglect, 12,* 343-354.

Outcomes

Acceptance: Health Status

DEFINITION: Reconciliation to health circumstances

ACCEPTANCE: HEALTH STATUS	None 1	Limited 2	Moderate 3	Substantial 4	Extensive 5
INDICATORS:					
Peacefulness	1	2	3	4	5
Ability to tolerate quiet periods	1	2	3	4	5
Relinquishment of previous concept of health	1	2	3	4	5
Calmness	1	2	3	4	5
Demonstration of positive self-regard	1	2	3	4	5
Deepening of intimacy	1	2	3	4	5
Expressed reactions to health status	1	2	3	4	5
Expressed feelings about health status	1	2	3	4	5
Recognition of reality of health situation	1	2	3	4	5
Pursuit of information	1	2	3	4	5
Coping with health situation	1	2	3	4	5
Health-related decision making	1	2	3	4	5
Clarification of values	1	2	3	4	5
Renewal of a sense of meaning	1	2	3	4	5
Performance of self-care tasks	1	2	3	4	5
Other _____ Specify	1	2	3	4	5

Outcomes

BACKGROUND READINGS:

Clayton, J.W. (1993). Paving the way to acceptance: Psychological adaptation to death and dying in cancer. *Professional Nurse, 8*(4), 206-211.

Kelley, M.P., & Henry, P. (1993). Open discussion can lead to acceptance: The psychosocial effects of stoma surgery. *Professional Nurse, 9*(2), 101-110.

Kübler-Ross, E. (1977). *On death and dying.* London: Tavistock Press.

Lazarus, R.S., & Folkman, S. (1984). *Stress, appraisal and coping.* New York: Springer.

Longo, M.B. (1993). Facilitating acceptance of a patient's decision to stop treatment. *Clinical Nurse Specialist, 7*(3), 233-243.

Melamed, S., Groswasser, Z., & Stern, M. (1992). Acceptance of disability, work involvement and subjective rehabilitation status of traumatic brain-injured (TBI) patients. *Brain Injury, 6*(3), 233-243.

Peplau, H. (1969). Professional closeness. *Nursing Forum, 8*(4), 346.

Pellegrino, E. (1989). Withholding and withdrawing treatment: Ethics at the bedside. *Clinical Neurosurgery, 35,* 164-184.

Roger, C.R. (1951). *Client-centered therapy.* Boston: Houghton Mifflin.

Wright, B.A. (1960). *Physical disability—a psychological approach.* New York: Harper & Row.

Adherence Behavior

DEFINITION: Self-initiated action taken to promote wellness, recovery, and rehabilitation

ADHERENCE BEHAVIOR	Never demonstrated 1	Rarely demonstrated 2	Sometimes demonstrated 3	Often demonstrated 4	Consistently demonstrated 5
INDICATORS:					
Asks questions when appropriate	1	2	3	4	5
Seeks health-related information from a variety of sources	1	2	3	4	5
Uses health-related information from a variety of sources to develop health strategies	1	2	3	4	5
Weighs risks/benefits of health behavior	1	2	3	4	5
Describes strategies to eliminate unhealthy behavior	1	2	3	4	5
Describes strategies to maximize health	1	2	3	4	5
Provides rationale for adopting a regimen	1	2	3	4	5
Reports using strategies to eliminate unhealthy behavior	1	2	3	4	5
Reports using strategies to maximize health	1	2	3	4	5
Uses health services congruent with need	1	2	3	4	5
Performs ADLs* consistent with energy and tolerance	1	2	3	4	5
Performs self-screening	1	2	3	4	5
Describes rationale for deviating from a recommended regimen	1	2	3	4	5
Performs self-monitoring	1	2	3	4	5
Other _____ Specify	1	2	3	4	5

*ADL = Activities of daily living.

BACKGROUND READINGS:

Barotsky, I., Sergenbaker, P., & Mills, M. (1979). Compliance and quality of life assessment. In J. Cohen (Ed.), *New directions in patient compliance* (pp. 59-74). Lexington, MA: D.C. Health.

Epstein, L., & Cluss, P.A. (1982). A behavioral perspective on adherence to long-term medical regimens. *Journal of Consulting and Clinical Psychology, 50,* 950-971.

Epstein, L., & Masek, B. (1978). Behavioral control of medicine compliance. *Journal of Applied Behavioral Analysis, 11,* 1-10.

Folden, S.L. (1993). Definitions of health and health goals of participants in a community-based pulmonary rehabilitation program. *Public Health Nursing, 10*(1), 31-35.

Gochman, D.S. (Ed.). (1988). *Health behavior: Emerging research perspectives.* New York: Plenum Press.

Heiby, E., & Carlson, J. (1986). The health compliance model. *The Journal of Compliance in Health Care, 1*(2), 135-152.

Jensen, L., & Allen, M. (1993). Wellness: The dialect of illness. *IMAGE-The Journal of Nursing Scholarship, 25*(3), 220-224.

Kravits, R. et al. (1993). Recall of recommendations and adherence to advice among patients with chronic medical conditions. *Archives of Internal Medicine, 153*(16), 1869-1878.

Miller, P., Wikoff, R., & Hiatt, A. (1972). Fishbein's model of measured behavior of hypertensive patients. *Nursing Research, 41*(2), 104-109.

Oldridge, N. (1982). Compliance in primary and secondary prevention of coronary heart disease: A review. *Preventive Medicine, 11,* 56-70.

Pender, N.J. (1990). Expressing health through lifestyle patterns. *Nursing Science Quarterly, 3*(3), 115-122.

Pender, N.J., & Pender, A.R. (1986). Attitudes, subjective norms, and intentions of engagement in health behaviors. *Nursing Research, 35*(1), 15-18.

Shumaker, S.A., Schron, E.B., & Ockene, J.K. (1990). *The handbook of health behavior change.* New York: Springer.

Woods, N. (1989). Conceptualization of self-care: Toward health oriented models. *Advances in Nursing Science, 12*(1), 1-13.

Outcomes

Aggression Control

DEFINITION: Ability to restrain assaultive, combative, or destructive behavior toward others

AGGRESSION CONTROL	Never demonstrated 1	Rarely demonstrated 2	Sometimes demonstrated 3	Often demonstrated 4	Consistently demonstrated 5
INDICATORS:					
Refrains from verbal outbursts	1	2	3	4	5
Refrains from violating others' personal space	1	2	3	4	5
Refrains from striking others	1	2	3	4	5
Refrains from harming others	1	2	3	4	5
Refrains from harming animals	1	2	3	4	5
Refrains from destroying property	1	2	3	4	5
Communicates needs appropriately	1	2	3	4	5
Communicates feelings appropriately	1	2	3	4	5
Verbalizes control of impulses	1	2	3	4	5
Identifies when angry	1	2	3	4	5
Identifies when frustrated	1	2	3	4	5
Identifies situations which precipitate hostility	1	2	3	4	5
Identifies responsibility to maintain control	1	2	3	4	5
Identifies when feeling aggressive	1	2	3	4	5
Identifies alternatives to aggression	1	2	3	4	5
Identifies alternatives to verbal outbursts	1	2	3	4	5
Vents negative feelings appropriately	1	2	3	4	5
Upholds contract to restrain aggressive behaviors	1	2	3	4	5

Outcomes

AGGRESSION CONTROL	Never demonstrated 1	Rarely demonstrated 2	Sometimes demonstrated 3	Often demonstrated 4	Consistently demonstrated 5
Maintains self-control without supervision	1	2	3	4	5
Other _____ Specify	1	2	3	4	5

Outcomes

BACKGROUND READINGS:

Grancola, P.R., & Zeichner, A. (1993). Aggressive behavior in the elderly: A critical review. *Clinical Gerontologist, 13*(2), 3-22.

Maxfield, M.C., Lewis, R.E., & Connor, S. (1996). Training staff to prevent aggressive behavior of cognitively impaired elderly patients during bathing and grooming. *Journal of Gerontological Nursing, 22*(1), 37-43.

Rantz, M.J., & McShane, R.E. (1995). Nursing interventions for chronically confused nursing home residents. *Geriatric Nursing, 16*(1), 22-27.

Ryden, M.B. (1992). Aggressive behavior in persons with dementia who live in the community. *Alzheimer Disease and Associated Disorders, 2*(4), 342-355.

Ambulation: Walking

DEFINITION: Ability to walk from place to place

AMBULATION: WALKING	Dependent, does not participate	Requires assistive person & device	Requires assistive person	Independent with assistive device	Completely independent
	1	2	3	4	5
INDICATORS:					
Bears weight	1	2	3	4	5
Walks with effective gait	1	2	3	4	5
Walks at slow pace	1	2	3	4	5
Walks at moderate pace	1	2	3	4	5
Walks at fast pace	1	2	3	4	5
Walks up steps	1	2	3	4	5
Walks down steps	1	2	3	4	5
Walks up inclines	1	2	3	4	5
Walks down inclines	1	2	3	4	5
Walks short distance (< 1 block)	1	2	3	4	5
Walks moderate distance (> 1 block < 5 blocks)	1	2	3	4	5
Walks long distance (5 blocks or >)	1	2	3	4	5
Other _____ Specify	1	2	3	4	5

BACKGROUND READINGS:

Dittmar, S. (1989). *Rehabilitation nursing: Process and application.* St. Louis: Mosby.

Jirovec, M.M. (1991). The impact of daily exercise on the mobility, balance, and urine control of cognitively impaired nursing home residents. *International Journal of Nursing Studies, 28*(2), 145-151.

Mikulic, M.A., Griffith, E.R., & Jebsen, R.H. (1976). Clinical application of a standardized mobility test. *Archives of Physical Medicine and Rehabilitation, 57*(3), 143-146.

Pomeroy, V. (1990). Development of an ADL-oriented assessment-of-mobility scale suitable for use for elderly people with dementia. *Physiotherapy, 76*(8), 446-448.

Tinetti, M.E. (1986). Performance-oriented assessment of mobility problems in elderly patients. *Journal of the American Geriatric Society, 34*, 119-126.

Ambulation: Wheelchair

DEFINITION: Ability to move from place to place in a wheelchair

AMBULATION: WHEELCHAIR	Dependent, does not participate	Requires assistive person & device	Requires assistive person	Independent with assistive device	Completely independent
	1	**2**	**3**	**4**	**5**
INDICATORS:					
Transfers to and from wheelchair	1	2	3	4	5
Propels wheelchair safely	1	2	3	4	5
Propels wheelchair short distance	1	2	3	4	5
Propels wheelchair moderate distance	1	2	3	4	5
Propels wheelchair long distance	1	2	3	4	5
Maneuvers curbs	1	2	3	4	5
Manuevers doorways	1	2	3	4	5
Maneuvers ramps	1	2	3	4	5
Other _____ Specify	1	2	3	4	5

BACKGROUND READINGS:

Dittmar, S. (1989). *Rehabilitation nursing: Process and application.* St. Louis: Mosby.

Kane, R.L., & Kane, R.A. (1981). *Assessing the elderly: A practical guide to measurement.* Lexington, MA: Lexington Books.

Mikulic, M.A., Griffith, E.R., & Jebsen, R.H. (1976). Clinical application of a standardized mobility test. *Archives of Physical Medicine and Rehabilitation, 57*(3), 143-146.

Outcomes

Anxiety Control

DEFINITION: Ability to eliminate or reduce feelings of apprehension and tension from an unidentifiable source

ANXIETY CONTROL	Never demonstrated 1	Rarely demonstrated 2	Sometimes demonstrated 3	Often demonstrated 4	Consistently demonstrated 5
INDICATORS:					
Monitors intensity of anxiety	1	2	3	4	5
Eliminates precursors of anxiety	1	2	3	4	5
Decreases environmental stimuli when anxious	1	2	3	4	5
Seeks information to reduce anxiety	1	2	3	4	5
Plans coping strategies for stressful situations	1	2	3	4	5
Uses effective coping strategies	1	2	3	4	5
Uses relaxation techniques to reduce anxiety	1	2	3	4	5
Reports decreased duration of episodes	1	2	3	4	5
Reports increased length of time between episodes	1	2	3	4	5
Maintains role performance	1	2	3	4	5
Maintains social relationships	1	2	3	4	5
Maintains concentration	1	2	3	4	5
Reports absence of sensory perceptual distortions	1	2	3	4	5
Reports adequate sleep	1	2	3	4	5
Reports absence of physical manifestations of anxiety	1	2	3	4	5
Behavioral manifestations of anxiety absent	1	2	3	4	5
Controls anxiety response	1	2	3	4	5
Other _____ Specify	1	2	3	4	5

BACKGROUND READINGS:

Laraia, M.T., Stuart, G.W., & Best, C.L. (1989). Behavioral treatment of panic-related disorders: A review. *Archives of Psychiatric Nursing, 3*(3), 125-133.

Stuart, G.W., & Sundeen, S.J. (1995). *Principles and practice of psychiatric nursing* (5th ed.). St. Louis: Mosby.

Waddell, K.L., & Demi, A.S. (1993). Effectiveness of an intensive partial hospitalization program for treatment of anxiety disorders. *Archives of Psychiatric Nursing, 7*(1), 2-10.

Outcomes

Balance

DEFINITION: Ability to maintain body equilibrium

BALANCE	Dependent, does not participate	Requires assistive person & device	Requires assistive person	Independent with assistive device	Completely independent
	1	**2**	**3**	**4**	**5**
INDICATORS:					
Standing balance	1	2	3	4	5
Sitting balance	1	2	3	4	5
Walking balance	1	2	3	4	5
Other _____ Specify	1	2	3	4	5

BACKGROUND READINGS:

Dittmar, S. (1989). *Rehabilitation nursing: Process and application.* St. Louis: Mosby.

Pomeroy, V. (1990). Development of an ADL-oriented assessment-of-mobility scale suitable for use with elderly people with dementia. *Physiotherapy, 76*(8), 446-448.

Roberts, B.L. (1989). Effects of walking on balance among elders. *Nursing Research, 38*(3), 180-182.

Tinetti, M.E. (1986). Performance-oriented assessment of mobility problems in elderly patients. *Journal of the American Geriatric Society, 34,* 119-126.

Blood Transfusion Reaction Control

DEFINITION: Extent to which complications of blood transfusions are minimized

BLOOD TRANSFUSION REACTION CONTROL	Not at all	To a slight extent	To a moderate extent	To a great extent	To a very great extent
	1	**2**	**3**	**4**	**5**
INDICATORS:					
Respiratory status IER*	1	2	3	4	5
Gastrointestinal status IER	1	2	3	4	5
Urine output IER	1	2	3	4	5
Heart rate IER	1	2	3	4	5
BP* IER	1	2	3	4	5
Skin color IER	1	2	3	4	5
Free of fever	1	2	3	4	5
Free of chills	1	2	3	4	5
Free of itching	1	2	3	4	5
Free of rash	1	2	3	4	5
Free of restlessness	1	2	3	4	5
Free of reported anxiety	1	2	3	4	5
Free of reported malaise	1	2	3	4	5
Free of chest pain	1	2	3	4	5
Free of lumbar pain	1	2	3	4	5
Free of IV site inflammation	1	2	3	4	5
Free of hemoglobinuria	1	2	3	4	5
Free of muscle spasms and twitching	1	2	3	4	5
Other _____ Specify	1	2	3	4	5

*IER = In expected range; BP = blood pressure.

BACKGROUND READINGS:

Luckmann J., & Sorenson, K.C. (1993). *Medical-surgical nursing: A psychophysiologic approach* (4th ed.). Philadelphia: W.B. Saunders.

McCance, K.L., & Huether, S.E. (1994). *Pathophysiology: The biologic basis for disease in adults and children* (2nd ed.). St. Louis: Mosby.

Body Image

DEFINITION: Positive perception of own appearance and body functions

BODY IMAGE	Never positive 1	Rarely positive 2	Sometimes positive 3	Often positive 4	Consistently positive 5
INDICATORS:					
Internal picture of self	1	2	3	4	5
Congruence between body reality, body ideal and body presentation	1	2	3	4	5
Description of affected body part	1	2	3	4	5
Willingness to touch affected body part	1	2	3	4	5
Satisfaction with body appearance	1	2	3	4	5
Satisfaction with body function	1	2	3	4	5
Adjustment to changes in physical appearance	1	2	3	4	5
Adjustment to changes in body function	1	2	3	4	5
Adjustment to changes in health status	1	2	3	4	5
Willingness to use strategies to enhance appearance and function	1	2	3	4	5
Other _____ Specify	1	2	3	4	5

BACKGROUND READINGS:

Comunale, D.L. (1992). Collaborative care planning with the arthritic client at home. *Journal of Home Health Care Practice, 4*(2), 8-15.

LeMone, P. (1991). Analysis of human phenomenon: Self-concept. *Nursing Diagnosis, 2*(3), 129-130.

Low, M.B. (1993). Women's body image: The nurse's role in promotion of self-acceptance. *AWONN's Clinical Issues, 4*(2), 213-219.

MacGinley, K.J. (1993). Nursing care of the patient with altered body image. *British Journal of Nursing, 2*(22), 1098-1102.

Newell, R. (1991). Body-image disturbance: Cognitive behavioral formulation and intervention. *Journal of Advanced Nursing, 16*, 1400-1405.

Price, B. (1990). A model for body image care. *Journal of Advanced Nursing, 15,* 585-593.

Price, B. (1992). Living with altered body image: The cancer experience. *British Journal of Nursing, 1*(13), 641-645.

Price, B. (1993). Profiling the high-risk altered body image patient. *Senior Nurse, 13*(4), 17-21.

Van Deusen, J., Harlowe, D., & Baker, L. (1989). Body image perceptions of the community-based elderly. *The Occupational Therapy Journal of Research, 9*(4), 243-248.

Wasson, D. & Anderson, M.A. (1995). Chemical dependency and adolescent self-esteem. *Clinical Nursing Research, 4*(3):274-289.

Outcomes

Body Positioning: Self-Initiated

DEFINITION: Ability to change own body positions

BODY POSITIONING: SELF-INITIATED	Dependent, does not participate 1	Requires assistive person & device 2	Requires assistive person 3	Independent with assistive device 4	Completely independent 5
INDICATORS:					
Lying to lying	1	2	3	4	5
Lying to sitting	1	2	3	4	5
Sitting to lying	1	2	3	4	5
Sitting to standing	1	2	3	4	5
Standing to sitting	1	2	3	4	5
Standing to kneeling	1	2	3	4	5
Kneeling to standing	1	2	3	4	5
Standing to squatting	1	2	3	4	5
Squatting to standing	1	2	3	4	5
Bending at waist while standing	1	2	3	4	5
Other _____ Specify	1	2	3	4	5

BACKGROUND READINGS:

Mikulic, M.A., Griffith, E.R., & Jebsen, R.H. (1976). Clinical application of a standardized mobility test. *Archives of Physical Medicine and Rehabilitation, 57*(3), 143-146.

Outcomes

Bone Healing

DEFINITION: The extent to which cells and tissues have regenerated following bone injury					
BONE HEALING	**None** **1**	**Slight** **2**	**Moderate** **3**	**Substantial** **4**	**Complete** **5**
INDICATORS:					
Hematoma formation WNL*	1	2	3	4	5
Cellular proliferation WNL	1	2	3	4	5
Callus formation WNL	1	2	3	4	5
Ossification, consolidation, and remodeling WNL	1	2	3	4	5
Circulation IER*	1	2	3	4	5
Bone function return	1	2	3	4	5
Resolution of pain	1	2	3	4	5
Resolution of edema	1	2	3	4	5
Degree of immobilization IER	1	2	3	4	5
Free of infection in surrounding tissue	1	2	3	4	5
Free of infection in bone	1	2	3	4	5
Other _____ Specify	1	2	3	4	5

*WNL = Within normal limits; IER = In expected range.

BACKGROUND READINGS:

Porth, C.M. (1994). *Pathophysiology: Concepts of altered health states* (4th ed.). Philadelphia: J.B. Lippincott.

Potter, P.A., & Perry, A.G. (1993). *Fundamentals of nursing: Concepts, process, and practice* (3rd ed.). St. Louis: Mosby.

Bowel Continence

DEFINITION: Control of passage of stool from the bowel

BOWEL CONTINENCE	Never demonstrated 1	Rarely demonstrated 2	Sometimes demonstrated 3	Often demonstrated 4	Consistently demonstrated 5
INDICATORS:					
Predictable evacuation of stool	1	2	3	4	5
Maintains control of passage of stool	1	2	3	4	5
Regular evacuation of stool at least q 3 days	1	2	3	4	5
Diarrhea not present	1	2	3	4	5
Constipation not present	1	2	3	4	5
Sphincter tone adequate to control defecation	1	2	3	4	5
Sphincter innervation functional	1	2	3	4	5
Identifies urge to defecate	1	2	3	4	5
Responds to urge in timely manner	1	2	3	4	5
Uses aids appropriately to achieve continence	1	2	3	4	5
Manages bowel appliance independently	1	2	3	4	5
Reaches toilet facility independently before defecating	1	2	3	4	5
Ingests adequate amount of fluid	1	2	3	4	5
Ingests adequate amount of fiber	1	2	3	4	5
Knows relationship of intake to evacuation pattern	1	2	3	4	5
Other _____ Specify	1	2	3	4	5

Outcomes

BACKGROUND READINGS:

Hogstel, M.O., & Nelson, M. (1992, January/February). Anticipation and early detection can reduce bowel elimination complications. *Geriatric Nursing*, 28-33.

Maas, M., & Specht, J. (1991). Bowel incontinence. In Maas, M., Buckwalter, K.C., & Hardy, M. (Eds). *Nursing diagnoses and interventions for the elderly.* Redwood City, CA: Addison-Wesley.

McLane, A. (1987). *Classification of nursing diagnoses: Proceedings of the 7th conference.* St. Louis: Mosby.

Bowel Elimination

DEFINITION: Ability of the gastrointestinal tract to form and evacuate stool effectively

BOWEL ELIMINATION	Extremely compromised 1	Substantially compromised 2	Moderately compromised 3	Mildly compromised 4	Not compromised 5
INDICATORS:					
Elimination pattern IER*	1	2	3	4	5
Control of bowel movements	1	2	3	4	5
Stool color WNL*	1	2	3	4	5
Stool amount for diet	1	2	3	4	5
Stool soft and formed	1	2	3	4	5
Stool odor WNL	1	2	3	4	5
Fat in stool WNL	1	2	3	4	5
Stool free of blood	1	2	3	4	5
Stool free of mucus	1	2	3	4	5
Constipation not present	1	2	3	4	5
Diarrhea not present	1	2	3	4	5
Ease of stool passage	1	2	3	4	5
Comfort of stool passage	1	2	3	4	5
Visible peristalsis not present	1	2	3	4	5
Painful cramps not present	1	2	3	4	5
Bloating not present	1	2	3	4	5
Bowel sounds	1	2	3	4	5
Sphincter tone	1	2	3	4	5
Muscle tone to evacuate stool	1	2	3	4	5
Manages bowel appliance independently	1	2	3	4	5
Passes stool without aids	1	2	3	4	5
Intervention for stool passage	1	2	3	4	5
Abuse of aids not present	1	2	3	4	5
Ingests adequate fluids	1	2	3	4	5
Ingests adequate fiber	1	2	3	4	5
Exercises adequate amount	1	2	3	4	5
Other _____ Specify	1	2	3	4	5

*IER = In expected range; WNL = Within normal limits.

Outcomes

BACKGROUND READINGS:

Heading, C. (1987). Factors affecting bowel functions. *Nursing, 21,* 773-783.

Hogstel, M.O. & Nelson, M. (1992, January/February). Anticipation and early detection can reduce bowel elimination complications. *Geriatric Nursing,* 28-33.

Lepshy, M.S., & Michael, A. (1993). Chronic diarrhea: Evaluation and treatment. *American Family Physician, 48*(8), 1461-1466.

Loening-Baucke, V. (1994). Management of chronic constipation in infants and toddlers. *American Family Physician, 46*(2), 397-406.

McLane, A.M., & McShane, R.E. (1991). Constipation. In Maas, M., Buckwalter, K., & Hardy, M. (Eds), *Nursing diagnoses and interventions for the elderly.* Redwood City, CA: Addison-Wesley Nursing.

McShane, R.E., & McLane, A.M. (1988). Constipation: Impact of etiological factors. *Journal of Gerontological Nursing, 14*(4), 31-34.

Morton, P.G. (1989). *Health assessment in nursing.* Springhouse, PA: Springhouse.

Palmer, M.H., McCormick, K.A., Langford, A., Langlais, J., & Alvaran, M. (1992). Continence outcomes: Documentation on medical records in the nursing home environment. *Journal of Nursing Care Quality, 6*(3), 36-43.

Potter, P., & Potter, A. (1993). *Fundamentals of nursing: Concepts, process, & practice* (3rd ed.). St. Louis: Mosby.

Outcomes

Breastfeeding Establishment: Infant

DEFINITION: Proper attachment of an infant to and sucking from the mother's breast for nourishment during the first 2-3 weeks

BREASTFEEDING ESTABLISHMENT: INFANT	Not adequate 1	Slightly adequate 2	Moderately adequate 3	Substantially adequate 4	Totally adequate 5
INDICATORS:					
Proper alignment and latch on	1	2	3	4	5
Proper areolar grasp	1	2	3	4	5
Proper areolar compression	1	2	3	4	5
Correct suck and tongue placement	1	2	3	4	5
Audible swallow	1	2	3	4	5
Swallowing a minimum of 5-10 minutes per breast	1	2	3	4	5
Minimum 8 feedings per day (on demand)	1	2	3	4	5
6 or more urinations per day (after infant 2-3 days of age)	1	2	3	4	5
2 or more loose, yellow, seedy stools per day	1	2	3	4	5
Age appropriate weight gain	1	2	3	4	5
Infant contentment after feeding	1	2	3	4	5
Other _____ Specify	1	2	3	4	5

BACKGROUND READINGS:

Lawrence, R. (1994). *Breastfeeding: A guide for the medical professional* (4th ed.). St. Louis: Mosby.

Minchin, M.K. (1989). Positioning for breastfeeding. *Birth: Issues in Perinatal Care and Education, 16*(2), 67-80.

Neifert, M.R., & Seacat, J.M. (1986). A guide to successful breastfeeding. *Contemporary Pediatrics, 3*, 1-14.

Page-Goertz, S. (1989). Discharge planning for the breastfeeding dyad. *Pediatric Nursing, 15*, 543-544.

Righard, L., & Alade, M.O. (1992). Sucking technique and its effect on success of breastfeeding. *Birth: Issues in Perinatal Care and Education, 19*, 185-189.

Riordan, J., & Auerbach, K.G. (1993). *Breastfeeding and human lactation.* Boston: Jones and Bartlett.

Shrago, L., & Bocar, D. (1990). The infant's contribution to breastfeeding. *Journal of Obstetric, Gynecologic, & Neonatal Nursing, 19*, 209-213.

Walker, M. (1989). Functional assessment of infant breastfeeding patterns. *Birth: Issues in Perinatal Care and Education, 16*, 140-147.

Breastfeeding Establishment: Maternal

DEFINITION: Maternal establishment of proper attachment of an infant to and sucking from the breast for nourishment during the first 2-3 weeks

BREASTFEEDING ESTABLISHMENT: MATERNAL	Not adequate 1	Slightly adequate 2	Moderately adequate 3	Substantially adequate 4	Totally adequate 5
INDICATORS:					
Comfort of position during nursing	1	2	3	4	5
Supports breast through "C" hold (cupping)	1	2	3	4	5
Breast fullness prior to feeding	1	2	3	4	5
Milk ejection (let-down) reflex	1	2	3	4	5
Contralateral breast leaking	1	2	3	4	5
Recognition of infant swallowing	1	2	3	4	5
Breaking of suction before removing infant from breast	1	2	3	4	5
Freedom from nipple tenderness	1	2	3	4	5
Avoidance of artificial nipple use with infant	1	2	3	4	5
Avoidance of giving water to infant	1	2	3	4	5
Supplementation appropriate to infant's age and health status	1	2	3	4	5
Understanding of infant's temperament	1	2	3	4	5
Recognition of early hunger cues	1	2	3	4	5
Ability to hand express or use pump	1	2	3	4	5
Appropriate storage of milk	1	2	3	4	5
Recognition of community and family support	1	2	3	4	5
Use of community and family support as needed	1	2	3	4	5
Satisfaction with breastfeeding process	1	2	3	4	5
Other _____ Specify	1	2	3	4	5

BACKGROUND READINGS:

Lawrence, R. (1994). *Breastfeeding: A guide for the medical professional* (4th ed.). St. Louis: Mosby.

Minchin, M.K. (1989). Positioning for breastfeeding. *Birth: Issues in Perinatal Care and Education, 16*(2), 67-80.

Neifert, M.R., & Seacat, J.M. (1986). A guide to successful breastfeeding. *Contemporary Pediatrics, 3*, 1-14.

Page-Goertz, S. (1989). Discharge planning for the breastfeeding dyad. *Pediatric Nursing, 15*, 543-544.

Righard, L., & Alade, M.O. (1992). Sucking technique and its effect on success of breastfeeding. *Birth: Issues in Perinatal Care and Education, 19*, 185-189.

Continued.

Outcomes

Outcomes

Riordan, J., & Auerbach, K.G. (1993). *Breastfeeding and human lactation.* Boston: Jones and Bartlett.

Shrago, L., & Bocar, D. (1990). The infant's contribution to breastfeeding. *Journal of Obstetric, Gynecologic, & Neonatal Nursing, 19,* 209-213.

Walker, M. (1989). Functional assessment of infant breastfeeding patterns. *Birth: Issues in Perinatal Care and Education, 16,* 140-147.

Breastfeeding Maintenance

DEFINITION: Continued nourishment of an infant through breastfeeding

BREASTFEEDING MAINTENANCE	Not adequate 1	Slightly adequate 2	Moderately adequate 3	Substantially adequate 4	Totally adequate 5
INDICATORS:					
Infant's growth in normal range	1	2	3	4	5
Infant's development in normal range	1	2	3	4	5
Family understanding of infant growth spurts	1	2	3	4	5
Family knowledge of benefits from continued breastfeeding	1	2	3	4	5
Mother's ability to safely collect and store breastmilk, if desired	1	2	3	4	5
Care provider's ability to safely thaw, warm and feed stored breastmilk	1	2	3	4	5
Mother's freedom from breast tenderness	1	2	3	4	5
Recognition of signs of decreased milk supply	1	2	3	4	5
Recognition of signs of plugged ducts and mastitis	1	2	3	4	5
Mother's avoidance of self-medication without checking with health care provider	1	2	3	4	5
Mother's continuation of lactation on return to work or school	1	2	3	4	5
Written material reinforcing all care instructions	1	2	3	4	5
Family recognition of community and health provider support	1	2	3	4	5
Family expression of satisfaction with support available	1	2	3	4	5
Family expression of satisfaction with breastfeeding process	1	2	3	4	5
Other _____ Specify	1	2	3	4	5

BACKGROUND READINGS:

Bear, K., & Tigges, B.B. (1993). Management strategies for promoting successful breastfeeding. *Nurse Practitioner: American Journal of Primary Health Care, 18,* 50, 53-54, 56-58, 60.

Coreil, J., & Murphy, J.E. (1988). Maternal commitment, lactation practices, and breastfeeding duration. *Journal of Obstetric, Gynecologic, & Neonatal Nursing, 17,* 273-278.

Lawrence, R. (1994). *Breastfeeding: A guide for the medical professional* (4th ed.). St. Louis: Mosby.

Rentschler, D.D. (1991). Correlates of successful breastfeeding. *IMAGE-The Journal of Nursing Scholarship, 23,* 151-154.

Riordan, J., & Auerbach, K.G. (1993). *Breastfeeding and human lactation.* Boston: Jones and Bartlett.

Outcomes

Breastfeeding Weaning

DEFINITION: Process leading to the eventual discontinuation of breastfeeding

BREASTFEEDING WEANING	Not adequate 1	Slightly adequate 2	Moderately adequate 3	Substantially adequate 4	Totally adequate 5
INDICATORS:					
Awareness that breastfeeding can continue beyond infancy	1	2	3	4	5
Recognition of infant weaning readiness cues	1	2	3	4	5
Family understanding of weaning options	1	2	3	4	5
Knowledge of benefits of gradual weaning	1	2	3	4	5
Knowledge of guidelines for rapid "emergency" weaning	1	2	3	4	5
Mother's freedom from plugged ducts or mastitis	1	2	3	4	5
Avoidance of solids before infant is 4 to 6 months old	1	2	3	4	5
Replacement of one breast feeding every few days	1	2	3	4	5
Introduction of solid foods one at a time	1	2	3	4	5
Introduction of solid foods using a spoon	1	2	3	4	5
Additional touch and attention to infant during time of weaning	1	2	3	4	5
Written material reinforcing all weaning information	1	2	3	4	5
Recognition of resources available for support	1	2	3	4	5
Use of available resources	1	2	3	4	5
Family expression of satisfaction with support received	1	2	3	4	5
Family expression of satisfaction with weaning process	1	2	3	4	5
Other _____ Specify	1	2	3	4	5

BACKGROUND READINGS:

Barness, L.A. (Ed.). (1993). *Pediatric nutrition handbook* (3rd ed.). Elk Grove Village, IL: American Academy of Pediatrics.

Castiglia, P.T. (1992). Weaning. *Journal of Pediatric Health Care, 6,* 38-39.

Hendricks, K.M., & Badruddin, S.H. (1992). Weaning recommendations: The scientific basis. *Nutrition Reviews, 50*(5), 125-133.

Outcomes

Hervada, A.R. (1992). Weaning: Historical perspectives, practical recommendations, and current controversies. *Current Problems in Pediatrics, 22*, 223-241.

Huggins, K., & Ziedrich, L. (1994). *The Nursing Mother's Guide to Weaning.* Boston: The Harvard Common Press.

Lawrence, R. (1994). *Breastfeeding: A guide for the medical professional* (4th ed.). St. Louis: Mosby.

Riordan, J., & Auerbach, K.G. (1993). *Breastfeeding and human lactation.* Boston: Jones and Bartlett.

Rogers, C.S., Morris, S., & Taper, L.J. (1987). Weaning from the breast: Influences on maternal decisions. *Pediatric Nursing, 13*, 341-345.

Spangler, A. (1992). *Amy Spangler's breastfeeding: A parent's guide.* Atlanta: Amy Spangler.

Walker, C. (1995). When to wean: Whose advice do mothers find helpful? *Health Visitor, 68*, 109-111.

Outcomes

Cardiac Pump Effectiveness

DEFINITION: Extent to which blood is ejected from the left ventricle per minute to support systemic perfusion pressure

CARDIAC PUMP EFFECTIVENESS	Extremely compromised 1	Substantially compromised 2	Moderately compromised 3	Mildly compromised 4	Not compromised 5
INDICATORS:					
BP IER*	1	2	3	4	5
Heart rate IER	1	2	3	4	5
Cardiac index IER	1	2	3	4	5
Ejection fraction IER	1	2	3	4	5
Activity tolerance IER	1	2	3	4	5
Peripheral pulses strong	1	2	3	4	5
Heart size normal	1	2	3	4	5
Skin color	1	2	3	4	5
Neck vein distension not present	1	2	3	4	5
Dysrhythmia not present	1	2	3	4	5
Abnormal heart sounds not present	1	2	3	4	5
Angina not present	1	2	3	4	5
Peripheral edema not present	1	2	3	4	5
Pulmonary edema not present	1	2	3	4	5
Profuse diaphoresis not present	1	2	3	4	5
Nausea not present	1	2	3	4	5
Extreme fatigue not present	1	2	3	4	5
Other _____ Specify	1	2	3	4	5

*BP = Blood pressure; IER = In expected range.

BACKGROUND READINGS:

Bumann, R., & Speltz, M. (1989). Decreased cardiac output: A nursing diagnosis. *Dimensions of Critical Care Nursing, 8*(1), 6-15.

Dalton, J. (1985). A descriptive study: Defining characteristics of the nursing diagnosis cardiac output, alterations in: Decreased. *IMAGE-The Journal of Nursing Scholarship, 17*(4), 113-117.

Dougherty, C. (1986). Decreased cardiac output: Validation of a nursing diagnosis. *Dimensions of Critical Care Nursing, 5*(3), 182-188.

Futrell, A. (1990). Decreased cardiac output: Case for a collaborative diagnosis. *Dimensions of Critical Care Nursing, 9*(4), 202-209.

U.S. Department of Health and Human Services. (1994). *Unstable angina: Diagnosis and management* (AHCPR Publication No 94-0602) Rockville, MD: Public Health Service Agency for Health Care Policy and Research.

U.S. Department of Health and Human Services. (1994). *Heart failure: Evaluation and care of patients with left-ventricular systolic dysfunction* (AHCPR Publication No. 94-0612). Rockville, MD: Public Health Service Agency for Health Care Policy and Research.

Outcomes

Caregiver Adaptation to Patient Institutionalization

DEFINITION: Family caregiver adaptation of role when the care recipient is transferred outside the home

CAREGIVER ADAPTATION TO PATIENT INSTITUTIONALIZATION	None 1	Limited 2	Moderate 3	Substantial 4	Extensive 5
INDICATORS:					
Trust in non-family caregiver(s)	1	2	3	4	5
Maintenance of desired control over care	1	2	3	4	5
Participation in care as desired	1	2	3	4	5
Maintenance of caregiver-care recipient relationship	1	2	3	4	5
Communication with agency caregiver(s)	1	2	3	4	5
Caregiver(s)' expression of feelings about change	1	2	3	4	5
Caregiver(s)' resolution of guilt	1	2	3	4	5
Caregiver(s)' resolution of anger	1	2	3	4	5
Caregiver(s)' use of conflict resolution methods	1	2	3	4	5
Caregiver(s)' comfort with role transition	1	2	3	4	5
Caregiver(s)' availability to provide consent for treatment(s)	1	2	3	4	5
Caregiver(s)' provision of information about patient's routine	1	2	3	4	5
Caregiver(s)' provision of patient's comfort items	1	2	3	4	5
Caregiver(s)' communication of nonverbal care recipient's needs	1	2	3	4	5
Other _____ Specify	1	2	3	4	5

BACKGROUND READINGS:

Bendorf, K., & Lyman, B. (1993). Transition from the hospital to the home for the infant requiring total parenteral nutrition. *Journal of Perinatal and Neonatal Nursing, 6*(4), 80-90.

Hardgrove, C., & Healy, D. (1984). The care-through-parent program at Moffitt Hospital. *Nursing Clinics of North America, 19*(1), 145-160.

Kaus, K.J. (1990). Fostering family integrity. In M. Craft & J.A. Denehy (Eds.), *Nursing interventions for infants and children* (pp. 181-200). Philadelphia: W.B. Saunders.

Lindsay, J.K., Roman, L., DeWys, M., Eager, M., Levick, J., & Quinn, M. (1993). Creative caring in the NICU: Parent to parent support. *Neonatal Network, 12*(4), 37-44.

Olson, R.K., Heater, B.S., & Becker, A.M. (1990). A meta-analysis of the effects of nursing interventions on children and parents. *Maternal-Child Nursing, 15*(2), 104-108.

Palmer, S.J. (1993). Care of sick children by parents: A meaningful role. *Journal of Advanced Nursing, 18,* 85-191.

Spicher, C.M., & Yund, C. (1989). Effects of preadmission preparation on compliance with home care instructions. *Journal of Pediatric Nursing, 4*(4), 255-262.

Tse, A.M., & Perez-Woods, R.C. (1990). Providing support. In M. Craft & J.A. Denehy (Eds.), *Nursing interventions for infants and children* (pp. 181-200). Philadelphia: W.B. Saunders.

Wolfer, J.A., & Visintainer, M.A. (1975). Pediatric surgical patients' and parents' stress responses and adjustment as a function of psychologic preparation and stress-point nursing care. *Nursing Research, 24*(4), 244-255.

Outcomes

Caregiver Emotional Health

DEFINITION: Feelings, attitudes and emotions of a family care provider while caring for a family member or significant other over an extended period of time

CAREGIVER EMOTIONAL HEALTH	Extremely compromised 1	Substantially compromised 2	Moderately compromised 3	Mildly compromised 4	Not compromised 5
INDICATORS:					
Satisfaction with life	1	2	3	4	5
Sense of control	1	2	3	4	5
Self-esteem	1	2	3	4	5
Free of anger	1	2	3	4	5
Free of resentfulness	1	2	3	4	5
Free of guilt	1	2	3	4	5
Free of depression	1	2	3	4	5
Free of frustration	1	2	3	4	5
Free of ambivalence concerning situation	1	2	3	4	5
Certainty about future	1	2	3	4	5
Perceived social connectedness	1	2	3	4	5
Perceived spiritual well-being	1	2	3	4	5
Free of perceived burden	1	2	3	4	5
Perceived adequacy of resources	1	2	3	4	5
Use of psychotropic drugs	1	2	3	4	5
Other _____ Specify	1	2	3	4	5

BACKGROUND READINGS:

Brown, M.A., & Powell-Cope, G.M. (1991). AIDS family caregiving: Transitions through uncertainty. *Nursing Research, 40*(6), 338-345.

Bull, M.J. (1990). Factors influencing family caregiver burden and health. *Western Journal of Nursing Research, 12*(6), 758-776.

Fruewirth, S.E. (1989). An application of Johnson's behavioral model: A case study. *Journal of Community Health Nursing, 6*(2), 61-71.

Lindgren, C.L. (1990). Burnout and social support in family caregivers. *Western Journal of Nursing Research, 12*(4), 469-487.

Romeis, J.C. (1989). Caregiver strain. *Journal of Aging and Health, 1*(2), 188-208.

Thompson, E.H., Futterman, A.M., Gallagher-Thompson, D., Rose, J.M., & Lovett, S.B. (1993). Social support and caregiving burden in family caregivers of frail elders. *Journal of Gerontology, 48*, S245-S254.

Outcomes

Caregiver Home Care Readiness

Outcomes

DEFINITION: Preparedness to assume responsibility for the health care of a family member or significant other in the home

CAREGIVER HOME CARE READINESS	None 1	Limited 2	Moderate 3	Substantial 4	Extensive 5
INDICATORS:					
Willingness to assume caregiving role	1	2	3	4	5
Knowledge about caregiving role	1	2	3	4	5
Demonstration of positive regard for care recipient	1	2	3	4	5
Participation in home care decisions	1	2	3	4	5
Knowledge of care recipient's disease process	1	2	3	4	5
Knowledge of recommended treatment regimen	1	2	3	4	5
Knowledge of recommended treatment procedures	1	2	3	4	5
Knowledge of prescribed activity	1	2	3	4	5
Knowledge of follow-up care	1	2	3	4	5
Knowledge of emergency care	1	2	3	4	5
Knowledge of financial resources	1	2	3	4	5
Adequacy of financial resources	1	2	3	4	5
Knowledge of when to contact health professionals	1	2	3	4	5
Social support	1	2	3	4	5
Confidence in ability to manage care at home	1	2	3	4	5
Caregiver well-being	1	2	3	4	5
Involvement of care recipient in planning care	1	2	3	4	5
Evidence of plans for caregiver backup	1	2	3	4	5
Knowledge of where to obtain needed equipment	1	2	3	4	5
Knowledge of equipment operation	1	2	3	4	5
Other _____ Specify	1	2	3	4	5

BACKGROUND READINGS:

Baginski, Y. (1994). Roadblocks to home care. *Caring, 13*(12), 18-20, 22, 24. From (1994, July/August) *Continuing Care, 13*(8).

Gennaro, S., & Bakewell-Sachs, S. (1992). Discharge planning and home care for low-birth weight infants. *NAACOGS Clinical Issues in Perinatal & Womens Health Nursing, 3*(1), 129-145.

Magilvy, J.K., & Lakomy, J.M. (1991). Transitions of older adults to home care. *Home Health Care Services Quarterly, 12*(4), 59-70.

Titler, M.G., & Pettit, D.M. (1995). Discharge readiness assessment. *Journal of Cardiovascular Nursing, 9*(4), 64-74.

Caregiver Lifestyle Disruption

DEFINITION: Disturbances in the lifestyle of a family member due to caregiving

CAREGIVER LIFESTYLE DISRUPTION	Severe 1	Substantial 2	Moderate 3	Slight 4	None 5
INDICATORS:					
Dissatisfaction with life circumstances	1	2	3	4	5
Role performance impaired	1	2	3	4	5
Role flexibility compromised	1	2	3	4	5
Opportunities for privacy compromised	1	2	3	4	5
Relationships with other family members disrupted	1	2	3	4	5
Social interactions disrupted	1	2	3	4	5
Social support compromised	1	2	3	4	5
Diversional activities compromised	1	2	3	4	5
Work productivity compromised	1	2	3	4	5
Role responsibilities compromised	1	2	3	4	5
Financial resources consumed	1	2	3	4	5
Relationships with friends impaired	1	2	3	4	5
Relationships with pets compromised	1	2	3	4	5
Other _____ Specify	1	2	3	4	5

BACKGROUND READINGS:

Baldwin, B.A., Kleeman, K.M., Stevens, G.L., & Rasin, J. (1989). Family caregiver stress: Clinical assessment and management. *International Psychogeriatrics, 1*(2), 183-193.

Gaynor, S.E. (1990). The long haul: The effects of home care on caregivers. *IMAGE-The Journal of Nursing Scholarship, 22*(4), 208-212.

Given, B.A., & Given, C.W. (1991). Family caregiving for the elderly. *Annual Review of Nursing Research, 9,* 77-101.

Kuhlman, G.J., Wilson, H.S., Hutchison, S.A., & Wallhagen, M. (1991). Alzheimer's disease and family caregiving: Critical syntheses of the literature and research agenda. *Nursing Research, 40*(6), 331-337.

Lindgren, C.L. (1990). Burnout and social support in family caregivers. *Western Journal of Nursing Research, 12*(4), 469-487.

Lindgren, C.L. (1993). The caregiver career. *IMAGE-The Journal of Nursing Scholarship, 25*(3), 214-219.

Oberst, M.T., Thomas, S.E., Gass, K.A., & Ward, S.E. (1989). Caregiving demands and appraisal of stress among family caregivers. *Cancer Nursing, 12*(4), 209-215.

Robinson, K.M. (1989). Predictors of depression among wife caregivers. *Nursing Research, 38*(8), 359-363.

Robinson, K. (1990). The relationships between social skills, social support, self-esteem and burden in adult caregivers. *Journal of Advanced Nursing, 15,* 788-795.

Stevenson, J.E. (1990). Family stress related to home care of Alzheimer's disease patients and implications for support. *Journal of Neuroscience Nursing, 22*(3), 179-188.

Thompson, E.H., Futterman, A.M., Gallagher-Thompson, D., Rose, J.M., & Lovette, S.B. (1993). Social support and caregiving burden in family caregivers of frail elders. *Journal of Gerontology, 48,* S245-S254.

Outcomes

Caregiver-Patient Relationship

DEFINITION: Positive interactions and connections between the caregiver and care recipient

CAREGIVER-PATIENT RELATIONSHIP	Extremely compromised 1	Substantially compromised 2	Moderately compromised 3	Mildly compromised 4	Not compromised 5
INDICATORS:					
Effective communication	1	2	3	4	5
Patience	1	2	3	4	5
Harmony	1	2	3	4	5
Calmness	1	2	3	4	5
Nurturance and affirmation	1	2	3	4	5
Companionship	1	2	3	4	5
Caring	1	2	3	4	5
Long-term commitment	1	2	3	4	5
Mutual acceptance	1	2	3	4	5
Mutual respect	1	2	3	4	5
Collaborative problem solving	1	2	3	4	5
Sense of responsibility	1	2	3	4	5
Mutual sense of attachment	1	2	3	4	5
Other _____ Specify	1	2	3	4	5

BACKGROUND READINGS:

Caldwell, S.M. (1993). Measuring family well-being: Conceptual model, reliability, validity and use. In C.F. Waltz & O.L. Strickland (Eds.), *Measuring client outcomes*. New York: Springer.

Clemen-Stone, S., Eigsti, D., & McGuire, S. (1991). *Comprehensive family and community health nursing*, St. Louis: Mosby.

Craft, M.J., & Willadsen, J.A. (1992). Interventions related to family. *Nursing Clinics of North America*, 27(20), 517-540.

Gaynor, S.E. (1990). The long haul: The effects of home care on caregivers. *IMAGE-The Journal of Nursing Scholarship*, 22(4), 208-212.

Hooyman, M., Gonyea, J., & Montgomery, R. (1985). Impact of in-home services termination on family caregivers. *The Gerontologist*, 25(2), 141-145.

O'Neill, C., & Sorenson, E.S. (1991). Home care of the elderly: A family perspective. *Advances in Nursing Science*, 13, 28-37.

Phillips, L.R. (1988). The fit of elder abuse with the family violence paradigm, and the implications of a paradigm shift for clinical practice. *Public Health Nursing*, 5(4), 222-229.

Printz-Feddersen, V. (1990). Group process effect on caregiver burden. *Journal of Neuroscience Nursing*, 22(3), 164-168.

Caregiver Performance: Direct Care

DEFINITION: Provision by family care provider of appropriate personal and health care for a family member or significant other

CAREGIVER PERFORMANCE: DIRECT CARE	Not adequate 1	Slightly adequate 2	Moderately adequate 3	Substantially adequate 4	Totally adequate 5
INDICATORS:					
Provision of emotional support to care recipient	1	2	3	4	5
Assists with activities of daily living	1	2	3	4	5
Knowledge of disease process	1	2	3	4	5
Knowledge of treatment plan	1	2	3	4	5
Adherence to treatment plan	1	2	3	4	5
Assists with instrumental activities of daily living	1	2	3	4	5
Performance of treatments	1	2	3	4	5
Monitoring of health status of care recipient	1	2	3	4	5
Monitoring of behavior of care recipient	1	2	3	4	5
Anticipation of care recipient's needs	1	2	3	4	5
Demonstration of unconditional positive regard for care recipient	1	2	3	4	5
Demonstration of competence in monitoring own caregiving skill level	1	2	3	4	5
Confidence in performing needed tasks	1	2	3	4	5
Other _____ Specify	1	2	3	4	5

BACKGROUND READINGS:

Given, B.A., & Given, C.W. (1991). Family caregiving for the elderly. *Annual Review of Nursing Research, 9,* 77-101.

Oberst, M.T., Thomas, S.E., Gass, K.A., & Ward, S.E. (1989). Caregiving demands and appraisal of stress among family caregivers. *Cancer Nursing, 12*(4), 209-215.

Pierson, M.A., & Irons, K. (1992). Identification of a cluster of nursing diagnoses for a caregiver support group. *Nursing Diagnosis, 3*(1), 36-41.

Printz-Feddersen, V. (1990). Group process effect on caregiver burden. *Journal of Neuroscience Nursing, 22*(3), 164-168.

Thomas, V.M., Ellison, K., Howell, E.V., & Winters, K. (1992). Caring for the person receiving ventilatory support at home: Caregivers' needs and involvement. *Heart and Lung, 21*(2), 180-186.

Wallhagen, M.I., & Kagan, S.H. (1993). Staying within bounds: Perceived control and the experience of elderly caregivers. *Journal of Aging Studies, 7*(2), 197-213.

Outcomes

Caregiver Performance: Indirect Care

DEFINITION: Arrangement and oversight of appropriate care for a family member or significant other by family care provider

CAREGIVER PERFORMANCE: INDIRECT CARE	Not adequate 1	Slightly adequate 2	Moderately adequate 3	Substantially adequate 4	Totally adequate 5
INDICATORS:					
Confidence in problem solving	1	2	3	4	5
Recognition of changes in health status of care recipient	1	2	3	4	5
Recognition of changes in behavior of care recipient	1	2	3	4	5
Demonstration of ability to anticipate care recipient's needs	1	2	3	4	5
Obtaining needed services for care recipient	1	2	3	4	5
Skill in overseeing needed services	1	2	3	4	5
Demonstration of regard for care recipient's needs	1	2	3	4	5
Skill in pursuing care problems with direct care providers	1	2	3	4	5
Confidence in performing needed tasks	1	2	3	4	5
Other _____ Specify	1	2	3	4	5

BACKGROUND READINGS:

Bowers, B.J. (1987). Intergenerational caregiving: Adult caregivers and their aging parents. *Advances in Nursing Science, 9*(2), 20-31.

Given, B.A., & Given, C.W. (1991). Family caregiving for the elderly. *Annual Review of Nursing Research, 9,* 77-101.

Oberst, M.T., Thomas, S.E., Gass, K.A., & Ward, S.E. (1989). Caregiving demands and appraisal of stress among family caregivers. *Cancer Nursing, 12*(4), 209-215.

Pierson, M.A., & Irons, K. (1992). Identification of a cluster of nursing diagnoses for a caregiver support group. *Nursing Diagnosis, 3*(1), 36-41.

Printz-Feddersen, V. (1990). Group process effect on caregiver burden. *Journal of Neuroscience Nursing, 22*(3), 164-168.

Thomas, V.M., Ellison, K., Howell, E.V., & Winters, K. (1992). Caring for the person receiving ventilatory support at home: Caregivers' needs and involvement. *Heart and Lung, 21*(2), 180-186.

Wallhagen, M.I., & Kagan, S.H. (1993). Staying within bounds: Perceived control and the experience of elderly caregivers. *Journal of Aging Studies, 7*(2), 197-213.

Outcomes

Caregiver Physical Health

DEFINITION: Physical well-being of a family care provider while caring for a family member or significant other over an extended period of time

CAREGIVER PHYSICAL HEALTH	Extremely compromised 1	Substantially compromised 2	Moderately compromised 3	Mildly compromised 4	Not compromised 5
INDICATORS:					
Physical health	1	2	3	4	5
Sleep pattern	1	2	3	4	5
BP IER*	1	2	3	4	5
Energy level	1	2	3	4	5
Physical comfort	1	2	3	4	5
Mobility level	1	2	3	4	5
Resistance to infection	1	2	3	4	5
Physical function	1	2	3	4	5
Weight IER	1	2	3	4	5
Gastrointestinal function	1	2	3	4	5
Medication use	1	2	3	4	5
Perceived general health	1	2	3	4	5
Use of health providers	1	2	3	4	5
Other _____ Specify	1	2	3	4	5

*BP = Blood pressure; IER = In expected range.

BACKGROUND READINGS:

Collins, C.E., Given, B.A., & Given, C.W. (1994). Interventions with family caregivers of persons with Alzheimer's disease. *Nursing Clinics of North America, 29*(1), 127-131.

Given, B.A., & Given, C.W. (1991). Family caregiving for the elderly. *Annual Review of Nursing Research, 9,* 77-101.

Pepin, J.I. (1992). Family caring and caring in nursing: *IMAGE-The Journal of Nursing Scholarship, 24*(2), 127-131.

Springer, D., & Brubaker, T.H. (1984). *Caregiving and the dependent elderly.* Newbury, CA: Sage.

Winslow, B., & O'Brien, R. (1992). Use of formal community resources by spouse caregivers of chronically ill adults. *Public Health Nursing, 9*(27), 128-132.

Zeisel, J., Hyde, J., & Levkoff, S. (1994, March/April). Best practices: An environment-behavior (E-B) model for Alzheimer special care units. *The American Journal of Alzheimer's Care and Related Disorders & Research,* 4-21.

Caregiver Stressors

DEFINITION: The extent of biopsychosocial pressure on a family care provider caring for a family member or significant other over an extended period of time

CAREGIVER STRESSORS	Extensive 1	Substantial 2	Moderate 3	Limited 4	None 5
INDICATORS:					
Reported stressors of caregiving	1	2	3	4	5
Physical limitations for caregiving	1	2	3	4	5
Psychological limitations for caregiving	1	2	3	4	5
Cognitive limitations for caregiving	1	2	3	4	5
Impairment of usual role performance	1	2	3	4	5
Impairment of social interactions	1	2	3	4	5
Perceived lack of social support	1	2	3	4	5
Perceived lack of health care system support	1	2	3	4	5
Lack of usual diversional activity	1	2	3	4	5
Impairment of usual work performance	1	2	3	4	5
Severity of care recipient illness	1	2	3	4	5
Amount of care or oversight required	1	2	3	4	5
Impairment of caregiver-patient relationship	1	2	3	4	5
Other _____ Specify	1	2	3	4	5

BACKGROUND READINGS:

Brown, M.A., & Powell-Cope, G.M. (1991). AIDS family caregiving: Transitions through uncertainty. *Nursing Research, 40*(6), 338-345.

Given, C.W., Given, B., Stommel, M., Collins, C., King, S., & Franklin, S. (1992). The caregiver reaction assessment (CRA) for caregivers to persons with chronic physical and mental impairments. *Research in Nursing & Health, 15*(4), 271-283.

Stevenson, J.E. (1990). Family stress related to home care of Alzheimer's disease patients and implications for support. *Journal of Neuroscience Nursing, 22*(3), 179-188.

Thompson, E.H., Futterman, A.M., Gallagher-Thompson, D., Rose, J.M., & Lovett, S.B. (1993). Social support and caregiving burden in family caregivers of frail elders. *Journal of Gerontology, 48*, S245-S254.

Wallhagen, M.I. (1992). Caregiving demands: Their difficulty and effects on the well-being of elderly caregivers. *Scholarly Inquiry for Nursing Practice: An International Journal, 6*(2), 111-133.

Outcomes

Outcomes

Caregiver Well-Being

DEFINITION: Primary care provider's satisfaction with health and life circumstances

CAREGIVER WELL-BEING	Extremely compromised 1	Substantially compromised 2	Moderately compromised 3	Mildly compromised 4	Not compromised 5
INDICATORS:					
Satisfaction with physical health	1	2	3	4	5
Satisfaction with emotional health	1	2	3	4	5
Satisfaction with lifestyle	1	2	3	4	5
Satisfaction with performance of usual roles	1	2	3	4	5
Satisfaction with social support	1	2	3	4	5
Satisfaction with instrumental support	1	2	3	4	5
Satisfaction with professional support	1	2	3	4	5
Satisfaction with social relationships	1	2	3	4	5
Satisfaction with caregiver role	1	2	3	4	5
Other _____ Specify	1	2	3	4	5

BACKGROUND READINGS:

Brown, M.A., & Powell-Cope, G.M. (1991). AIDS family caregiving: Transitions through uncertainty. *Nursing Research, 40*(6), 338-345.

Given, C.W., Given, B., Stommel, M., Collins, C., King, S., & Franklin, S. (1992). The caregiver reaction assessment (CRA) for caregivers to persons with chronic physical and mental impairments. *Research in Nursing & Health, 15*(4), 271-283.

Pender, N. (1996). *Health promotion in nursing practice* (3rd ed.). Stanford, CT: Appleton & Lange.

Stevenson, J.E. (1990). Family stress related to home care of Alzheimer's disease patients and implications for support. *Journal of Neuroscience Nursing, 22*(3), 179-188.

Thompson, E.H., Futterman, A.M., Gallagher-Thompson, D., Rose, J.M., & Lovett, S.B. (1993). Social support and caregiving burden in family caregivers of frail elders. *Journal of Gerontology, 48,* S245-S254.

Wallhagen, M.I. (1992). Caregiving demands: Their difficulty and effects on the well-being of elderly caregivers. *Scholarly Inquiry for Nursing Practice: An International Journal, 6*(2), 111-133.

Caregiving Endurance Potential

DEFINITION: Factors that promote family care provider continuance over an extended period of time

CAREGIVING ENDURANCE POTENTIAL	Not adequate 1	Slightly adequate 2	Moderately adequate 3	Substantially adequate 4	Totally adequate 5
INDICATORS:					
Mutually satisfying care recipient-caregiver relationship	1	2	3	4	5
Mastery of direct care activities	1	2	3	4	5
Mastery of indirect care activities	1	2	3	4	5
Services needed for the care recipient	1	2	3	4	5
Social support for caregiver	1	2	3	4	5
Health care system support for caregiver	1	2	3	4	5
Resources to provide care	1	2	3	4	5
Respite for caregiver	1	2	3	4	5
Opportunities for caregiver leisure activities	1	2	3	4	5
Other _____ Specify	1	2	3	4	5

Outcomes

BACKGROUND READINGS:

Given, B.A., Stommel, M., Collins, C., King, S., & Given, C.W. (1990). Responses of elderly spouse caregivers. *Research in Nursing & Health, 13,* 77-85.

Nolan, M.R., Grant, G., & Ellis, N.C. (1990). Stress is in the eye of the beholder: Reconceptualizing the measurement of career burden. *Journal of Advanced Nursing, 15,* 544-555.

Oberst, M.T., Thomas, S.E., Gass, K.A., & Ward, S.E. (1989). Caregiving demands and appraisal of stress among family caregivers. *Cancer Nursing, 12*(4), 209-215.

Pierson, M.A., & Irons, K. (1992). Identification of a cluster of nursing diagnoses for a caregiver support group. *Nursing Diagnosis, 3*(1), 36-41.

Rawlins, S.R. (1991). Using the connecting process to meet family caregiver needs. *Journal of Professional Nursing, 7,* 213-220.

Romeis, J.C. (1989). Caregiver strain. *Journal of Aging and Health, 1*(2), 188-208.

Stevenson, J.E. (1990). Family stress related to home care of Alzheimer's disease patients and implications for support. *Journal of Neuroscience Nursing, 22*(3), 179-188.

Thompson, E.H., Futterman, A.M., Gallagher-Thompson, D., Rose, J.M., & Lovett, S.B. (1993). Social support and caregiving burden in family caregivers of frail elders. *Journal of Gerontology, 48,* S245-S254.

Wallhagen, M.I. (1992). Caregiving demands: Their difficulty and effects on the well-being of elderly caregivers. *Scholarly Inquiry for Nursing Practice: An International Journal, 6*(2), 111-133.

Winslow, B., & O'Brien, R. (1992). Use of formal community resources by spouse caregivers of chronically ill adults. *Public Health Nursing, 9*(27), 128-132.

Child Adaptation to Hospitalization

DEFINITION: Child's adaptive response to hospitalization

CHILD ADAPTATION TO HOSPITALIZATION	None 1	Limited 2	Moderate 3	Substantial 4	Extensive 5
INDICATORS:					
Resolution of agitation	1	2	3	4	5
Resolution of separation anxiety	1	2	3	4	5
Resolution of regressive behavior(s)	1	2	3	4	5
Resolution of anxiety	1	2	3	4	5
Resolution of fear	1	2	3	4	5
Resolution of anger	1	2	3	4	5
Resolution of behavioral disturbances	1	2	3	4	5
Sense of control	1	2	3	4	5
Responsiveness to comfort measures	1	2	3	4	5
Responsiveness to diversional therapy	1	2	3	4	5
Participation in social interaction	1	2	3	4	5
Maintenance of parent-child attachment	1	2	3	4	5
Recognition of need for hospitalization	1	2	3	4	5
Self-control	1	2	3	4	5
Participation in decision-making	1	2	3	4	5
Reported understanding of illness and treatment	1	2	3	4	5
Maintenance of pre-admission self-care behaviors	1	2	3	4	5
Cooperation with procedures	1	2	3	4	5
Maintenance of social relationships	1	2	3	4	5
Other _____ Specify	1	2	3	4	5

Outcomes

BACKGROUND READINGS:

Coucouvanis, J.A. (1990). Behavior management. In M. Craft & J.A. Denehy (Eds.), *Nursing interventions for infants and children* (pp. 151-165). Philadelphia: W.B. Saunders.

Manion, J. (1990). Preparing children for hospitalization, procedures, or surgery. In M. Craft & J.A. Denehy (Eds.), *Nursing interventions for infants and children* (pp. 74-90). Philadelphia: W.B. Saunders.

Olson, R.K., Heater, B.S., & Becker, A.M. (1990). A meta-analysis of the effects of nursing interventions on children and parents. *Maternal-Child Nursing, 15*(2), 104-108.

Whaley, L.F., & Wong, D.L. (1987). *Nursing care of infants and children* (pp. 1053-1100). St. Louis: Mosby.

Wolfer, J.A., & Visintainer, M.A. (1975). Pediatric surgical patients' and parents' stress responses and adjustment as a function of psychologic preparation and stress-point nursing care. *Nursing Research, 24*(4), 244-255.

Ziegler, D.B., & Prior, M.M. (1994). Preparation for surgery and adjustment to hospitalization. *Nursing Clinics of North America, 29*(4), 655-669.

Child Development: 2 Months

DEFINITION: Milestones of physical, cognitive, and psychosocial progression by 2 months of age

CHILD DEVELOPMENT: 2 MONTHS	Extreme delay from expected range	Substantial delay from expected range	Moderate delay from expected range	Mild delay from expected range	No delay from expected range
	1	2	3	4	5
INDICATORS:					
Posterior fontanel closed	1	2	3	4	5
Crawling reflex disappearance	1	2	3	4	5
Lifts head, neck, and upper chest with support on forearms while in prone position	1	2	3	4	5
Some head control in upright position	1	2	3	4	5
Hands frequently open	1	2	3	4	5
Grasp reflex fading	1	2	3	4	5
Coos and vocalizes	1	2	3	4	5
Shows interest in auditory stimuli	1	2	3	4	5
Shows interest in visual stimuli	1	2	3	4	5
Smiles	1	2	3	4	5
Shows pleasure in interactions, especially with primary caregivers	1	2	3	4	5
Other _____ Specify	1	2	3	4	5

BACKGROUND READINGS:

Bricker, D. (Ed). (1993). *AEPS measurement for birth-three years* (Vol. 1). Baltimore: Paul H. Brookes Publishing.

Green, M. (Ed.). (1994). *Bright futures: Guidelines for health supervision of infants, children and adolescents.* Arlington, VA: National Center for Education in Maternal and Child Health.

Outcomes

Child Development: 4 Months

DEFINITION: Milestones of physical, cognitive, and psychosocial progression by 4 months of age

CHILD DEVELOPMENT: 4 MONTHS	Extreme delay from expected range 1	Substantial delay from expected range 2	Moderate delay from expected range 3	Mild delay from expected range 4	No delay from expected range 5
INDICATORS:					
In prone position holds head erect and raises body on hands	1	2	3	4	5
Controls head well	1	2	3	4	5
Rolls over from prone to supine	1	2	3	4	5
Holds own hands	1	2	3	4	5
Grasps rattle	1	2	3	4	5
Reaches for objects	1	2	3	4	5
Bats at objects	1	2	3	4	5
Babbles and coos	1	2	3	4	5
Recognizes parents' voices	1	2	3	4	5
Recognizes parents' touch	1	2	3	4	5
Looks at and becomes excited by mobile	1	2	3	4	5
Smiles, laughs, and squeals	1	2	3	4	5
Sleeps for at least 6 hours	1	2	3	4	5
Comforts self (e.g., falls asleep by self without breast or bottle)	1	2	3	4	5
Other _____ Specify	1	2	3	4	5

BACKGROUND READINGS:

Green, M. (Ed.). (1994). *Bright futures: Guidelines for health supervision of infants, children and adolescents.* Arlington, VA: National Center for Education in Maternal and Child Health.

Outcomes

Child Development: 6 Months

DEFINITION: Milestones of physical, cognitive, and psychosocial progression by 6 months of age

CHILD DEVELOPMENT: 6 MONTHS	Extreme delay from expected range	Substantial delay from expected range	Moderate delay from expected range	Mild delay from expected range	No delay from expected range
	1	2	3	4	5
INDICATORS:					
No head lag when pulled to sit	1	2	3	4	5
Rolls over	1	2	3	4	5
Sits with support	1	2	3	4	5
Stands when placed and bears weight	1	2	3	4	5
Grasps and mouths objects	1	2	3	4	5
Gestures (e.g., points, shakes head)	1	2	3	4	5
Starts to self-feed	1	2	3	4	5
Shows interest in toys	1	2	3	4	5
Transfers small objects from hand to hand	1	2	3	4	5
Vocalizes/sings syllables (dada, baba)	1	2	3	4	5
Babbles reciprocally	1	2	3	4	5
Smiles, laughs, squeals, imitates noise	1	2	3	4	5
Turns to sounds	1	2	3	4	5
Beginning signs of stranger anxiety	1	2	3	4	5
Comforts self	1	2	3	4	5
Other _____ Specify	1	2	3	4	5

BACKGROUND READINGS:

Bricker, D. (Ed.) (1993). *AEPS measurement for birth-three years* (Vol. 1). Baltimore: Paul H. Brookes Publishing.

Green, M. (Ed.). (1994). *Bright futures: Guidelines for health supervision of infants, children and adolescents.* Arlington, VA: National Center for Education in Maternal and Child Health.

Rossetti, L.M. (1990). *Infant-toddler assessment: An interdisciplinary approach.* Boston: Little, Brown.

Outcomes

Child Development: 12 Months

DEFINITION: Milestones of physical, cognitive, and psychosocial progression by 12 months of age

CHILD DEVELOPMENT: 12 MONTHS	Extreme delay from expected range 1	Substantial delay from expected range 2	Moderate delay from expected range 3	Mild delay from expected range 4	No delay from expected range 5
INDICATORS:					
Pulls to stand	1	2	3	4	5
Cruises around furniture	1	2	3	4	5
Attempts to take steps alone	1	2	3	4	5
Precise pincer grasp	1	2	3	4	5
Points with index fingers	1	2	3	4	5
Bangs blocks together	1	2	3	4	5
Drinks from cup	1	2	3	4	5
Feeds self finger foods	1	2	3	4	5
Feeds self with spoon	1	2	3	4	5
Uses vocabulary of one to three words in addition to mama, dada	1	2	3	4	5
Imitates vocalizations	1	2	3	4	5
Looks for dropped or hidden object	1	2	3	4	5
Plays social games	1	2	3	4	5
Waves bye-bye	1	2	3	4	5
Other _____ Specify	1	2	3	4	5

BACKGROUND READINGS:

Bricker, D. (Ed). (1993). *AEPS measurement for birth-three years* (Vol. 1). Baltimore: Paul H. Brookes Publishing.

Green, M. (Ed.). (1994). *Bright futures: Guidelines for health supervision of infants, children and adolescents.* Arlington, VA: National Center for Education in Maternal and Child Health.

Rossetti L.M. (1990). *Infant-toddler assessment: An interdisciplinary approach.* Boston: Little, Brown.

Outcomes

Child Development: 2 Years

DEFINITION: Milestones of physical, cognitive, and psychosocial progression by 2 years of age

CHILD DEVELOPMENT: 2 YEARS	Extreme delay from expected range	Substantial delay from expected range	Moderate delay from expected range	Mild delay from expected range	No delay from expected range
	1	2	3	4	5
INDICATORS:					
Walks quickly	1	2	3	4	5
Stoops well	1	2	3	4	5
Walks up and down stairs one step at a time	1	2	3	4	5
Walks backwards	1	2	3	4	5
Kicks a ball	1	2	3	4	5
Throws a ball	1	2	3	4	5
Makes circular and horizontal strokes with crayon	1	2	3	4	5
Stacks five to six blocks	1	2	3	4	5
Feeds self with spoon and fork	1	2	3	4	5
Follows two-step commands	1	2	3	4	5
Indicates wants verbally	1	2	3	4	5
Uses phrases of two to three words	1	2	3	4	5
Listens to story looking at pictures	1	2	3	4	5
Points to some body parts	1	2	3	4	5
Parallel play	1	2	3	4	5
Imitates adults	1	2	3	4	5
Interacts with adults in simple games	1	2	3	4	5
Other _____ Specify	1	2	3	4	5

BACKGROUND READINGS:

Bricker, D. (Ed). (1993). *AEPS measurement for birth-three years* (Vol. 1). Baltimore: Paul H. Brookes Publishing.

Green, M. (Ed.). (1994). *Bright futures: Guidelines for health supervision of infants, children and adolescents.* Arlington, VA: National Center for Education in Maternal and Child Health.

Rossetti, L.M. (1990). *Infant-toddler assessment: An interdisciplinary approach.* Boston: Little, Brown.

Outcomes

Child Development: 3 Years

DEFINITION: Milestones of physical, cognitive, and psychosocial progression by 3 years of age

CHILD DEVELOPMENT: 3 YEARS	Extreme delay from expected range	Substantial delay from expected range	Moderate delay from expected range	Mild delay from expected range	No delay from expected range
	1	2	3	4	5
INDICATORS:					
Balances on one foot	1	2	3	4	5
Pedals a riding toy	1	2	3	4	5
Dresses self	1	2	3	4	5
Control of writing/coloring instruments	1	2	3	4	5
Copies a circle	1	2	3	4	5
Copies a cross	1	2	3	4	5
Control of bowel in daytime	1	2	3	4	5
Control of bladder in daytime	1	2	3	4	5
Distinguishes gender differences	1	2	3	4	5
Gives own first name	1	2	3	4	5
Gives own age	1	2	3	4	5
Engages in magical thinking/ fantasy	1	2	3	4	5
Plays interactive games with peers	1	2	3	4	5
Begins cooperative group play	1	2	3	4	5
Uses sentences of three or four words	1	2	3	4	5
Speech understood by strangers	1	2	3	4	5
Other _____ Specify	1	2	3	4	5

BACKGROUND READINGS:

Bricker, D. (Ed). (1993). *AEPS measurement for birth-three years* (Vol. 1). Baltimore: Paul H. Brookes Publishing.

Green, M. (Ed.). (1994). *Bright futures: Guidelines for health supervision of infants, children and adolescents.* Arlington, VA: National Center for Education in Maternal and Child Health.

Outcomes

Child Development: 4 Years

DEFINITION: Milestones of physical, cognitive, and psychosocial progression by 4 years of age

CHILD DEVELOPMENT: 4 YEARS	Extreme delay from expected range	Substantial delay from expected range	Moderate delay from expected range	Mild delay from expected range	No delay from expected range
	1	**2**	**3**	**4**	**5**
INDICATORS:					
Walks, climbs, runs	1	2	3	4	5
Goes up and down stairs	1	2	3	4	5
Hops and jumps on one foot	1	2	3	4	5
Rides tricycle or bicycle with training wheels	1	2	3	4	5
Throws overhand ball	1	2	3	4	5
Builds tower of 10 blocks	1	2	3	4	5
Draws person with three parts	1	2	3	4	5
Gives first and last name	1	2	3	4	5
Uses sentences of four to five words, short paragraphs	1	2	3	4	5
Vocabulary includes past tense	1	2	3	4	5
Describes a recent experience	1	2	3	4	5
Can sing a song	1	2	3	4	5
Distinguishes fantasy from reality	1	2	3	4	5
Describes use of items used in the home (e.g., food and appliances)	1	2	3	4	5
Other _____ Specify	1	2	3	4	5

BACKGROUND READINGS:

Green, M. (Ed.). (1994). *Bright futures: Guidelines for health supervision of infants, children and adolescents.* Arlington, VA: National Center for Education in Maternal and Child Health.

Outcomes

Child Development: 5 Years

DEFINITION: Milestones of physical, cognitive, and psychosocial progression by 5 years of age

CHILD DEVELOPMENT: 5 YEARS	Extreme delay from expected range	Substantial delay from expected range	Moderate delay from expected range	Mild delay from expected range	No delay from expected range
	1	**2**	**3**	**4**	**5**
INDICATORS:					
Walks, climbs, runs with coordination	1	2	3	4	5
Able to skip	1	2	3	4	5
Dresses self without help	1	2	3	4	5
Draws a person with head, body, arms, and legs	1	2	3	4	5
Copies a triangle or square	1	2	3	4	5
Counts using fingers	1	2	3	4	5
Recognizes most letters of alphabet	1	2	3	4	5
Prints some letters	1	2	3	4	5
Uses complete sentence of five words	1	2	3	4	5
Vocabulary includes future tense	1	2	3	4	5
Speaks short paragraphs	1	2	3	4	5
Gives own address	1	2	3	4	5
Gives own phone number	1	2	3	4	5
Follows rules of interactive games with peers	1	2	3	4	5
Other _____ Specify	1	2	3	4	5

BACKGROUND READINGS:

Green, M. (Ed.). (1994). *Bright futures: Guidelines for health supervision of infants, children and adolescents.* Arlington, VA: National Center for Education in Maternal and Child Health.

Child Development: Middle Childhood (6-11 Years)

DEFINITION: Milestones of physical, cognitive, and psychosocial progression between 6 and 11 years of age

CHILD DEVELOPMENT: MIDDLE CHILDHOOD (6-11 YEARS)	Extreme delay from expected range	Substantial delay from expected range	Moderate delay from expected range	Mild delay from expected range	No delay from expected range
	1	**2**	**3**	**4**	**5**
INDICATORS:					
Practices good health habits	1	2	3	4	5
Plays in groups	1	2	3	4	5
Develops close friendships	1	2	3	4	5
Identifies with same sex peer group	1	2	3	4	5
Assumes responsibility for selected household tasks	1	2	3	4	5
Follows through with commitments to extracurricular activities	1	2	3	4	5
Expresses feelings constructively	1	2	3	4	5
Displays self-confidence	1	2	3	4	5
Understands right and wrong	1	2	3	4	5
Follows safety rules	1	2	3	4	5
Expresses increasingly complex thoughts	1	2	3	4	5
Shows creativity	1	2	3	4	5
Comprehends increasingly complex ideas	1	2	3	4	5
Assumes responsibility for homework	1	2	3	4	5
Performs in school to level of ability	1	2	3	4	5
Other _____ Specify	1	2	3	4	5

BACKGROUND READINGS:

Green, M. (Ed.). (1994). *Bright futures: Guidelines for health supervision of infants, children and adolescents.* Arlington, VA: National Center for Education in Maternal and Child Health.

Outcomes

Child Development: Adolescence (12-17 Years)

DEFINITION: Milestones of physical, cognitive, and psychosocial progression between 12 and 17 years of age

CHILD DEVELOPMENT: ADOLESCENCE (12-17 YEARS)	Extreme delay from expected range	Substantial delay from expected range	Moderate delay from expected range	Mild delay from expected range	No delay from expected range
	1	2	3	4	5
INDICATORS:					
Practices good health habits	1	2	3	4	5
Describes sexual development	1	2	3	4	5
Expresses comfort with own sexual identity	1	2	3	4	5
Uses social interaction skills	1	2	3	4	5
Uses conflict resolution skills	1	2	3	4	5
Maintains good peer relationships with same gender	1	2	3	4	5
Maintains good peer relationships with the opposite gender	1	2	3	4	5
Demonstrates capacity for intimacy	1	2	3	4	5
Practices responsible sexual behaviors	1	2	3	4	5
Avoids alcohol, tobacco, and drugs	1	2	3	4	5
Demonstrates coping	1	2	3	4	5
Displays increasing levels of autonomy	1	2	3	4	5
Describes personal value system	1	2	3	4	5
Uses formal operational thinking	1	2	3	4	5
Sets academic goals	1	2	3	4	5
Performs in school to level of ability	1	2	3	4	5
Other _____ Specify	1	2	3	4	5

BACKGROUND READINGS:

Green, M. (Ed.). (1994). *Bright futures: Guidelines for health supervision of infants, children and adolescents.* Arlington, VA: National Center for Education in Maternal and Child Health.

Outcomes

Circulation Status

DEFINITION: Extent to which blood flows unobstructed, unidirectionally, and at an appropriate pressure through large vessels of the systemic and pulmonary circuits

CIRCULATION STATUS	Extremely compromised 1	Substantially compromised 2	Moderately compromised 3	Mildly compromised 4	Not compromised 5
INDICATORS:					
Systolic BP IER*	1	2	3	4	5
Diastolic BP IER	1	2	3	4	5
Pulse pressure IER	1	2	3	4	5
Mean BP IER	1	2	3	4	5
Central venous pressure IER	1	2	3	4	5
Pulmonary wedge pressure IER	1	2	3	4	5
Orthostatic hypotension not present	1	2	3	4	5
Heart rate IER	1	2	3	4	5
Abnormal heart sounds not present	1	2	3	4	5
Angina not present	1	2	3	4	5
Blood gases IER	1	2	3	4	5
Arterial-venous O_2 difference IER	1	2	3	4	5
Adventitious breath sounds not present	1	2	3	4	5
24-hour intake and output balanced	1	2	3	4	5
Peripheral tissue perfusion	1	2	3	4	5
Peripheral pulses strong	1	2	3	4	5
Peripheral pulses symmetrical	1	2	3	4	5
Large vessel bruits not present	1	2	3	4	5
Neck vein distention not present	1	2	3	4	5
Peripheral edema not present	1	2	3	4	5
Ascites not present	1	2	3	4	5
Cognitive status IER	1	2	3	4	5

*BP = Blood pressure; IER = In expected range.   *Continued.*

Outcomes

Outcomes

CIRCULATION STATUS—cont'd	Extremely compromised 1	Substantially compromised 2	Moderately compromised 3	Mildly compromised 4	Not compromised 5
Extreme fatigue not present	1	2	3	4	5
Other _____ Specify	1	2	3	4	5

BACKGROUND READINGS:

Andreoli, K.G., Zipes, D.P., Wallace, A.G., Kinney, M.R., & Fowkes, V.K. (Eds.). (1987). *Comprehensive cardiac care* (6th ed.). St. Louis: Mosby.

Cullen, L. (1992). Interventions related to circulatory care. *Nursing Clinics of North America, 27*(2), 445-477.

Douglas, M.K., & Shinn, J.A. (1985). *Advances in cardiovascular nursing,* Rockville, MD: Aspen.

Fahey, V.A. (Ed.). (1988). *Vascular nursing.* Philadelphia: W.B. Saunders.

Luckman, J., & Sorenson, K.C. (1987). *Medical-surgical nursing: A psychophysiological approach* (3rd ed.). Philadelphia: W.B. Saunders.

McCloskey, J.C., & Bulechek, G.M. (Eds.). (1992). *Nursing interventions classification (NIC).* St. Louis: Mosby.

Murphy, T.G., & Bennett, E.J. (1992). Low-tech, high-touch perfusion assessment. *American Journal of Nursing, May,* 36-46.

Sheehy, S.B. (1990). *Manual of emergency care* (3rd ed.). St. Louis: Mosby.

Smith, S.L. (1990). Postoperative perfusion deficits. *Critical Care Nursing Clinics of North America, 2*(4), 567-578.

Cognitive Ability

DEFINITION: Ability to execute complex mental processes

COGNITIVE ABILITY	Extremely compromised 1	Substantially compromised 2	Moderately compromised 3	Mildly compromised 4	Not compromised 5
INDICATORS:					
Communicates clearly and appropriately for age and ability	1	2	3	4	5
Demonstrates control over selected events and situations	1	2	3	4	5
Attentiveness	1	2	3	4	5
Concentration	1	2	3	4	5
Orientation	1	2	3	4	5
Demonstrates immediate memory	1	2	3	4	5
Demonstrates recent memory	1	2	3	4	5
Demonstrates remote memory	1	2	3	4	5
Processes information	1	2	3	4	5
Weighs alternatives when making decisions	1	2	3	4	5
Makes appropriate decisions	1	2	3	4	5
Other _____ Specify	1	2	3	4	5

Outcomes

BACKGROUND READINGS:

Abraham, I., & Reel, S. (1993). Cognitive nursing interventions with long-term care residents: Effects on neurocognitive dimensions. *Archives of Psychiatric Nursing, VI*(6), 356-365.

Agostinelli, B., Demers, K., Garrigan, D., & Waszynski, C. (1994). Targeted interventions: Use of the mini-mental state exam. *Journal of Gerontological Nursing, 20*(8), 15-23.

Dellasega, C. (1992). Home health nurses' assessments of cognition. *Applied Nursing Research, 5*(3), 127-133.

Foreman, M., Theis, S., & Anderson, M.A. (1993). Adverse events in the hospitalized elderly. *Clinical Nursing Research, 2*(3) 360-370.

Foreman, M., Gilles, D., & Wagner, D. (1989). Impaired cognition in the critically ill elderly patient: Clinical implications. *Critical Care Nursing Quarterly, 12*(1), 61-73.

Inaba-Roland, K., & Maricle, R. (1992). Assessing delirium in the acute care setting. *Heart and Lung, 21*(1), 48-55.

Jubeck, M. (1992). Are you sensitive to the cognitive needs of the elderly? *Home Healthcare Nurse, 10*(5), 20-25.

Continued.

Kupferer, S., Uebele, J., & Levin, D. (1988). Geriatric ambulatory surgery patients: Assessing cognitive functions. *AORN Journal, 47*(3), 752-766.

Mason, P. (1989). Cognitive assessment parameters and tools for the critically injured adult. *Critical Care Nursing Clinics of North America, 1*(1), 45-53.

Strub, R., & Black, W. (1993). *The mental status examination in neurology* (3rd ed.). Philadelphia: F. A. Davis.

Outcomes

Cognitive Orientation

DEFINITION: Ability to identify person, place, and time

COGNITIVE ORIENTATION	Never demonstrated 1	Rarely demonstrated 2	Sometimes demonstrated 3	Often demonstrated 4	Consistently demonstrated 5
INDICATORS:					
Identifies self	1	2	3	4	5
Identifies significant other	1	2	3	4	5
Identifies current place	1	2	3	4	5
Identifies correct day	1	2	3	4	5
Identifies correct month	1	2	3	4	5
Identifies correct year	1	2	3	4	5
Identifies correct season	1	2	3	4	5
Other _____ Specify	1	2	3	4	5

BACKGROUND READINGS:

Abraham, I., & Reel, S. (1993). Cognitive nursing interventions and long-term care residents: Effects on neurocognitive dimensions. *Archives of Psychiatric Nursing, VI*(6), 356-365.

Agostinelli, B., Demers, K., Garrigan, D., & Waszynski, C. (1994). Targeted interventions: Use of the mini-mental state exam. *Journal of Gerontological Nursing, 20*(8), 15-23.

Dellasega, C. (1992). Home health nurses' assessments of cognition. *Applied Nursing Research, 5*(3), 127-133.

Foreman, M., Theis, S., & Anderson, M.A. (1993). Adverse events in the hospitalized elderly. *Clinical Nursing Research, 2*(3) 360-370.

Foreman, M., Gilles, D., & Wagner, D. (1989). Impaired cognition in the critically ill elderly patient: Clinical implications. *Critical Care Nursing Quarterly, 12*(1), 61-73.

Inaba-Roland, K., & Maricle, R. (1992). Assessing delirium in the acute care setting. *Heart and Lung, 21*(1), 48-55.

Jubeck, M. (1992). Are you sensitive to the cognitive needs of the elderly? *Home Healthcare Nurse, 10*(5), 20-25.

Kupferer, S., Uebele, J., & Levin, D. (1988). Geriatric ambulatory surgery patients: Assessing cognitive functions. *AORN Journal, 47*(3), 752-766.

Mason, P. (1989). Cognitive assessment parameters and tools for the critically injured adult. *Critical Care Nursing Clinics of North America, 1*(1), 45-53.

Strub, R., & Black, W. (1993). *The mental status examination in neurology* (3rd ed.). Philadelphia: F.A. Davis.

Comfort Level

DEFINITION: Feelings of physical and psychological ease

COMFORT LEVEL	None 1	Limited 2	Moderate 3	Substantial 4	Extensive 5
INDICATORS:					
Reported physical well-being	1	2	3	4	5
Reported satisfaction with symptom control	1	2	3	4	5
Reported psychological well-being	1	2	3	4	5
Expressed contentment with physical surroundings	1	2	3	4	5
Expressed contentment with social relationships	1	2	3	4	5
Expressed spiritual contentment	1	2	3	4	5
Reported satisfaction with level of independence	1	2	3	4	5
Expressed satisfaction with pain control	1	2	3	4	5
Other _____ Specify	1	2	3	4	5

BACKGROUND READINGS:

Fleming, C., Scanlon, C., & D'Agostino, N.S. (1987). A study of the comfort needs of patients with advanced cancer. *Cancer Nursing, 10*(5), 237-243.

Gropper, E.I. (1992). Promoting health by promoting comfort. *Nursing Forum, 27*(2), 5-8.

Hamilton, J. (1989). Comfort and the hospitalized chronically ill. *Journal of Gerontological Nursing, 15*(4), 28-33.

Kennedy, G.T. (1991). *A nursing investigation of comfort and comforting care of the acutely ill patient.* Unpublished doctoral dissertation, The University of Texas, Austin.

Kolcaba, K.Y. (1992). Holistic comfort: Operationalizing the construct as a nurse-sensitive outcome. *Advances in Nursing Science, 15*(1), 1-10.

Slater, K. (1985). *Human comfort.* Springfield, IL: Charles C Thomas.

Communication Ability

DEFINITION: Ability to receive, interpret, and express spoken, written and non-verbal messages

COMMUNICATION ABILITY	Extremely compromised 1	Substantially compromised 2	Moderately compromised 3	Mildly compromised 4	Not compromised 5
INDICATORS:					
Use of written language	1	2	3	4	5
Use of spoken language	1	2	3	4	5
Use of pictures and draw-ings	1	2	3	4	5
Use of sign language	1	2	3	4	5
Use of non-verbal lan-guage	1	2	3	4	5
Acknowledgment of mes-sages received	1	2	3	4	5
Directs message appropri-ately	1	2	3	4	5
Exchanges messages with others	1	2	3	4	5
Other _____ Specify	1	2	3	4	5

BACKGROUND READINGS:

Arnold, E., & Boggs, K. (1995). *Interpersonal relationships: Professional communications skills for nurses* (2nd ed.). Philadelphia: W.B. Saunders.

Potter, P.A., & Perry, A.G. (1993). *Fundamentals of nursing: Concepts, process and practice* (3rd ed.). St. Louis: Mosby.

Strub, R.L. & Black, F.W. (1993). *The mental status examination in neurology* (3rd ed.). Philadelphia: F.A. Davis.

Communication: Expressive Ability

DEFINITION: Ability to express and interpret verbal and/or non-verbal messages

COMMUNICATION: EXPRESSIVE ABILITY	Extremely compromised 1	Substantially compromised 2	Moderately compromised 3	Mildly compromised 4	Not compromised 5
INDICATORS:					
Use of written language	1	2	3	4	5
Use of spoken language: vocal	1	2	3	4	5
Use of spoken language: esophageal	1	2	3	4	5
Use of clarity of speech	1	2	3	4	5
Use of pictures and drawings	1	2	3	4	5
Use of sign language	1	2	3	4	5
Use of non-verbal language	1	2	3	4	5
Directs message appropriately	1	2	3	4	5
Other _____ Specify	1	2	3	4	5

BACKGROUND READINGS:

Arnold, E., & Boggs, K. (1995). *Interpersonal relationships: Professional communications skills for nurses* (2nd ed.). Philadelphia: W.B. Saunders.

Potter, P.A., & Perry, A.G. (1993). *Fundamentals of nursing: Concepts, process, and practice* (3rd ed.). St. Louis: Mosby.

Strub, R.L., & Black, F.W. (1993). *The mental status examination in neurology* (3rd ed.). Philadelphia: F.A. Davis.

Outcomes

Communication: Receptive Ability

DEFINITION: Ability to receive and interpret verbal and/or non-verbal messages

COMMUNICATION: RECEPTIVE ABILITY	Extremely compromised 1	Substantially compromised 2	Moderately compromised 3	Mildly compromised 4	Not compromised 5
INDICATORS:					
Use of written language	1	2	3	4	5
Use of spoken language	1	2	3	4	5
Use of pictures and drawings	1	2	3	4	5
Use of sign language	1	2	3	4	5
Use of non-verbal language	1	2	3	4	5
Acknowledgment of messages received	1	2	3	4	5
Other _____ Specify	1	2	3	4	5

BACKGROUND READINGS:

Arnold, E., & Boggs, K. (1995). *Interpersonal relationships: Professional communications skills for nurses* (2nd ed.). Philadelphia: W.B. Saunders.

Potter, P.A., & Perry, A.G. (1993). *Fundamentals of nursing: Concepts, process, and practice* (3rd ed.). St. Louis: Mosby.

Strub, R.L., & Black, F.W. (1993). *The mental status examination in neurology* (3rd ed.). Philadelphia: F. A. Davis.

Compliance Behavior

DEFINITION: Actions taken on the basis of professional advice to promote wellness, recovery, and rehabilitation

COMPLIANCE BEHAVIOR	Never demonstrated 1	Rarely demonstrated 2	Sometimes demonstrated 3	Often demonstrated 4	Consistently demonstrated 5
INDICATORS:					
Relies on health professional for current information	1	2	3	4	5
Requests prescribed regimen	1	2	3	4	5
Reports following prescribed regimen	1	2	3	4	5
Accepts health professional's diagnosis	1	2	3	4	5
Keeps appointments with a health professional	1	2	3	4	5
Modifies regimen as directed by a health professional	1	2	3	4	5
Performs self-screening when directed	1	2	3	4	5
Performs ADLs* as prescribed	1	2	3	4	5
Seeks external reinforcement for performance of health behaviors	1	2	3	4	5
Other _____ Specify	1	2	3	4	5

*ADL = Activities of daily living.

BACKGROUND READINGS:

Barotsky, I., Sergenbaker, P., & Mills, M. (1979). Compliance and quality of life assessment. In J. Cohen (Ed.), *New directions in patient compliance* (pp. 59-74). Lexington, MA: D.C. Health.

Coates, T., Martin, R. Gerbert, B., & Cummings, L. (1979). Physician and dentist compliance with smoking cessation counseling. In S. Shumaker, E. Schron & J. Ockene (Eds.), *The handbook of health behavior change* (pp. 231-240). New York: Springer.

Epstein, L., & Cluss, P.A. (1982). A behavioral perspective on adherence to long-term medical regimens. *Journal of Consulting and Clinical Psychology, 50,* 950-971.

Epstein, L., & Masek, B. (1978). Behavioral control of medicine compliance. *Journal of Applied Behavioral Analysis, 11,* 1-10.

Folden, S.L. (1993). Definitions of health and health goals of participants in a community-based pulmonary rehabilitation program. *Public Health Nursing, 10*(1), 31-35.

Gochman, D.S. (Ed.). (1988). *Health behavior: Emerging research perspectives.* New York: Plenum Press.

Heiby, E., & Carlson, J. (1986). The health compliance model. *The Journal of Compliance in Health Care, 1*(2), 135-152.

Jensen, L., & Allen, M. (1993). Wellness: The dialect of illness. *IMAGE-The Journal of Nursing Scholarship, 25*(3), 220-224.

King, I.M. (1988). Measuring health goal attainment in patients. In C.F. Waltz & O.L. Strickland (Eds.), *Measurement of nursing outcomes* (Ch. 6.). New York: Springer.

Kravits, R. et al. (1993, August 23). Recall of recommendations and adherence to advice among patients with chronic medical conditions. *Archives of Internal Medicine, 153,* 1869-1878.

Oldridge, N. (1982). Compliance in primary and secondary prevention of coronary heart disease: A review. *Preventive Medicine, 11,* 56-70.

Pender, N.J. (1990). Expressing health through lifestyle patterns. *Nursing Science Quarterly, 3*(3), 115-122.

Pender, N.J., & Pender, A.R. (1986). Attitudes, subjective norms, and intentions to engage in health behaviors. *Nursing Research, 35*(1), 15-18.

Sacket, D., & Haynes, R. (1976). *Compliance with therapeutic regimens.* Baltimore: The Johns Hopkins University Press.

Woods, N. (1989). Conceptualization of self-care: Toward health oriented models. *Advances in Nursing Science, 12*(1), 1-13.

Outcomes

Concentration

DEFINITION: Ability to focus on a specific stimulus				
CONCENTRATION	Never demonstrated 1	Rarely demonstrated 2	Sometimes demonstrated 3	Often demonstrated 4	Consistently demonstrated 5
INDICATORS:					
Maintains attention	1	2	3	4	5
Maintains focus without being distracted	1	2	3	4	5
Responds appropriately to visual cues	1	2	3	4	5
Responds appropriately to auditory cues	1	2	3	4	5
Responds appropriately to tactile cues	1	2	3	4	5
Responds appropriately to olfactory cues	1	2	3	4	5
Responds appropriately to language cues	1	2	3	4	5
Spells 'world' backwards	1	2	3	4	5
Counts backward from 20 by 3s, or from 100 by 7s	1	2	3	4	5
Names the months of the year backward, starting with January	1	2	3	4	5
Draws a circle	1	2	3	4	5
Draws a pentagon	1	2	3	4	5
Other _____ Specify	1	2	3	4	5

BACKGROUND READINGS:

Abraham, I., & Reel, S. (1993). Cognitive nursing interventions with long-term care residents: Effects on neurocognitive dimensions. *Archives of Psychiatric Nursing, VI*(6), 356-365.

Agostinelli, B., Demers, K., Garrigan, D., & Waszynski, C. (1994). Targeted interventions: Use of the mini-mental state exam. *Journal of Gerontological Nursing, 20*(8), 15-23.

Dellasega, C. (1992). Home health nurses' assessments of cognition. *Applied Nursing Research, 5*(3), 127-133.

Foreman, M., Theis, S., & Anderson, M.A. (1993). Adverse events in the hospitalized elderly. *Clinical Nursing Research, 2*(3), 360-370.

Foreman, M., Gilles, D., & Wagner, D. (1989). Impaired cognition in the critically ill elderly patient: Clinical implications. *Critical Care Nursing Quarterly, 12*(1), 61-73.

Inaba-Roland, K., & Maricle, R. (1992). Assessing delirium in the acute care setting. *Heart and Lung, 21*(1), 48-55.

Jubeck, M. (1992). Are you sensitive to the cognitive needs of the elderly? *Home Healthcare Nurse, 10*(5), 20-25.

Kupferer, S., Uebele, J., & Levin, D. (1988). Geriatric ambulatory surgery patients: Assessing cognitive functions. *AORN Journal, 47*(3), 752-766.

Mason, P. (1989). Cognitive assessment parameters and tools for the critically injured adult. *Critical Care Nursing Clinics of North America, 1*(1), 45-53.

Strub, R., & Black, W. (1993). *The mental status examination in neurology* (3rd ed.). Philadelphia: F.A. Davis.

Outcomes

Coping

DEFINITION: Actions to manage stressors that tax an individual's resources

COPING	Never demonstrated 1	Rarely demonstrated 2	Sometimes demonstrated 3	Often demonstrated 4	Consistently demonstrated 5
INDICATORS:					
Identifies effective coping patterns	1	(2)	3	4	5
Identifies ineffective coping patterns	1	2	3	4	(5)
Verbalizes sense of control	1	2	(3)	4	5
Reports decrease in stress	1	(2)	3	4	5
Verbalizes acceptance of situation	1	2	3	4	(5)
Seeks information concerning illness and treatment	1	2	3	4	(5)
Modifies lifestyle as needed	1	(2)	3	4	5
Adapts to developmental changes	1	2	3	4	(5)
Uses available social support	1	2	3	4	(5)
Employs behaviors to reduce stress	1	(2)	3	4	5
Identifies multiple coping strategies	1	2	3	4	(5)
Uses effective coping strategies	1	(2)	3	4	5
Avoids unduly stressful situations	1	(2)	3	4	5
Verbalizes need for assistance	1	2	3	4	(5)
Seeks professional help as appropriate	1	2	3	4	5
Reports decrease in physical symptoms of stress	1	2	3	4	5
Reports decrease in negative feelings	1	2	3	4	(5)
Reports increase in psychological comfort	1	2	3	4	5
Other _____ Specify	1	2	3	4	5

BACKGROUND READINGS:

Baldree, K., Murphy, S., & Powers, M. (1982). Stress identification and coping patterns in patients on hemodialysis. *Nursing Research, 31*(2), 107-112.

Folkman, S., Lazarus, R., Gruen, R., & Delongis, A. (1986). Appraisal, coping, health status, and psychological symptoms. *Journal of Personality and Social Psychology, 50*(3), 571-579.

McHaffie, H. (1992). The assessment of coping. *Clinical Nursing Research, 1*(1), 67-79.

Panzarine, S. (1985). Coping: Conceptual and methodological issues. *Advances in Nursing Science, 7*(4), 49-57.

Outcomes

Decision Making

DEFINITION: Ability to choose between two or more alternatives

DECISION MAKING	Never demonstrated 1	Rarely demonstrated 2	Sometimes demonstrated 3	Often demonstrated 4	Consistently demonstrated 5
INDICATORS:					
Identifies relevant information	1	2	3	4	5
Identifies alternatives	1	2	3	4	5
Identifies potential consequences of each alternative	1	2	3	4	5
Identifies resources necessary to support each alternative	1	2	3	4	5
Recognizes contradiction with others' desires	1	2	3	4	5
Acknowledges social context of the situation	1	2	3	4	5
Acknowledges relevant legal implications	1	2	3	4	5
Weighs alternatives	1	2	3	4	5
Chooses among alternatives	1	2	3	4	5
Other _____ Specify	1	2	3	4	5

BACKGROUND READINGS:

Abraham, I., & Reel, S. (1993). Cognitive nursing interventions with long-term care residents: Effects on neurocognitive dimensions. *Archives of Psychiatric Nursing, VI*(6), 356-365.

Agostinelli, B., Demers, K., Garrigan, D., & Waszynski, C. (1994). Targeted interventions: Use of the mini-mental state exam. *Journal of Gerontological Nursing, 20*(8), 15-23.

Dellasega, C. (1992). Home health nurses' assessments of cognition. *Applied Nursing Research, 5*(3), 127-133.

Foreman, M., Theis, S., & Anderson, M.A. (1993). Adverse events in the hospitalized elderly. *Clinical Nursing Research, 2*(3) 360-370.

Foreman, M., Gilles, D., & Wagner, D. (1989). Impaired cognition in the critically ill elderly patient: Clinical implications. *Critical Care Nursing Quarterly, 12*(1), 61-73.

Inaba-Roland, K., & Maricle, R. (1992). Assessing delirium in the acute care setting. *Heart and Lung, 21*(1), 48-55.

Jubeck, M. (1992). Are you sensitive to the cognitive needs of the elderly? *Home Healthcare Nurse, 10*(5), 20-25.

Kupferer, S., Uebele, J., & Levin, D. (1988). Geriatric ambulatory surgery patients: Assessing cognitive functions. *AORN Journal, 47*(3), 752-766.

Mason, P. (1989). Cognitive assessment parameters and tools for the critically injured adult. *Critical Care Nursing Clinics of North America, 1*(1), 45-53.

Strub, R., & Black, W. (1993). *The mental status examination in neurology* (3rd ed.). Philadelphia: F. A. Davis.

Dignified Dying

DEFINITION: Maintaining personal control and comfort with the approaching end of life

DIGNIFIED DYING	Not at all	To a slight extent	To a moderate extent	To a great extent	To a very great extent
	1	**2**	**3**	**4**	**5**
INDICATORS:					
Expresses readiness for death	1	2	3	4	5
Resolves important issues and concerns	1	2	3	4	5
Shares feelings about dying	1	2	3	4	5
Reconciles previous relationships	1	2	3	4	5
Completes meaningful goals	1	2	3	4	5
Maintains sense of control of remaining time	1	2	3	4	5
Exchanges affection with others	1	2	3	4	5
Disengages gradually from significant others	1	2	3	4	5
Recalls lifetime memories	1	2	3	4	5
Reviews life's accomplishments	1	2	3	4	5
Discusses spiritual experiences	1	2	3	4	5
Discusses spiritual concerns	1	2	3	4	5
Appears calm and tranquil	1	2	3	4	5
Verbalizes comfort	1	2	3	4	5
Expresses pain relief	1	2	3	4	5
Expresses symptom control (e.g., nausea, anxiety, dyspnea)	1	2	3	4	5
Maintains personal hygiene	1	2	3	4	5
Maintains physical independence	1	2	3	4	5
Expresses hopefulness	1	2	3	4	5
Participates in decisions	1	2	3	4	5
Controls treatment choices	1	2	3	4	5
Chooses food/drink intake	1	2	3	4	5
Controls personal possessions	1	2	3	4	5
Puts affairs in order	1	2	3	4	5
Other _____ Specify	1	2	3	4	5

Continued.

Outcomes

Outcomes

BACKGROUND READINGS:

Barbus, A.J. (1975). The dying person's bill of rights. *American Journal of Nursing, 75*(1), 99.

Callanan, M., & Kelley, P. (1992). *Final gifts.* New York: Poseidon Press.

Ferrell B.R. (1993). To know suffering. *Oncology Nursing Forum, 20*(10), 1471-1477.

McCanse, R.P. (1995). The McCanse Readiness for Death Instrument (MRDI): A reliable and valid measure for hospice care. *Hospice Journal, 10*(1), 15-26.

Potter, P.A., & Perry, A.G. (1993). *Fundamentals of nursing: Concepts, process, and practice* (3rd ed.). St. Louis: Mosby.

Quill, T.E. (1993). *Death and dignity: Making choices and taking charge.* New York: W. W. Norton & Co.

Schmele, J.A. (1995). Perceptions of a dying patient of the quality of care and caring: An interview wth Ivan Hanson. *Journal of Nursing Care Quality, 9*(4), 31-42.

Distorted Thought Control

DEFINITION: Ability to self-restrain disruption in perception, thought processes, and thought content

DISTORTED THOUGHT CONTROL	Never demonstrated 1	Rarely demonstrated 2	Sometimes demonstrated 3	Often demonstrated 4	Consistently demonstrated 5
INDICATORS:					
Recognizes hallucinations or delusions are occurring	1	2	3	4	5
Refrains from attending to hallucinations or delusions	1	2	3	4	5
Refrains from responding to hallucinations or delusions	1	2	3	4	5
Verbalizes frequency of hallucinations or delusions	1	2	3	4	5
Describes content of hallucinations or delusions	1	2	3	4	5
Reports decrease in hallucinations or delusions	1	2	3	4	5
Asks for validation of reality	1	2	3	4	5
Maintains affect consistent with mood	1	2	3	4	5
Interacts with others appropriately	1	2	3	4	5
Behaviors indicate accurate interpretation of environment	1	2	3	4	5
Exhibits logical thought flow patterns	1	2	3	4	5
Exhibits reality based thinking	1	2	3	4	5
Exhibits appropriate thought content	1	2	3	4	5
Exhibits ability to grasp ideas of others	1	2	3	4	5
Other _____ Specify	1	2	3	4	5

Outcomes

Continued.

Outcomes

BACKGROUND READINGS:

Andreasen, N.C., & Black, D. (1991). *Introductory textbook of psychiatry.* Washington DC: American Psychiatric Press.

Grimaldi, D., & Cousins, A. (1985). Paranoia. *Journal of Emergency Nursing, 11*(4), 201-204.

Rosenthal, T.T., & McGuinness, T.M. (1986). Dealing with delusional patients: Discovering the distorted truth. *Issues in Mental Health Nursing, 8,* 143-154.

Stuart, G.W., & Sundeen, S.J. (1991). *Principles and practice of psychiatric nursing* (4th ed.). St. Louis: Mosby.

Electrolyte & Acid/Base Balance

DEFINITION: Balance of electrolytes and non-electrolytes in the intracellular and extracellular compartments of the body

ELECTROLYTE & ACID/BASE BALANCE	Extremely compromised 1	Substantially compromised 2	Moderately compromised 3	Mildly compromised 4	Not compromised 5
INDICATORS:					
Heart rate IER*	1	2	3	4	5
Heart rhythm IER	1	2	3	4	5
Respiratory rate IER	1	2	3	4	5
Respiratory rhythm IER	1	2	3	4	5
Serum sodium WNL*	1	2	3	4	5
Serum potassium WNL	1	2	3	4	5
Serum chloride WNL	1	2	3	4	5
Serum calcium WNL	1	2	3	4	5
Serum magnesium WNL	1	2	3	4	5
Serum pH WNL	1	2	3	4	5
Serum albumin WNL	1	2	3	4	5
Serum creatinine WNL	1	2	3	4	5
Serum bicarbonate WNL	1	2	3	4	5
BUN* WNL	1	2	3	4	5
Urine pH WNL	1	2	3	4	5
Mental alertness	1	2	3	4	5
Cognitive orientation	1	2	3	4	5
Muscle strength	1	2	3	4	5
Neuromuscular non-irritability	1	2	3	4	5
Tingling in extremities not present	1	2	3	4	5
Other _____ Specify	1	2	3	4	5

*IER = In expected range; WNL = Within normal limits; BUN = Blood urea nitrogen.

BACKGROUND READINGS:

Cherry, R. (1992). Furosemide facts. *Emergency Medical Services, 21*(9), 79.

Cullen, L. (1992). Interventions related to fluid and electrolytes. *Nursing Clinics of North America, 27*(2), 60, 62, 79.

Innerarity, S.A., & Stark, J.L. (1994). *Fluids and electrolytes* (2nd ed.). Springhouse, PA: Springhouse.

Joy, C. (Ed.). (1989). *Pediatric trauma nursing.* Rockville, MD: Aspen.

McCance, K.L., & Huether, E.E. (1994). *Pathophysiology: The biological basis for disease in adults and children.* St. Louis: Mosby.

Continued.

Methany, N. (1992). *Fluid and electrolyte balance: Nursing considerations* (2nd ed.). Philadelphia: J.B. Lippincott.

Norris, C. (1982). *Concept classification in nursing.* Rockville, MD: Aspen.

Schuller, D., Mitchell, J., Calendrino, F., & Schuster, D. (1991). Fluid balance during pulmonary edema: Is fluid gain a marker or a cause of post-operative outcome? *Chest, 100*(4), 1068-1075.

Outcomes

Endurance

DEFINITION: Extent that energy enables a person's activity

ENDURANCE	Extremely compromised 1	Substantially compromised 2	Moderately compromised 3	Mildly compromised 4	Not compromised 5
INDICATORS:					
Performance of usual routine	1	2	3	4	5
Activity	1	2	3	4	5
Rested appearance	1	2	3	4	5
Concentration	1	2	3	4	5
Interest in surroundings	1	2	3	4	5
Muscle endurance	1	2	3	4	5
Eating pattern	1	2	3	4	5
Libido	1	2	3	4	5
Energy restored after rest	1	2	3	4	5
Exhaustion not present	1	2	3	4	5
Lethargy not present	1	2	3	4	5
Blood oxygen level WNL*	1	2	3	4	5
Hemoglobin WNL	1	2	3	4	5
Hematocrit WNL	1	2	3	4	5
Blood glucose WNL	1	2	3	4	5
Serum electrolytes WNL	1	2	3	4	5
Other _____ Specify	1	2	3	4	5

*WNL = Within normal limits.

BACKGROUND READINGS:

Ellis, J.R., & Nowlis, E.A. (1994). *Providing nursing care within the nursing process* (5th ed.). Philadelphia: J.B. Lippincott.

Johns, M.E. (1991). Activity and exercise. In S. Wingate (Ed.), *Cardiac nursing: A clinical management and patient care resource* (pp. 141-145). Gaithersburg, MD: Aspen.

Lubkin, I.M. (1990). *Chronic illness: Impact and interventions* (2nd ed.). Boston: Jones and Bartlett.

Potter, P.A., & Perry, A. (1989). *Fundamentals of nursing: Concepts, process, and practice* (2nd ed.). St. Louis: Mosby.

Pugh, L.C., & Milligan, R. (1993). A framework for the study of childbearing fatigue. *Advances in Nursing Science, 15*(4), 60-70.

Topf, M. (1992). Effects of personal control over hospital noise on sleep. *Research in Nursing and Health, 15,* 19-22.

Outcomes

Energy Conservation

DEFINITION: Extent of active management of energy to initiate and sustain activity

ENERGY CONSERVATION	Not at all	To a slight extent	To a moderate extent	To a great extent	To a very great extent
	1	2	3	4	5
INDICATORS:					
Balances activity and rest	1	2	3	4	5
Naps IER*	1	2	3	4	5
Recognizes energy limitations	1	2	3	4	5
Uses energy conservation techniques	1	2	3	4	5
Adapts lifestyle to energy level	1	2	3	4	5
Maintains adequate nutrition	1	2	3	4	5
Endurance level adequate for activity	1	2	3	4	5
Other _____ Specify	1	2	3	4	5

*IER = In expected range.

BACKGROUND READINGS:

Dixon, J.K., Dixon, J.P., & Hickey, M. (1993). Energy as a central factor in the self assessment of health. *Advances in Nursing Science, 15*(4), 1-12.

Lubkin, I.M. (1990). *Chronic illness: Impact and Interventions* (2nd ed.). Boston: Jones and Bartlett.

McCance, K.L., & Huether, K.L. (1994). *Pathophysiology: The biological basis for disease in adults and children.* St. Louis: Mosby.

Potter, P.A., & Perry, A. (1989). *Fundamentals of nursing: Concepts, process, and practice* (2nd ed.). St. Louis: Mosby.

Outcomes

Fear Control

DEFINITION: Ability to eliminate or reduce disabling feelings of alarm aroused by an identifiable source

FEAR CONTROL	Never demonstrated 1	Rarely demonstrated 2	Sometimes demonstrated 3	Often demonstrated 4	Consistently demonstrated 5
INDICATORS:					
Monitors intensity of fear	1	2	3	4	5
Eliminates precursors of fear	1	2	3	4	5
Seeks information to reduce fear	1	2	3	4	5
Avoids source of fear when possible	1	2	3	4	5
Plans coping strategies for fearful situations	1	2	3	4	5
Uses effective coping strategies	1	2	3	4	5
Uses relaxation techniques to reduce fear	1	2	3	4	5
Reports decreased duration of episodes	1	2	3	4	5
Reports increased length of time between episodes	1	2	3	4	5
Maintains role performance	1	2	3	4	5
Maintains social relationships	1	2	3	4	5
Maintains concentration	1	2	3	4	5
Maintains control over life	1	2	3	4	5
Maintains physical functioning	1	2	3	4	5
Maintains a sense of purpose despite fear	1	2	3	4	5
Remains productive	1	2	3	4	5
Controls fear response	1	2	3	4	5
Other _____ Specify	1	2	3	4	5

BACKGROUND READINGS:

McFarland, G.K. & McFarlane, E.A. (1993). *Nursing diagnosis & intervention: Planning for patient care* (2nd ed.). St. Louis: Mosby.

Stuart, G.W., & Sundeen, S.J. (1991). *Principles and practice of psychiatric nursing* (4th ed.). St. Louis: Mosby.

Outcomes

Fluid Balance

DEFINITION: Balance of water in the intracellular and extracellular compartments of the body

FLUID BALANCE	Extremely compromised 1	Substantially compromised 2	Moderately compromised 3	Mildly compromised 4	Not compromised 5
INDICATORS:					
BP IER*	1	2	3	4	5
Mean arterial pressure IER	1	2	3	4	5
Central venous pressure IER	1	2	3	4	5
Pulmonary wedge pressure IER	1	2	3	4	5
Peripheral pulses palpable	1	2	3	4	5
Orthostatic hypotension not present	1	2	3	4	5
24-hour intake and output balanced	1	2	3	4	5
Adventitious breath sounds not present	1	2	3	4	5
Body weight stable	1	2	3	4	5
Ascites not present	1	2	3	4	5
Neck vein distention not present	1	2	3	4	5
Peripheral edema not present	1	2	3	4	5
Sunken eyes not present	1	2	3	4	5
Confusion not present	1	2	3	4	5
Abnormal thirst not present	1	2	3	4	5
Skin hydration	1	2	3	4	5
Moist mucous membranes	1	2	3	4	5
Serum electrolytes WNL*	1	2	3	4	5
Hematocrit WNL	1	2	3	4	5
Urine specific gravity WNL	1	2	3	4	5
Other _____ Specify	1	2	3	4	5

*BP = Blood pressure; IER = In expected range; WNL = Within normal limits.

BACKGROUND READINGS:

Bosquet, G.L. (1990). Congestive heart failure: A review of nonpharmacologic therapies. *Journal of Cardiovascular Nursing, 4*(3), 35-46.

Coats, A.J.S., Adamopoulos, S., Meyer, T.E., Conway, J., & Sleight, P. (1990). Effects of physical training in chronic heart failure. *The Lancet, 335,* 63-66.

Fukada, N. (1990). Outcome standards for the client with congestive heart failure. *Journal of Cardiovascular Nursing, 4*(3), 59-70.

Johanson, B.C. et al. (1988). *Standards for critical care* (3rd ed.). St. Louis: Mosby.

Reuther, M.A. & Hansen, C.B. (1985). *Cardiovascular nursing.* New Hyde Park, NY: Medical Examination Publishing.

Sadler, D. (1984). *Nursing for cardiovascular health.* Norwalk, CT: Appleton-Century-Crofts.

Outcomes

Grief Resolution

DEFINITION: Adjustment to actual or impending loss

GRIEF RESOLUTION	Not at all	To a slight extent	To a moderate extent	To a great extent	To a very great extent
	1	2	3	4	5

INDICATORS:

Expresses feelings about loss	1	2	3	4	5
Expresses spiritual beliefs about death	1	2	3	4	5
Verbalizes reality of loss	1	2	3	4	5
Verbalizes acceptance of loss	1	2	3	4	5
Describes meaning of the loss or death	1	2	3	4	5
Participates in planning funeral	1	2	3	4	5
Maintains current will	1	2	3	4	5
Maintains advance directives	1	2	3	4	5
Discusses unresolved conflict(s)	1	2	3	4	5
Reports absence of somatic distress	1	2	3	4	5
Reports decreased preoccupation with loss	1	2	3	4	5
Maintains living environment	1	2	3	4	5
Maintains grooming and hygiene	1	2	3	4	5
Reports absence of sleep disturbance	1	2	3	4	5
Reports adequate nutritional intake	1	2	3	4	5
Reports normal sexual desire	1	2	3	4	5
Seeks social support	1	2	3	4	5
Shares loss with significant others	1	2	3	4	5
Reports involvement in social activities	1	2	3	4	5
Progresses through stages of grief	1	2	3	4	5
Expresses positive expectations about the future	1	2	3	4	5
Other _____ Specify	1	2	3	4	5

BACKGROUND READINGS:

Batemen, A., Broderick, D., Gleason, L., Kardon, R., Flaherty, C., & Anderson, S. (1992). Dysfunctional grieving. *Journal of Psychosocial Nursing, 30*(12), 5-9.

Cooley, M.E. (1992). Bereavement care: A role for nurses. *Cancer Nursing, 15*(2), 125-129.

Freitag-Koontz, M.J. (1988). Parents' grief reaction to the diagnosis of their infants' severe neurologic impairment and static encephalopathy. *Journal of Perinatal and Neonatal Nursing, 2*(2), 45-57.

Gibbons, M.B. (1992). A child dies, a child survives: The impact of sibling loss. *Journal of Pediatric Health Care, 6*(2), 45-57.

Harrigan, R., Naber, M., Jensen, K., Tse, A., & Perez, D. (1993). Perinatal grief: Response to the loss of an infant. *Neonatal Network, 12*(5), 25-31.

Kallenberg, K., & Soderfeldt, B. (1992). Three years later: Grief, view of life, and personal crisis after the death of a family member. *Journal of Palliative Care, 8*(4), 13-19.

Kirschling, J.M., & McBride, A.B. (1989). Effects of age and sex on the experience of widowhood. *Western Journal of Nursing Research, 11*(2), 207-218.

Kuntz, B. (1991). Exploring the grief of adolescents after the death of a parent. *Journal of Child and Adolescent Psychiatric and Mental Health Nursing, 4*(3), 105-109.

Outcomes

Growth

DEFINITION: A normal increase in body size and weight					
GROWTH	Extreme deviation from expected range 1	Substantial deviation from expected range 2	Moderate deviation from expected range 3	Mild deviation from expected range 4	No deviation from expected range 5

INDICATORS:

Weight percentile for sex	1	2	3	4	5
Weight percentile for age	1	2	3	4	5
Weight percentile for height	1	2	3	4	5
Rate of weight gain	1	2	3	4	5
Rate of height gain	1	2	3	4	5
Length/height percentile for age	1	2	3	4	5
Length/height percentile for sex	1	2	3	4	5
Head circumference percentile for age	1	2	3	4	5
Bone mass index	1	2	3	4	5
Mean body mass	1	2	3	4	5
Other _____ Specify	1	2	3	4	5

BACKGROUND READINGS:

Allen, K.D., Warzak, W.J., Greger, N.G., Bernotas, T.D., & Huseman, C.A. (1993). Psychosocial adjustment of children with isolated growth hormone deficiency, *Children's Health Care, 22*(1), 61-72.

Blinkin, N.J., Yip, R., Fleshood, L., & Trowbridge, F.L. (1988). Birth weight and childhood growth. *Pediatrics, 82*(6), 828-834.

Dietz, W., & Gortmaker, S. (1985). Do we fatten our children at the television set? Obesity and television viewing in children and adolescents. *Pediatrics, 107*(5), 807-812.

Georgieff, M.K., Hoffman, J.S., Pereira, G.R., Bernbaum, J., & Hoffman-Williamson, M. (1985). Effect of neonatal caloric deprivation on head growth and 1-year developmental status in preterm infants. *Journal of Pediatrics, 107*, 581-587.

Jung, E., & Czajka-Narins, D.M. (1985). Birth weight doubling and tripling times: An updated look at the effects of birth weight, sex, race and type of feeding. *The American Journal of Clinical Nutrition, 42*(8), 182-189.

Sapala, S. (1994). Pediatric management problems. *Pediatric Nursing, 20*(1), 54-55.

Tanner, J.M., & Davies, P.S.W. (1985). Clinical longitudinal standards for height and height velocity for North American children. *The Journal of Pediatrics, 107*(3), 317-329.

Whaley, L., & Wong, D. (1991). *Nursing care of infants and children.* St. Louis: Mosby.

Health Beliefs

DEFINITION: Personal convictions that influence health behaviors					
HEALTH BELIEFS	Very weak **1**	Weak **2**	Moderate **3**	Strong **4**	Very strong **5**
INDICATORS:					
Perceived importance of taking action	1	2	3	4	5
Perceived threat from inaction	1	2	3	4	5
Perceived benefits of action	1	2	3	4	5
Perceived internal control of action	1	2	3	4	5
Perceived control of health outcome	1	2	3	4	5
Perceived reduction of threat from action	1	2	3	4	5
Perceived improvement in lifestyle from action	1	2	3	4	5
Perceived ability to perform action	1	2	3	4	5
Perceived resources to perform action	1	2	3	4	5
Perceived absence of barriers to action	1	2	3	4	5
Other _____ Specify	1	2	3	4	5

BACKGROUND READINGS:

Gillis, A.J. (1993). Determinants of health promoting lifestyle: An integrative review. *Journal of Advanced Nursing, 18,* 345-353.

Hayes, D., & Ross, C. (1987). Concern with appearance, health beliefs, and eating habits. *Journal of Health and Social Behavior, 28*(6), 120-130.

Thompson, J., McFarland, G.K., Hirsch, J.E., & Tucker, S.M. (Eds.). *Mosby's clinical nursing* (3rd ed.). St. Louis: Mosby.

Robertson, D., & Keller, C. (1992). Relationships among health beliefs, self-efficacy, and exercise adherence in patients with coronary artery disease. *Heart and Lung, 21*(1), 56-63.

Sechrist, K., Walker, S., & Pender, N. (1967). Development and psychometric evaluation of the exercise benefits/barriers scale. *Research in Nursing and Health, 10,* 357-365.

Outcomes

Health Beliefs: Perceived Ability to Perform

DEFINITION: Personal conviction that one can carry out a given health behavior

HEALTH BELIEFS: PERCEIVED ABILITY TO PERFORM	Very weak 1	Weak 2	Moderate 3	Strong 4	Very strong 5
INDICATORS:					
Perception that health behavior is not too complex	1	2	3	4	5
Perception that health behavior requires reasonable effort	1	2	3	4	5
Perception that the frequency of health behavior is not excessive	1	2	3	4	5
Perception of likelihood of performing health behavior over time	1	2	3	4	5
Confidence related to past experience with health behavior	1	2	3	4	5
Confidence related to past experience with similar health behaviors	1	2	3	4	5
Confidence related to observation or anecdotal experiences of others	1	2	3	4	5
Confidence in ability to perform health behavior	1	2	3	4	5
Other _____ Specify	1	2	3	4	5

BACKGROUND READINGS:

Hayes, D., & Ross, C. (1987). Concern with appearance, health beliefs, and eating habits. *Journal of Health and Social Behavior, 28*(6), 120-130.

Jemmot, L., & Jemmot, J. (1992). Increasing condom-use intentions among sexually active black adolescent women. *Nursing Research, 41*(5), 273-278.

Jensen, K., Banwart, L., Venhaus, R., Popkess-Vawter, S., & Perkins, S.B. (1993). Advanced rehabilitation nursing care of coronary angioplasty patients using self-efficacy theory. *Journal of Advanced Nursing, 18,* 926-931.

Kim, K., Horan, M., Gendler, P., & Patel, M. (1991). Development and evaluation of the osteoporosis health belief scale. *Research in Nursing and Health, 14,* 155-163.

Lowe, N.K. (1993). Maternal confidence for labor: Development of the childbirth self-efficacy inventory. *Research in Nursing and Health, 16*(2), 141-149.

Robertson, D., & Keller, C. (1992). Relationships among health beliefs, self-efficacy, and exercise adherence in patients with coronary artery disease. *Heart and Lung, 21*(1), 56-63.

Sechrist, K., Walker, S., & Pender, N. (1967). Development and psychometric evaluation of the exercise benefits/barriers scale. *Research in Nursing and Health, 10,* 357-365.

De Weerdt, I., Visser, A., & Van der Veen, E. (1989). Attitude behavior theories and diabetes education programs. *Patient Education and Counseling, 14,* 3-19.

Health Beliefs: Perceived Control

DEFINITION: Personal conviction that one can influence a health outcome

HEALTH BELIEFS: PERCEIVED CONTROL	Very weak 1	Weak 2	Moderate 3	Strong 4	Very strong 5
INDICATORS:					
Perceived responsibility for health decisions	1	2	3	4	5
Requested involvement in health decisions	1	2	3	4	5
Efforts at gathering information	1	2	3	4	5
Belief that own decisions control health outcomes	1	2	3	4	5
Belief that own actions control health outcomes	1	2	3	4	5
Willingness to designate surrogate decision maker	1	2	3	4	5
Willingness to have current living will	1	2	3	4	5
Other _____ Specify	1	2	3	4	5

BACKGROUND READINGS:

Calnan, M., & Moss, S. (1984). The health belief model and compliance with education given at a class in breast self-examination. *Journal of Health and Social Behavior, 25,* 198-210.

Gillis, A.J. (1993). Determinants of health promoting lifestyle: An integrative review. *Journal of Advanced Nursing, 18,* 345-353.

Hayes, D., & Ross, C. (1987). Concern with appearance, health beliefs, and eating habits. *Journal of Health and Social Behavior, 28*(6), 120-130.

Outcomes

Health Beliefs: Perceived Resources

DEFINITION: Personal conviction that one has adequate means to carry out a health behavior

HEALTH BELIEFS: PERCEIVED RESOURCES	Very weak 1	Weak 2	Moderate 3	Strong 4	Very strong 5
INDICATORS:					
Perceived support of significant others	1	2	3	4	5
Perceived support of friends	1	2	3	4	5
Perceived support of neighbors	1	2	3	4	5
Perceived support of health care worker	1	2	3	4	5
Perceived support from self-help groups	1	2	3	4	5
Perceived functional ability	1	2	3	4	5
Perceived energy level	1	2	3	4	5
Perceived comfort level	1	2	3	4	5
Perceived adequacy of time	1	2	3	4	5
Perceived adequacy of personal finances	1	2	3	4	5
Perceived adequacy of health insurance	1	2	3	4	5
Perceived access to equipment	1	2	3	4	5
Perceived access to supplies	1	2	3	4	5
Perceived access to services	1	2	3	4	5
Perceived access to transportation	1	2	3	4	5
Perceived access to physical assistance	1	2	3	4	5
Other _____ Specify	1	2	3	4	5

BACKGROUND READINGS:

Gillis, A.J. (1993). Determinants of health promoting lifestyle: An integrative review. *Journal of Advanced Nursing, 18,* 345-353.

Kim, K., Horan, M., Gendler, P., & Patel, M. (1991). Development and evaluation of the osteoporosis health belief scale. *Research in Nursing and Health, 14,* 155-163.

Robertson, D., & Keller, C. (1992). Relationships among health beliefs, self-efficacy, and exercise adherence in patients with coronary artery disease. *Heart and Lung, 21*(1), 56-63.

Sechrist, K., Walker, S., & Pender, N. (1967). Development and psychometric evaluation of the exercise benefits/barriers scale. *Research in Nursing and Health, 10,* 357-365.

Outcomes

Health Beliefs: Perceived Threat

DEFINITION: Personal conviction that a health problem is serious and has potential negative consequences for lifestyle

HEALTH BELIEFS: PERCEIVED THREAT	Very weak 1	Weak 2	Moderate 3	Strong 4	Very strong 5
INDICATORS:					
Perceived threat to health	1	2	3	4	5
Perceived dissatisfaction with current health status	1	2	3	4	5
Perceived vulnerability to health problem	1	2	3	4	5
Concern regarding illness or injury	1	2	3	4	5
Concern regarding complications	1	2	3	4	5
Perceived severity of illness or injury	1	2	3	4	5
Perceived severity of complications	1	2	3	4	5
Perceived discomfort	1	2	3	4	5
Perception that condition may be of long duration	1	2	3	4	5
Perceived impact on current lifestyle	1	2	3	4	5
Perceived impact on future lifestyle	1	2	3	4	5
Perceived impact on functional status	1	2	3	4	5
Other _____ Specify	1	2	3	4	5

BACKGROUND READINGS:

Calnan, M., & Moss, S. (1984). The health belief model and compliance with education given at a class in breast self-examination. *Journal of Health and Social Behavior, 25,* 198-210.

Dunn, S., Beeney, L., Hoskins, P., & Turtle, J. (1990). Knowledge and attitude change as predictors of metabolic improvement in diabetes education. *Social Science Medicine, 31*(10), 1135-1141.

Kim, K., Horan, M., Gendler, P., & Patel, M. (1991). Development and evaluation of the osteoporosis health belief scale. *Research in Nursing and Health, 14,* 155-163.

Robertson, D., & Keller, C. (1992). Relationships among health beliefs, self-efficacy, and exercise adherence in patients with coronary artery disease. *Heart and Lung, 21*(1), 56-63.

Thompson, J., McFarland, G., Hirsch, J., & Tucker, S. (1993). *Mosby's clinical nursing* (3rd ed.). St. Louis: Mosby.

De Weerdt, I., Visser, A., & Van Der Veen, E. (1989). Attitude behavior theories and diabetes education programs. *Patient Education and Counseling, 14,* 3-19.

Outcomes

Health Orientation

DEFINITION: Personal view of health and health behaviors as priorities

HEALTH ORIENTATION	Very weak 1	Weak 2	Moderate 3	Strong 4	Very strong 5
INDICATORS:					
Focus on wellness	1	2	3	4	5
Focus on disease prevention and management	1	2	3	4	5
Focus on maintaining role performance	1	2	3	4	5
Focus on maintaining functional abilities	1	2	3	4	5
Focus on adjustment to life situations	1	2	3	4	5
Focus on overall well-being	1	2	3	4	5
Expectation that individual is responsible for choices	1	2	3	4	5
Perception that health behavior is relevant to self	1	2	3	4	5
Perception that health provider expectations are congruent with one's cultural background	1	2	3	4	5
Perception that health behaviors are congruent with one's cultural background	1	2	3	4	5
Perceived importance of following culturally expected health practices	1	2	3	4	5
Perception that health is a high priority in making lifestyle choices	1	2	3	4	5
Other _____ Specify	1	2	3	4	5

BACKGROUND READINGS:

Gillis, A.J. (1993). Determinants of health promoting lifestyle: An integrative review. *Journal of Advanced Nursing, 18,* 345-353.

Kulbok, P., & Baldwin, J. (1992). From preventive health behavior to health promotion: Advancing a positive construct of health. *Advances in Nursing Science, 14*(4), 50-64.

Palank, C. (1991). Determinants of health promoting behavior. *Nursing Clinics of North America, 26*(4), 815-832.

Pender, N.J. (1990). Expressing health through lifestyle patterns. *Nursing Science Quarterly, 3*(3), 115-122.

Health Promoting Behavior

HEALTH PROMOTING BEHAVIOR	Never demonstrated 1	Rarely demonstrated 2	Sometimes demonstrated 3	Often demonstrated 4	Consistently demonstrated 5
DEFINITION: Actions to sustain or increase wellness					
INDICATORS:					
Uses risk avoidance behaviors	1	2	3	4	5
Monitors environment for risks	1	2	3	4	5
Monitors personal behavior for risks	1	2	3	4	5
Seeks balance among exercise, work, leisure, rest and nutrition	1	2	3	4	5
Uses effective stress reduction behaviors	1	2	3	4	5
Maintains satisfactory social relationships	1	2	3	4	5
Performs health habits correctly	1	2	3	4	5
Supports healthful public policy	1	2	3	4	5
Uses financial and physical resources to promote health	1	2	3	4	5
Uses social support to promote health	1	2	3	4	5
Other _____ Specify	1	2	3	4	5

BACKGROUND READINGS:

Green, L., & Raeburn. (1990). Contemporary development in health promotion. In N. Bracht, (Ed.), *Health promotion at the community level* (pp. 29-44). Newberry Park, CA: Sage.

Kulbok, P., & Baldwin, J. (1992). From preventive health behavior to health promotion: Advancing a positive construct of health. *Advances in Nursing Science, 14*(4), 50-64.

Mechanic, D., & Cleary, P. (1980). Factors associated with maintenance of positive behavior. *Preventive Medicine, 9,* 805-814.

Simmons, M.D., Mullen, P., Mains, D., Tabak, E., & Green, L. (1992). Characteristics of controlled studies of patient education and counseling for preventive health behavior. *Patient Education and Counseling, 19,* 175-204.

Walker, S., Sechrist, K., & Pender, N. (1987). The health promoting lifestyle profile: Development and psychometric characteristics. *Nursing Research, 36*(2), 76-81.

Outcomes

Health Seeking Behavior

DEFINITION: Actions to promote optimal wellness, recovery, and rehabilitation

HEALTH SEEKING BEHAVIOR	Never demonstrated 1	Rarely demonstrated 2	Sometimes demonstrated 3	Often demonstrated 4	Consistently demonstrated 5
INDICATORS:					
Asks questions when indicated	1	2	3	4	5
Completes health-related tasks	1	2	3	4	5
Performs self-screening when indicated	1	2	3	4	5
Contacts health professionals when indicated	1	2	3	4	5
Performs ADLs* consistent with energy and tolerance	1	2	3	4	5
Describes strategies to eliminate unhealthy behavior	1	2	3	4	5
Adheres to self-developed strategies to eliminate unhealthy behavior	1	2	3	4	5
Performs prescribed health behavior when indicated	1	2	3	4	5
Seeks current health-related information	1	2	3	4	5
Describes strategies to maximize health	1	2	3	4	5
Adheres to self-developed strategies to maximize health	1	2	3	4	5
Other _____ Specify	1	2	3	4	5

*ADL = Activities of daily living.

Outcomes

BACKGROUND READINGS:

Folden, S.L. (1993). Definitions of health and health goals of participants in a community-based pulmonary rehabilitation program. *Public Health Nursing, 10*(1), 31-35.

Jensen, L., & Allen, M. (1993). Wellness: The dialect of illness. *IMAGE-The Journal of Nursing Scholarship, 25*(3), 220-224.

Pender, N.J. (1990). Expressing health through lifestyle patterns. *Nursing Science Quarterly, 3*(3), 115-122.

Pender, N.J., & Pender, A.R. (1986). Attitudes, subjective norms, and intentions of engage in health behaviors. *Nursing Research, 35*(1), 15-18.

Woods, N. (1989). Conceptualization of self-care: Toward health oriented models. *Advances in Nursing Science, 12*(1), 1-13.

Outcomes

Hope

DEFINITION: Presence of internal state of optimism that is personally satisfying and life-supporting

HOPE	None 1	Limited 2	Moderate 3	Substantial 4	Extensive 5
INDICATORS:					
Expression of a positive future orientation	1	2	3	4	5
Expression of faith	1	2	3	4	5
Expression of will to live	1	2	3	4	5
Expression of reasons to live	1	2	3	4	5
Expression of meaning in life	1	2	3	4	5
Expression of optimism	1	2	3	4	5
Expression of belief in self	1	2	3	4	5
Expression of belief in others	1	2	3	4	5
Expression of inner peace	1	2	3	4	5
Expression of sense of self-control	1	2	3	4	5
Demonstration of zest for life	1	2	3	4	5
Setting of goals	1	2	3	4	5
Other _____ Specify	1	2	3	4	5

BACKGROUND READINGS:

Hall, B. (1990). The struggle of the diagnosed terminally ill person to maintain hope. *Nursing Science Quarterly, 3*(4) 177-184.

Herth, K. (1993). Hope in the family caregiver of terminally ill people. *Journal of Advanced Nursing, 18,* 538-548.

Hunt-Raleigh, E. (1992). Sources of hope in chronic illness. *Oncology Nursing Forum, 3*(19), 443-448.

Owen, D. (1989). Nurses perspectives on the meaning of hope in patients with cancer: A qualitative study. *Oncology Nursing Forum, 1*(16), 75-79.

Stephenson, C. (1991). The concept of hope revisited for nursing. *Journal of Advanced Nursing, 16,* 1456-1461.

Outcomes

Hydration

DEFINITION: Amount of water in the intracellular and extracellular compartments of the body

HYDRATION	Extremely compromised 1	Substantially compromised 2	Moderately compromised 3	Mildly compromised 4	Not compromised 5
INDICATORS:					
Skin hydration	1	2	3	4	5
Moist mucous membranes	1	2	3	4	5
Peripheral edema not present	1	2	3	4	5
Ascites not present	1	2	3	4	5
Abnormal thirst not present	1	2	3	4	5
Adventitious breath sounds not present	1	2	3	4	5
Shortness of breath not present	1	2	3	4	5
Sunken eyes not present	1	2	3	4	5
Fever not present	1	2	3	4	5
Perspiration ability	1	2	3	4	5
Urine output WNL*	1	2	3	4	5
BP* WNL	1	2	3	4	5
Hematocrit WNL	1	2	3	4	5
Other _____ Specify	1	2	3	4	5

*WNL = Within normal limits; BP = blood pressure.

BACKGROUND READINGS:

Arieff, A. (1986). Hyponatremia, convulsions, respiratory arrest, and permanent brain damage after elective surgery in healthy women. *The New England Journal of Medicine, 314*(24), 1529-1534.

Carcillo, J.A., Davis, A.L., & Zaritsky, A. (1991). Role of early fluid resuscitation in pediatric septic shock. *Journal of the American Medical Association, 266*(9), 1242-1245.

Gilski, D. (1993). Controversies in patient management after cardiac surgery. *Journal of Cardiovascular Nursing, 7*(4), 1-13.

Hill, P., & Aldag, J. (1991). Potential indicators of insufficient milk supply. *Research in Nursing and Health, 14,* 11-19.

Innerarity, S.A., & Stark, J.L. (1994). *Fluids and electrolytes* (2nd ed.). Springhouse, PA: Springhouse.

Identity

DEFINITION: Ability to distinguish between self and non-self and to characterize one's essence				
IDENTITY	**Never demonstrated** **1**	**Rarely demonstrated** **2**	**Sometimes demonstrated** **3**	**Often demonstrated** **4**	**Consistently demonstrated** **5**

INDICATORS:

Verbalizes affirmations of personal identity	1	2	3	4	5
Exhibits congruent verbal and non-verbal behavior about self	1	2	3	4	5
Verbalizes clear sense of personal identity	1	2	3	4	5
Differentiates self from environment	1	2	3	4	5
Differentiates self from other human beings	1	2	3	4	5
Perceives environment accurately	1	2	3	4	5
Performs social roles	1	2	3	4	5
Verbalizes own value system	1	2	3	4	5
Challenges faulty beliefs about self	1	2	3	4	5
Challenges negative images of self	1	2	3	4	5
Recognizes interpersonal versus intrapersonal conflict	1	2	3	4	5
Establishes personal boundaries	1	2	3	4	5
Verbalizes trust in self	1	2	3	4	5
Other _____ Specify	1	2	3	4	5

BACKGROUND READINGS:

Barnard, D. (1990). Healing the damaged self: Identity, intimacy, and meaning in the lives of the chronically ill. *Perspectives in Biology & Medicine, 33*(4), 535-546.

Burns, R. (1982). *Self-concept development & education.* New York: Holt, Rinehart & Winston.

Erickson, E. (1968). *Identity, youth and crisis.* New York: W.W. Norton & Co.

Gara, M.A., Rosenberg, S., & Cohen, B. (1987). Personal identity and the schizophrenic process: An integration. *Psychiatry, 50,* 267-278.

Grotevant, H.D., & Adams, G.R. (1984). Development of an objective measure to assess ego identity in adolescence: Validation and replication. *Journal of Youth and Adolescence, 13*(5), 419-437.

Hernandez, J., & Diclemente, R. (1992). Self control and ego identity development as predictors of unprotected sex in late adolescent males. *Journal of Adolescence, 15,* 437-447.

Marcia, J.E. (1966). Development and validations of ego identity status. *Journal of Personality and Social Psychology, 3,* 551-558.

Marcia, J.E. (1967). Ego identity status: Relationships to change in self esteem, general adjustment, and authoritarianism. *Journal of Personality, 35,* 118-133.

McFarland, G.K., & McFarlane, E.A. (1993). *Nursing Diagnosis and Intervention: Planning for patient care* (2nd ed.). St. Louis: Mosby.

Mosby's Medical, Nursing & Allied Health Dictionary. (1994). (4th ed.). St. Louis: Mosby.

Oldaker, S. (1985). Identity confusion: Nursing diagnoses for adolescents. *Nursing Clinics of North America, 20*(4), 763-773.

Streitmatter, J. (1993). Gender differences in identity development: An examination of longitudinal data. *Adolescence, 28,*(109), 55-66.

Streitmatter, J. (1993). Identity status and identity style: A replication study. *Journal of Adolescence, 16,* 211-215.

Stuart, G.W. (1990). *Principles and practices of psychiatric nursing* (4th ed). St. Louis: Mosby.

Outcomes

Immobility Consequences: Physiological

DEFINITION: Compromise in physiological functioning due to impaired physical mobility

IMMOBILITY CONSEQUENCES: PHYSIOLOGICAL	Severe 1	Substantial 2	Moderate 3	Slight 4	None 5
INDICATORS:					
Pressure sore(s)	1	2	3	4	5
Constipation	1	2	3	4	5
Stool impaction	1	2	3	4	5
Decreased nutrition status	1	2	3	4	5
Hypoactive bowel	1	2	3	4	5
Paralytic ileus	1	2	3	4	5
Urinary calculi	1	2	3	4	5
Urinary retention	1	2	3	4	5
Fever	1	2	3	4	5
Urinary tract infection	1	2	3	4	5
Decreased muscle strength	1	2	3	4	5
Decreased muscle tone	1	2	3	4	5
Bone fracture	1	2	3	4	5
Impaired joint movement	1	2	3	4	5
Contracted joints	1	2	3	4	5
Ankylosed joints	1	2	3	4	5
Orthostatic hypotension	1	2	3	4	5
Venous thrombosis	1	2	3	4	5
Lung congestion	1	2	3	4	5
Decreased cough effectiveness	1	2	3	4	5
Decreased vital capacity	1	2	3	4	5
Pneumonia	1	2	3	4	5
Other _____ Specify	1	2	3	4	5

BACKGROUND READINGS:

Kottke, F.J., & Lehmann, J.F. (1990). *Krusen's handbook of physical medicine and rehabilitation* (4th ed.). Philadelphia: W.B. Saunders.

Maas, M. (1991). Impaired physical mobility. In M. Maas, K.C. Buckwalter, & M. Hardy (Eds.), *Nursing diagnoses and interventions for the elderly* (pp. 263-284). Redwood City, CA: Addison-Wesley Nursing.

Milde, F.K. (1981). Physiological immobilization. In L. Hart, J. Reese & M. Fearing (Eds.), *Concepts common to acute illness: Identification and management* (pp. 67-109). St. Louis: Mosby.

Olson, E.V., Johnson, B.J., Thompson, L.F., McCarthy, J.S., Edmonds, R.E., Schroeder, L.M., & Wade, M. (1967). The hazards of immobility. *American Journal of Nursing, 67*(4), 780-797.

Potter, P.A., & Petty, A.G. (1993). Mobility and immobility. In P.A. Potter & A.G. Perry (Eds.), *Fundamentals of nursing: Concepts, process, and practice* (3rd ed), (pp. 1460-1520). St. Louis: Mosby.

Rubin, M. (1988). The physiology of bedrest. *American Journal of Nursing, 88*(1), 50-55.

Immobility Consequences: Psycho-Cognitive

DEFINITION: Extent of compromise in psycho-cognitive functioning due to impaired physical mobility

IMMOBILITY CONSEQUENCES: PSYCHO-COGNITIVE	Severe 1	Substantial 2	Moderate 3	Slight 4	None 5
INDICATORS:					
Decreased alertness	1	2	3	4	5
Decreased orientation	1	2	3	4	5
Decreased attentiveness	1	2	3	4	5
Perceptual distortions	1	2	3	4	5
Decreased kinesthetic sense	1	2	3	4	5
Decreased interest and motivation	1	2	3	4	5
Exaggerated emotions	1	2	3	4	5
Sleep disturbances	1	2	3	4	5
Decreased self-esteem	1	2	3	4	5
Negative body image	1	2	3	4	5
Inability to act	1	2	3	4	5
Other _____ Specify	1	2	3	4	5

BACKGROUND READINGS:

Friedrich, R.M., & Lively, S.I. (1981). Psychological immobilization. In L. Hart, J. Reese, & M. Fearing (Eds.), *Concepts common to acute illness: Identification and management* (pp. 51-66). St. Louis: Mosby.

Maas, M. (1991). Impaired physical mobility. In M. Maas, K.C. Buckwalter, & M. Hardy (Eds.), *Nursing diagnoses and interventions for the elderly* (pp. 263-284). Redwood City, CA: Addison-Wesley Nursing.

Rubin, M. (1988). How bedrest changes perception. *American Journal of Nursing, 88*(1), 55-56.

Outcomes

Outcomes

Immune Hypersensitivity Control

DEFINITION: Extent to which inappropriate immune responses are suppressed

IMMUNE HYPERSENSITIVITY CONTROL	Not at all	To a slight extent	To a moderate extent	To a great extent	To a very great extent
	1	**2**	**3**	**4**	**5**
INDICATORS:					
Respiratory status IER*	1	2	3	4	5
Cardiac status IER	1	2	3	4	5
Gastrointestinal status IER	1	2	3	4	5
Renal status IER	1	2	3	4	5
Neurological status IER	1	2	3	4	5
Joint mobility IER	1	2	3	4	5
Skin integrity maintained	1	2	3	4	5
Mucosa integrity maintained	1	2	3	4	5
Free of allergic reactions	1	2	3	4	5
Free of localized inflammatory responses	1	2	3	4	5
Free of autoimmune events	1	2	3	4	5
Free of vasculitis	1	2	3	4	5
Free of transplant rejection	1	2	3	4	5
Free of graft versus host response	1	2	3	4	5
Free of itching	1	2	3	4	5
Free of jaundice	1	2	3	4	5
Absence of auto-antibodies or auto-antigens	1	2	3	4	5
Bilirubin-WNL*	1	2	3	4	5
CBC* WNL	1	2	3	4	5
Differential WBC* values WNL	1	2	3	4	5
Complement levels WNL	1	2	3	4	5
T4-cell level WNL	1	2	3	4	5
T8-cell level WNL	1	2	3	4	5
Other _____ Specify	1	2	3	4	5

*IER = In expected range; WNL = within normal limits; CBC = complete blood count; WBC = white blood (cell) count.

BACKGROUND READINGS:

Birney, M.H. (1991). Psychoneuroimmunology: A holistic framework for the study of stress and illness. *Holistic Nursing Practice, 5*(4), 32-38.

Brandt, B. (1990). Nursing protocol for the patient with neutropenia. *Oncology Nursing Forum, 17*(1) (Supplement), 9-15.

Flaskerud, J.H., & Ungvarski, P.J. (1992). *HIV/AIDS: A guide to nursing care* (2nd ed.). Philadelphia: W.B. Saunders.

Hymes, D.J. (1985). Primary immunodeficiency disorders in the neonate. *Neonatal Network-The Journal of Neonatal Nursing, 3*(4), 40-48.

McCance, K.L., & Huether, S.E. (1994). *Pathophysiology: The biological basis for disease in adults and children* (2nd ed.). St. Louis: Mosby.

Phillips, M.C., & Olson, L.R. (1993). The immunologic role of the gastrointestinal tract. *Critical Care Nursing Clinics of North America, 5*(1), 107-118.

Van Wynsberghe, D., Noback, C.R., & Carola, R. (1995). *Human anatomy and physiology* (3rd ed.). New York: McGraw-Hill.

Workman, M.L. (1993). The immune system: Your defensive partner and offensive foe. *AACN, 4*(3), 453-470.

Outcomes

Immune Status

DEFINITION: Adequacy of natural and acquired appropriately targeted resistance to internal and external antigens

IMMUNE STATUS	Extremely compromised 1	Substantially compromised 2	Moderately compromised 3	Mildly compromised 4	Not compromised 5
INDICATORS:					
Recurrent infections not present	1	2	3	4	5
Tumors not present	1	2	3	4	5
Gastrointestinal status IER*	1	2	3	4	5
Respiratory status IER	1	2	3	4	5
Genitourinary status IER	1	2	3	4	5
Weight IER	1	2	3	4	5
Body temperature IER	1	2	3	4	5
Skin integrity	1	2	3	4	5
Mucosa integrity	1	2	3	4	5
Chronic fatigue not present	1	2	3	4	5
Immunizations current	1	2	3	4	5
Antibody titers WNL*	1	2	3	4	5
Appropriate skin test reaction with exposure	1	2	3	4	5
Absolute WBC* values WNL	1	2	3	4	5
Differential WBC values WNL	1	2	3	4	5
T4-cell level WNL	1	2	3	4	5
T8-cell level WNL	1	2	3	4	5
Complement levels WNL	1	2	3	4	5
Thymus x-ray findings IER	1	2	3	4	5
Other _____ Specify	1	2	3	4	5

*IER = In expected range; WNL = within normal limits; WBC = white blood (cell) count.

BACKGROUND READINGS:

Birney, M.H. (1991). Psychoneuroimmunology: A holistic framework for the study of stress and illness. *Holistic Nursing Practice, 5*(4), 32-38.

Brandt, B. (1990). Nursing protocol for the patient with neutropenia. *Oncology Nursing Forum, 17*(1) (Supplement), 9-15.

Flaskerud, J.H., & Ungvarski, P.J. (1991). *HIV/AIDS: A guide to nursing care* (2nd ed.). Philadelphia: W.B. Saunders.

Outcomes

Hymes, D.J. (1985). Primary immunodeficiency disorders in the neonate. *Neonatal Network-The Journal of Neonatal Nursing, 3*(4), 40-48.

McCance, K.L., & Huether, S.E. (1994). *Pathophysiology: The biologic basis for disease in adults and children* (2nd ed.). St. Louis: Mosby.

Phillips, M.C., & Olson, L.R. (1993). The immunologic role of the gastrointestinal tract. *Critical Care Nursing Clinics of North America, 5*(1), 107-118.

Van Wynsberghe, D., Noback, C.R., & Carola, R. (1995). *Human anatomy and physiology* (3rd ed.). New York: McGraw-Hill.

Workman, M.L. (1993). The immune system: Your defensive partner and offensive foe. *AACN, 4*(3), 453-470.

Outcomes

Immunization Behavior

DEFINITION: Actions to obtain immunity from a preventable communicable disease

IMMUNIZATION BEHAVIOR	Never demonstrated 1	Rarely demonstrated 2	Sometimes demonstrated 3	Often demonstrated 4	Consistently demonstrated 5
INDICATORS:					
Acknowledges disease risk without immunization	1	2	3	4	5
Describes risks associated with specific immunization	1	2	3	4	5
Describes contraindications to specific immunization	1	2	3	4	5
Brings updated vaccination card to each visit	1	2	3	4	5
Obtains immunizations recommended for age by the AAP* or USPHS*	1	2	3	4	5
Describes relief measures for vaccine side effects	1	2	3	4	5
Acknowledges need to report any adverse reactions	1	2	3	4	5
Reports previous adverse reactions prior to immunization	1	2	3	4	5
Confirms date of next immunization	1	2	3	4	5
Obtains immunizations recommended with chronic illness by the AAP or USPHS	1	2	3	4	5
Obtains immunizations recommended for occupational risk by AAP or USPHS	1	2	3	4	5
Obtains immunizations recommended for travel by the AAP or USPHS	1	2	3	4	5
Identifies community resources for immunization	1	2	3	4	5
Other _____ Specify	1	2	3	4	5

*AAP = American Academy of Pediatrics; USPHS = United States Public Health Service.

Outcomes

BACKGROUND READINGS:

Selekman, J. (1994). The guidelines for immunizations have changed again! *Pediatric Nursing, 20*(4), 376-378.

Sharts-Hopko, N.C. (1994). Current immunization guidelines. *MCN: American Journal of Maternal Child Nursing, 19*(2), 82-84.

Smith, C., & Maurer, F. (1995). *Community health nursing: Theory and practice.* Philadelphia: W.B. Saunders.

U.S. Department of Health and Human Services. (1994). *Clinician's handbook of preventive service: Put prevention into practice.* Washington, DC: U.S. Government Printing Office.

Outcomes

Impulse Control

DEFINITION: Ability to self-restrain compulsive or impulsive behaviors

IMPULSE CONTROL	Never demonstrated 1	Rarely demonstrated 2	Sometimes demonstrated 3	Often demonstrated 4	Consistently demonstrated 5
INDICATORS:					
Identifies harmful impulsive behaviors	1	2	3	4	5
Identifies feelings that lead to impulsive actions	1	2	3	4	5
Identifies behaviors that lead to impulsive actions	1	2	3	4	5
Identifies consequences of impulsive actions to self or others	1	2	3	4	5
Recognizes risks in environment	1	2	3	4	5
Avoids high risk environments and situations	1	2	3	4	5
Verbalizes control of impulses	1	2	3	4	5
Seeks help when experiencing impulses	1	2	3	4	5
Identifies social support systems	1	2	3	4	5
Accepts referrals for treatment	1	2	3	4	5
Upholds contract to control behavior	1	2	3	4	5
Maintains self-control without supervision	1	2	3	4	5
Other _____ Specify	1	2	3	4	5

BACKGROUND READINGS:

American Psychiatric Association Practice Guidelines (1993). *American Journal of Psychiatry, 150*(2), 207-228.

Dyckoff, D., Goldstein, L., & Levine-Schacht, L. (1996). The investigation of behavioral contracting in patients with borderline personality disorder. *Journal of the American Psychiatric Nurses Association, 2*(3), 71-76.

Gallop, R. (1992). Self-destructive and impulsive behavior in the patient with borderline personality disorder: Rethinking hospital treatment and management. *Archives of Psychiatric Nursing, 6*(6), 366-373.

Gallop, R., McCay, E., & Esplen, M.T. (1992). The conceptualization of impulsivity for psychiatric nursing practice. *Archives of Psychiatric Nursing, 6*(6), 366-373.

Outcomes

Miller, L.J. (1990). The formal treatment contract in the inpatient management of borderline personality disorder. *Hospital and Community Psychiatry, 41*(9) 985-987.

Staples, N.R., & Schwartz, M. (1990). Anorexia nervosa support group: Providing transitional support. *Journal of Psychosocial Nursing and Mental Health Services, 28*(2), 6-10.

Stuart, G.W., & Sundeen, S.J. (1995). *Principles and practice of psychiatric nursing* (5th ed.). St. Louis: Mosby.

Outcomes

Infection Status

DEFINITION: Presence and extent of infection

INFECTION STATUS	Severe 1	Substantial 2	Moderate 3	Slight 4	None 5
INDICATORS:					
Rash	1	2	3	4	5
Uncrusted vesicles	1	2	3	4	5
Foul-smelling discharge	1	2	3	4	5
Purulent sputum	1	2	3	4	5
Purulent drainage	1	2	3	4	5
Pyuria	1	2	3	4	5
Fever	1	2	3	4	5
Pain/tenderness	1	2	3	4	5
Gastrointestinal symptoms	1	2	3	4	5
Lymphadenopathy	1	2	3	4	5
Malaise	1	2	3	4	5
Chilling	1	2	3	4	5
Unexplained cognitive impairment	1	2	3	4	5
Neonate: lethargy	1	2	3	4	5
Neonate: jitteriness	1	2	3	4	5
Neonate: hypothermia	1	2	3	4	5
Neonate: respiratory distress	1	2	3	4	5
Neonate: poor feeding	1	2	3	4	5
Chest x-ray infiltration	1	2	3	4	5
Blood culture colonization	1	2	3	4	5
Sputum culture colonization	1	2	3	4	5
Cerebrospinal fluid culture colonization	1	2	3	4	5
Wound site culture colonization	1	2	3	4	5
Urine culture colonization	1	2	3	4	5
Stool culture colonization	1	2	3	4	5
WBC* elevation	1	2	3	4	5
WBC depression	1	2	3	4	5
Other _____ Specify	1	2	3	4	5

*WBC = White blood (cell) count.

Outcomes

BACKGROUND READINGS:

Albrutyn, E., & Talbot, G.H. (1987). Surveillance strategies: A primer. *Infection Control, 8*(11), 459-464.

Birnbaum, D. (1987). Nosocomial infection surveillance programs. *Infection Control, 8*(11), 474-479.

Haley, R.W., Aber, R.C., & Bennett, J.V. (1986). Surveillance of nosocomial infections. In J.V. Bennett & D. S. Brachman (Eds.), *Hospital infections* (2nd ed., pp. 51-71). Boston: Little, Brown.

Hopkins, C.C. (1983). Epidemiologic principles in intensive care. In M.A. Roderick (Ed.), *Infection control in critical care* (pp. 3-12). Rockville, MD: Aspen.

Outcomes

Information Processing

DEFINITION: Ability to acquire, organize, and use information

INFORMATION PROCESSING	Never demonstrated 1	Rarely demonstrated 2	Sometimes demonstrated 3	Often demonstrated 4	Consistently demonstrated 5
INDICATORS:					
Correctly identifies common objects	1	2	3	4	5
Reads and understands a short sentence or paragraph	1	2	3	4	5
Verbalizes a coherent message	1	2	3	4	5
Exhibits organized thought processes	1	2	3	4	5
Exhibits logical thought processes	1	2	3	4	5
Explains similarity or dissimilarity between two items	1	2	3	4	5
Adds or subtracts several numbers	1	2	3	4	5
Other _____ Specify	1	2	3	4	5

BACKGROUND READINGS:

Abraham, I., & Reel, S. (1993). Cognitive nursing interventions with long-term care residents: Effects on neurocognitive dimensions. *Archives of Psychiatric Nursing, VI*(6), 356-365.

Agostinelli, B., Demers, K., Garrigan, D., & Waszynski, C. (1994). Targeted interventions: Use of the mini-mental state exam. *Journal of Gerontological Nursing, 20*(8), 15-23.

Dellasega, C. (1992). Home health nurses' assessments of cognition. *Applied Nursing Research, 5*(3), 127-133.

Foreman, M., Theis, S., & Anderson, M.A. (1993). Adverse events in the hospitalized elderly. *Clinical Nursing Research, 2*(3) 360-370.

Foreman, M., Gilles, D., & Wagner, D. (1989). Impaired cognition in the critically ill elderly patient: Clinical implications. *Critical Care Nursing Quarterly, 12*(1), 61-73.

Inaba-Roland, K., & Maricle, R. (1992). Assessing delirium in the acute care setting. *Heart and Lung, 21*(1), 48-55.

Jubeck, M. (1992). Are you sensitive to the cognitive needs of the elderly? *Home Healthcare Nurse, 10*(5), 20-25.

Kupferer, S., Uebele, J., & Levin, D. (1988). Geriatric ambulatory surgery patients: Assessing cognitive functions. *AORN Journal, 47*(3), 752-766.

Mason, P. (1989). Cognitive assessment parameters and tools for the critically injured adult. *Critical Care Nursing Clinics of North America, 1*(1), 45-53.

Strub, R., & Black, W. (1993). *The mental status examination in neurology* (3rd ed.). Philadelphia: F. A. Davis.

Outcomes

Joint Movement: Active

DEFINITION: Range of motion of joints with self-initiated movement

JOINT MOVEMENT: ACTIVE SPECIFY JOINT(S) _____	No motion 1	Limited motion 2	Moderate motion 3	Substantial` motion 4	Full motion 5
INDICATORS:					
Jaw	1	2	3	4	5
Neck	1	2	3	4	5
Fingers (right)	1	2	3	4	5
Fingers (left)	1	2	3	4	5
Thumb (right)	1	2	3	4	5
Thumb (left)	1	2	3	4	5
Wrist (right)	1	2	3	4	5
Wrist (left)	1	2	3	4	5
Elbow (right)	1	2	3	4	5
Elbow (left)	1	2	3	4	5
Shoulder (right)	1	2	3	4	5
Shoulder (left)	1	2	3	4	5
Ankle (right)	1	2	3	4	5
Ankle (left)	1	2	3	4	5
Knee (right)	1	2	3	4	5
Knee (left)	1	2	3	4	5
Hip (right)	1	2	3	4	5
Hip (left)	1	2	3	4	5
Other _____ Specify	1	2	3	4	5

BACKGROUND READINGS:

Bates, B. (1991). *A guide to the physical examination and history taking* (5th ed.). Philadelphia: J.B. Lippincott.

Dittmar, S. (1989). *Rehabilitation nursing: Process and application.* St. Louis: Mosby.

Seidel, H.M., Ball, J.W., Dains, J.E., & Benedict, G.W. (1987). *Mosby's guide to physical examination.* St. Louis: Mosby.

Outcomes

Joint Movement: Passive

DEFINITION: Range of motion of joints with assisted movement

JOINT MOVEMENT: PASSIVE SPECIFY JOINT(S) _____	No motion 1	Limited motion 2	Moderate motion 3	Substantial motion 4	Full motion 5
INDICATORS:					
Jaw	1	2	3	4	5
Neck	1	2	3	4	5
Fingers (right)	1	2	3	4	5
Fingers (left)	1	2	3	4	5
Thumb (right)	1	2	3	4	5
Thumb (left)	1	2	3	4	5
Wrist (right)	1	2	3	4	5
Wrist (left)	1	2	3	4	5
Elbow (right)	1	2	3	4	5
Elbow (left)	1	2	3	4	5
Shoulder (right)	1	2	3	4	5
Shoulder (left)	1	2	3	4	5
Ankle (right)	1	2	3	4	5
Ankle (left)	1	2	3	4	5
Knee (right)	1	2	3	4	5
Knee (left)	1	2	3	4	5
Hip (right)	1	2	3	4	5
Hip (left)	1	2	3	4	5
Other _____ Specify	1	2	3	4	5

BACKGROUND READINGS:

Bates, B. (1991). *A guide to the physical examination and history taking* (5th ed.). Philadelphia: J.B. Lippincott.

Dittmar, S. (1989). *Rehabilitation nursing: process and application.* St. Louis: Mosby.

Seidel, H.M., Ball, J.W., Dains, J.E., & Benedict, G.W. (1987). *Mosby's guide to physical examination.* St. Louis: Mosby.

Outcomes

Knowledge: Breastfeeding

DEFINITION: Extent of understanding conveyed about lactation and nourishment of infant through breastfeeding

KNOWLEDGE: BREASTFEEDING	None 1	Limited 2	Moderate 3	Substantial 4	Extensive 5
INDICATORS:					
Description of benefits of breastfeeding	1	2	3	4	5
Description of physiology of lactation	1	2	3	4	5
Description of breastmilk composition, letdown process, foremilk versus hindmilk	1	2	3	4	5
Description of early infant hunger cues	1	2	3	4	5
Description of proper technique for attaching infant to the breast	1	2	3	4	5
Description of proper infant positioning while nursing	1	2	3	4	5
Description of nutritive versus nonnutritive suck	1	2	3	4	5
Description of evaluation of infant swallowing	1	2	3	4	5
Description of proper technique to break infant suction	1	2	3	4	5
Description of signs of adequate milk supply	1	2	3	4	5
Description of signs of adequately nourished breastfed infant	1	2	3	4	5
Description of nipple evaluation	1	2	3	4	5
Description of signs of mastitis, blocked ducts, nipple trauma	1	2	3	4	5
Explanation of reasons for early avoidance of artificial nipples and supplements	1	2	3	4	5
Description of proper breastmilk expression and storage techniques	1	2	3	4	5
Description of passage of ingested substances through breastmilk	1	2	3	4	5
Description of weaning readiness	1	2	3	4	5
Description of how to access health care system	1	2	3	4	5
Other _____ Specify	1	2	3	4	5

BACKGROUND READINGS:

Lawrence, R. (1994). *Breastfeeding: A guide for the medical professional* (4th ed.). St. Louis: Mosby.

Minchin, M.K. (1989). Positioning for breastfeeding. *Birth: Issues in Perinatal Care and Education,* 16(2), 67-80.

Righard, L., & Alade, M. (1992). Sucking technique and its effect on success of breastfeeding. *Birth: Issues in Perinatal Care and Education, 19,* 185-189.

Continued.

Riordan, J., & Auerbach, K.G. (1993). *Breastfeeding and human lactation*. Boston: Jones and Bartlett.

Shrago, L., & Bocar, D. (1990). The infant's contribution to breastfeeding. *Journal of Obstetric, Gynecologic, and Neonatal Nursing, 19,* 209-213.

Spangler, A. (1992). *Amy Spangler's breastfeeding: A parent's guide*. Atlanta: A. Spangler Publications.

Walker, M. (1989). Functional assessment of infant breastfeeding patterns. *Birth: Issues in Perinatal Care and Education, 16,* 140-147.

Outcomes

Knowledge: Child Safety

DEFINITION: Extent of understanding conveyed about safely caring for a child

KNOWLEDGE: CHILD SAFETY	None 1	Limited 2	Moderate 3	Substantial 4	Extensive 5
INDICATORS:					
Description of appropriate activities for child's developmental level	1	2	3	4	5
Description of drowning hazards	1	2	3	4	5
Description of methods to prevent drowning	1	2	3	4	5
Description of methods to prevent electrical shock	1	2	3	4	5
Description of use of bicycle helmets	1	2	3	4	5
Description of methods to prevent choking on objects	1	2	3	4	5
Demonstration of first aid techniques	1	2	3	4	5
Description of correct use of safety seats and seat belts	1	2	3	4	5
Demonstration of CPR*	1	2	3	4	5
Demonstration of Heimlich maneuver	1	2	3	4	5
Description of methods to prevent farm and vehicle accidents	1	2	3	4	5
Description of methods to prevent falls	1	2	3	4	5
Description of methods to prevent playground accidents	1	2	3	4	5
Description of methods to prevent burns	1	2	3	4	5
Description of use of functioning smoke detectors	1	2	3	4	5
Description of proper surveillance of outdoor play	1	2	3	4	5
Description of teaching stranger awareness	1	2	3	4	5
Other _____ Specify	1	2	3	4	5

*CPR = Cardiopulmonary resuscitation.

BACKGROUND READINGS:

Eichelberger, M.R., Gotschall, C.S., Feely, H.B., Harstad, P., & Bowman, L.M. (1990). Parental attitudes and knowledge of child safety. *American Journal of Diseases of Children*, 144(6):714-720.

Gilk, D., Kronenfeld, J., & Jackson, K. (1993). Safety behaviors among parents of preschoolers. *Health Values*, 17(1), 18-25.

Grossman, D.C., & Rivera, F. P. (1992). Injury control in childhood. *Pediatric Clinics of North America*, 39(3), 471-484.

Rivera, F.P., & Howard, D. (1982). Parental knowledge of child development and injury risks. *Developmental and Behavioral Pediatrics*, 3(2), 103-105.

Wortel E., Geus, G.H., Kok, G., & van Woerkum, C. (1994). Injury control in pre-school children: A review of parental safety measures and the behavioral determinants. *Health Education Research*, 9(2), 201-213.

Knowledge: Diet

DEFINITION: Extent of understanding conveyed about diet

KNOWLEDGE: DIET	None 1	Limited 2	Moderate 3	Substantial 4	Extensive 5
INDICATORS:					
Description of recommended diet	1	2	3	4	5
Explanation of rationale for recommended diet	1	2	3	4	5
Description of advantages following recommended diet	1	2	3	4	5
Setting of goals for diet	1	2	3	4	5
Explanation of relationships among diet, exercise and body weight	1	2	3	4	5
Description of foods allowed in diet	1	2	3	4	5
Description of foods to be avoided	1	2	3	4	5
Interpretation of food labels	1	2	3	4	5
Description of guidelines for food preparation	1	2	3	4	5
Selection of foods recommended in diet	1	2	3	4	5
Planning of menus using diet guidelines	1	2	3	4	5
Development of strategies to change dietary habits	1	2	3	4	5
Development of diet plans for social situations	1	2	3	4	5
Performance of self-monitoring activities	1	2	3	4	5
Description of potential for food and medication interaction	1	2	3	4	5
Other _____ Specify	1	2	3	4	5

BACKGROUND READINGS:

Bloomgarden, Z.T., Karmally, W., Metzger, J., Brothers, M., Nechemias, C., Bookman, J., Faierman, D., Ginsberg-Fellner, F., Rayfield, E., & Brown, W.V. (1987). Randomized controlled trial of diabetic patient education: Improved knowledge without improved metabolic status. *Diabetes Care, 10*(3), 263-272.

Bushnell, F. (1992, October). Self-care teaching for congestive heart failure patients. *Journal of Gerontological Nursing,* 27-32.

Devins, G.M., Binik, Y.M., Mandin, H., Litourneau, P.K., Hollomby, D.J., Barre, P.E., & Prichard, S. (1990). The kidney disease questionnaire: A test for measuring patient knowledge about end-stage renal disease. *Journal of Clinical Epidemiology, 43*(3), 297-307.

Garrard, J., Joynes, J.O., Mullen, L., McNeil, L., Mensing, C., Feste, C., & Etzwiler, D.D. (1987). Psychometric study of patient knowledge test. *Diabetes Care, 10*(4), 500-509.

Gilden, J.L., Hendryx, M., Casia, C., & Singh, S.P. (1989). The effectiveness of diabetes education programs for older patients and their spouses. *Journal of American Geriatrics Society, 37*(11), 1023-1030.

Mazzuca, S.A., Moorman, N.H., Wheeler, M.L., Norton, J.A., Fineberg, N.S., Vinicor, F., Cohen, S.J., & Clark, C.M. (1986). The diabetes education study: A controlled trial of the effects of diabetes patient education. *Diabetes Care, 9*(1), 1-10.

Redman, B. (1993). Knowledge deficit (specify). In J.M. Thompson, G.K. McFarland, J.E. Hirsch, & S.M. Tucker (Eds.), *Mosby's clinical nursing* (pp. 1548-1552). St. Louis: Mosby.

Scherer, Y.K., Janelli, L.M., & Schmieder, L.E. (1992). A time-series perspective of effectiveness of a health teaching program on chronic obstructive pulmonary disease. *Journal of Healthcare Education and Training, 6*(3), 7-13.

Smith, M.M., Hicks, V.L., & Heyward, V.H. (1991). Coronary disease knowledge test: Developing a valid and reliable tool. *Nurse Practitioner, 16*(4), 28, 31, 35-38.

Knowledge: Disease Process

DEFINITION: Extent of understanding conveyed about a specific disease process

KNOWLEDGE: DISEASE PROCESS	None 1	Limited 2	Moderate 3	Substantial 4	Extensive 5
INDICATORS:					
Familiarity with disease name	1	2	3	4	5
Description of disease process	1	2	3	4	5
Description of cause or contributing factors	1	2	3	4	5
Description of risk factors	1	2	3	4	5
Description of effects of disease	1	2	3	4	5
Description of signs and symptoms	1	2	3	4	5
Description of usual disease course	1	2	3	4	5
Description of measures to minimize disease progression	1	2	3	4	5
Description of complications	1	2	3	4	5
Description of signs and symptoms of complications	1	2	3	4	5
Description of precautions to prevent complications	1	2	3	4	5
Other _____ Specify	1	2	3	4	5

BACKGROUND READINGS:

Bloomgarden, Z.T., Karmally, W., Metzger, J., Brothers, M., Nechemias, C., Bookman, J., Faierman, D., Ginsberg-Fellner, F., Rayfield, E., & Brown, W.V. (1987). Randomized controlled trial of diabetic patient education: Improved knowledge without improved metabolic status. *Diabetes Care, 10*(3), 263-272.

Bushnell, F. (1992, October). Self-care teaching for congestive heart failure patients. *Journal of Gerontological Nursing,* 27-32.

Devins, G.M., Binik, Y.M., Mandin, H., Litourneau, P.K., Hollomby, D.J., Barre, P.E., & Prichard, S. (1990). The kidney disease questionnaire: A test for measuring patient knowledge about end-stage renal disease. *Journal of Clinical Epidemiology, 43*(3), 297-307.

Garrard, J., Joynes, J.O., Mullen, L., McNeil, L., Mensing, C., Feste, C., & Etzwiler, D.D. (1987). Psychometric study of patient knowledge test. *Diabetes Care, 10*(4), 500-509.

Gilden, J.L., Hendryx, M., Casia, C., & Singh, S.P. (1989). The effectiveness of diabetes education programs for older patients and their spouses. *Journal of American Geriatrics Society, 37*(11), 1023-1030.

Mazzuca, S.A., Moorman, N.H., Wheeler, M.L., Norton, J.A., Fineberg, N.S., Vinicor, F., Cohen, S.J., & Clark, C.M. (1986). The diabetes education study: A controlled trial of the effects of diabetes patient education. *Diabetes Care, 9*(1), 1-10.

Redman, B. (1993). Knowledge deficit (specify). In J.M. Thompson, G.K. McFarland, J.E. Hirsch, & S.M. Tucker (Eds.), *Mosby's clinical nursing* (pp. 1548-1552). St. Louis: Mosby.

Scherer, Y.K., Janelli, L.M., & Schmieder, L.E. (1992). A time-series perspective of effectiveness of a health teaching program on chronic obstructive pulmomary disease. *Journal of Healthcare Education and Training, 6*(3), 7-13.

Smith, M.M., Hicks, V.L., & Heyward, V.H. (1991). Coronary disease knowledge test: Developing a valid and reliable tool. *Nurse Practitioner, 16*(4), 28, 31, 35-38.

Outcomes

Knowledge: Energy Conservation

DEFINITION: Extent of understanding conveyed about energy conservation techniques

KNOWLEDGE: ENERGY CONSERVATION	None 1	Limited 2	Moderate 3	Substantial 4	Extensive 5
INDICATORS:					
Description of recommended activity level	1	2	3	4	5
Description of activity restrictions	1	2	3	4	5
Description of appropriate activities	1	2	3	4	5
Description of conditions that increase energy expenditure	1	2	3	4	5
Description of conditions that decrease energy expenditure	1	2	3	4	5
Description of energy limitations	1	2	3	4	5
Description of how to balance rest and activity	1	2	3	4	5
Performance of methods to conserve energy	1	2	3	4	5
Performance of pulse taking	1	2	3	4	5
Performance of controlled breathing	1	2	3	4	5
Performance of proper body mechanics	1	2	3	4	5
Performance of work simplification techniques	1	2	3	4	5
Performance of use of assistive devices	1	2	3	4	5
Balancing rest and activity	1	2	3	4	5
Other _____ Specify	1	2	3	4	5

BACKGROUND READINGS:

Hart, L.K., & Freel, M.I. (1982). Fatigue. In C.M. Norris (Ed.), *Concept clarification in nursing* (pp. 251-261). Rockville, MD: Aspen.

Lubkin, I.M. (1990). *Chronic illness: Impact and interventions* (2nd ed.). Boston: Jones and Bartlett.

McFarlane, E.A. (1993). Activity intolerance. In J.M. Thompson, G.K. McFarland, J.E. Hirsch, & S.M. Tucker (Eds.), *Clinical nursing* (3rd ed., pp. 1498-1500). St. Louis: Mosby.

McFarlane, E.A. (1993). High risk for activity intolerance. In J.M. Thompson, G.K. McFarland, J.E. Hirsch, & S.M. Tucker (Eds.), *Clinical nursing* (3rd ed., pp. 1497-1498). St. Louis: Mosby.

Mock, V.L. (1993). Fatigue. In J.M. Thompson, G.K. McFarland, J.E. Hirsch, & S.M. Tucker (Eds.), *Clinical nursing* (3rd ed., pp. 1504-1506). St. Louis: Mosby.

Morris, M.L. (1982). Tiredness and fatigue. In C.M. Norris (Ed.), *Concept clarification in nursing* (pp. 263-275). Rockville, MD: Aspen.

Knowledge: Health Behaviors

DEFINITION: Extent of understanding conveyed about the promotion and protection of health

KNOWLEDGE: HEALTH BEHAVIORS	None	Limited	Moderate	Substantial	Extensive
	1	2	3	4	5
INDICATORS:					
Description of healthy nutritional practices	1	2	3	4	5
Description of benefits of activity and exercise	1	2	3	4	5
Description of effective stress management techniques	1	2	3	4	5
Description of effective sleep-wake patterns	1	2	3	4	5
Description of methods of family planning	1	2	3	4	5
Description of health effects of tobacco use	1	2	3	4	5
Description of health effects of alcohol use	1	2	3	4	5
Description of health effects of chemical substance use	1	2	3	4	5
Description of safe use of prescription drugs	1	2	3	4	5
Description of safe use of non-prescription drugs	1	2	3	4	5
Description of effect of caffeine use	1	2	3	4	5
Description of measures to reduce the risk of accidental injury	1	2	3	4	5
Description of how to avoid exposure to environmental hazards	1	2	3	4	5
Description of measures to prevent transmission of infectious disease	1	2	3	4	5
Description of health promotion and protection services	1	2	3	4	5
Description of appropriate use of self-screening	1	2	3	4	5
Other _____ Specify	1	2	3	4	5

BACKGROUND READINGS:

Simons-Morton, D.G., Mullen, P.D., Mains, D.A., Tabak, E.R., & Green, L.W. (1992). Characteristics of controlled studies of patient education and counseling for preventive health behaviors. *Patient Education and Counseling, 19*, 174-204.

Spellbring, A.M. (1991). Nursing's role in health promotion. *Nursing Clinics of North America, 16*(4), 805-814.

Tanner, E.K.W. (1991). Assessment of a health-promotive lifestyle. *Nursing Clinics of North America, 26*(4), 845-854.

U.S. Department of Health and Human Services. (1990). *Healthy people 2000. National health promotion and disease prevention objectives.* Washington, DC: U.S. Government Printing Office.

U.S. Department of Health and Human Services. (1994). *Clinician's handbook of preventive services: Put prevention into practice.* Washington, DC: U.S. Government Printing Office.

Outcomes

Knowledge: Health Resources

DEFINITION: Extent of understanding conveyed about health care resources

KNOWLEDGE: HEALTH RESOURCES	None 1	Limited 2	Moderate 3	Substantial 4	Extensive 5
INDICATORS:					
Description of resources that enhance health	1	2	3	4	5
Description of when to contact a health professional	1	2	3	4	5
Description of emergency measures	1	2	3	4	5
Description of resources for emergency care	1	2	3	4	5
Description of need for follow-up care	1	2	3	4	5
Description of plan for follow-up care	1	2	3	4	5
Description of community resources available for assistance	1	2	3	4	5
Description of how to connect with needed services	1	2	3	4	5
Other _____ Specify	1	2	3	4	5

BACKGROUND READINGS:

Bull, M.J. (1994). Patients' and professionals' perceptions of quality in discharge planning. *Journal of Nursing Care Quality, 8*(2), 47-61.

Main, C.C. (1988). Nursing care of the dysrhythmia patient hospitalized for electrophysiology testing. *Journal of Cardiovascular Nursing, 3*(1), 24-32.

Redman, B. (1993). Knowledge deficit (specify). In J.M. Thompson, G.K. McFarland, J.E. Hirsch, & S.M. Tucker (Eds.), *Mosby's clinical nursing* (3rd ed., pp. 548-1552). St. Louis: Mosby.

Wyness, M.A. (1990). Evaluation of an educational program for patients taking warfarin. *Journal of Advanced Nursing, 15,* 1052-1063.

Outcomes

Knowledge: Infection Control

DEFINITION: Extent of understanding conveyed about prevention and control of infection

KNOWLEDGE: INFECTION CONTROL	None 1	Limited 2	Moderate 3	Substantial 4	Extensive 5
INDICATORS:					
Description of mode of transmission	1	2	3	4	5
Description of factors contributing to transmission	1	2	3	4	5
Description of practices that reduce transmission	1	2	3	4	5
Description of signs and symptoms	1	2	3	4	5
Description of screening procedures	1	2	3	4	5
Description of monitoring procedures	1	2	3	4	5
Description of activities to increase resistance to infection	1	2	3	4	5
Description of treatment for diagnosed infection	1	2	3	4	5
Description of follow-up for diagnosed infection	1	2	3	4	5
Other _____ Specify	1	2	3	4	5

BACKGROUND READINGS:

Health Services, Centers for Disease Control. (1991). *Core curriculum on tuberculosis* (2nd ed.). Bethesda, MD: U.S. Department of Health and Human Services.

Flaskerud, J.H., & Ungvarski, P.J. (1995). *HIV/AIDS: A guide to nursing care* (3rd ed.). Philadelphia: W.B. Saunders.

National Center for Nursing Research. (1990). *HIV infection: Prevention and care.* Bethesda, MD: U.S. Department of Health and Human Services.

Rotheram, M.J., Reid, M.A., & Rosario, M. (1994). Factors mediating changes in sexual HIV risk behaviors among gay and bisexual male adolescents. *American Journal of Public Health, 84*(12), 1938-1946.

Simons-Morton, D.G., Mullen, P.D., Mains, D.A., Tabak, E.R., & Green, L.W. (1992). Characteristics of controlled studies of patient education and counseling for preventive health behaviors. *Patient Education and Counseling, 19,* 174-204.

Statton, P., & Alexander, N.J. (1993). Prevention of sexually transmitted infections: Physical and chemical barrier methods. *Infectious Disease Clinics of North America, 7*(4), 841-859.

Outcomes

Knowledge: Medication

DEFINITION: Extent of understanding conveyed about the safe use of medication

KNOWLEDGE: MEDICATION	None 1	Limited 2	Moderate 3	Substantial 4	Extensive 5
INDICATORS:					
Recognition of need to inform health provider of all medications being taken	1	2	3	4	5
Statement of correct medication name	1	2	3	4	5
Description of appearance of medication	1	2	3	4	5
Description of actions of medication	1	2	3	4	5
Description of side effects of medication	1	2	3	4	5
Description of medication precautions	1	2	3	4	5
Description of use of memory aids	1	2	3	4	5
Description of potential adverse reactions when taking multiple drugs	1	2	3	4	5
Description of potential for interaction with other agents	1	2	3	4	5
Description of correct administration of medication	1	2	3	4	5
Description of self-monitoring techniques	1	2	3	4	5
Description of proper medication storage	1	2	3	4	5
Description of proper care of administration devices	1	2	3	4	5
Description of how to obtain required medication and supplies	1	2	3	4	5
Description of proper disposal of unused medications	1	2	3	4	5
Identification of needed laboratory tests	1	2	3	4	5
Description of proper use of medication alert identification	1	2	3	4	5
Other _____ Specify	1	2	3	4	5

BACKGROUND READINGS:

Barry, K. (1993). Patient self-medication: An innovative approach to medication teaching. *Journal of Nursing Care Quality, 8*(1), 75-82.

Colley, C.A. (1993, May). Polypharmacy: The cure becomes the disease. *Journal of General Internal Medicine, 8*, 278-283.

Donnelly, D. (1987). Instilling eye drops: Difficulties experienced by patients following cataract surgery. *Journal of Advanced Nursing, 12*, 235-243.

Everitt, D.E., & Avorn, J. (1986). Drug prescribing for the elderly. *Archives of Internal Medicine, 146*, 2393-2396.

Continued.

Kleoppel, J.W., & Henry, D.W. (1987). Teaching patients, families, and communities about their medications. In C.E. Smith (Ed.), *Patient education: Nurses in partnership with other health professionals,* (pp. 271-296). Philadelphia: W.B. Saunders.

Proos, M., Reiley, P., Eagan, J., Stengrevics, S., Castile, J., & Arian, D. (1992). A study of the effects of self-medication on patients' knowledge of and compliance with their medication regimen (Special report). *Journal of Nursing Care Quality,* 18-26.

Simons-Morton, D.G., Mullen, P.D., Mains, D.A., Tabak, E.R., & Green, L.W. (1992). Characteristics of controlled studies of patient education and counseling for preventive health behaviors. *Patient Education and Counseling, 19,* 174-204.

Tettersell, M.J. (1993). Asthma patients' knowledge in relation to compliance with drug therapy. *Journal of Advanced Nursing, 18,* 103-113.

U.S. Department of Health and Human Services. (1990). *Healthy people 2000: National health promotion and disease prevention objectives.* Washington, DC: U.S. Government Printing Office.

U.S. Department of Health and Human Services. (1994). *Clinician's handbook of prevention services: Put prevention into practice.* Washington, DC: U.S. Government Printing Office.

Wyness, M.A. (1990). Evaluation of an educational program for patients taking warfarin. *Journal of Advanced Nursing, 15,* 1052-1063.

Outcomes

Knowledge: Personal Safety

DEFINITION: Extent of understanding conveyed about preventing unintentional injuries

KNOWLEDGE: PERSONAL SAFETY	None 1	Limited 2	Moderate 3	Substantial 4	Extensive 5
INDICATORS:					
Description of suffocation prevention measures	1	2	3	4	5
Description of measures to prevent falls	1	2	3	4	5
Description of measures to reduce risk of accidental injury	1	2	3	4	5
Description of home safety measures	1	2	3	4	5
Description of water safety precautions	1	2	3	4	5
Description of fire safety measures	1	2	3	4	5
Description of burn prevention measures	1	2	3	4	5
Description of electrocution prevention	1	2	3	4	5
Description of poison prevention measures	1	2	3	4	5
Description of bicycle safety guidelines	1	2	3	4	5
Description of pedestrian safety	1	2	3	4	5
Description of benefits of helmet use	1	2	3	4	5
Description of firearm safety measures	1	2	3	4	5
Description of measures to protect at-risk persons from unintentional injury	1	2	3	4	5
Description of safety measures for operating motor vehicles	1	2	3	4	5
Description of emergency procedures	1	2	3	4	5
Description of age-specific safety risks	1	2	3	4	5
Description of personal high-risk behaviors	1	2	3	4	5
Description of work safety risks	1	2	3	4	5
Description of community safety risks	1	2	3	4	5
Other _____ Specify	1	2	3	4	5

BACKGROUND READINGS:

Simons-Morton, D.G., Mullen, P.D., Mains, D.A., Tabak, E.R., & Green, L.W. (1992). Characteristics of controlled studies of patient education and counseling for preventive health behaviors. *Patient Education and Counseling, 19,* 174-204.

U.S. Department of Health and Human Services. (1990). *Healthy people 2000. National health promotion and disease prevention objectives.* Washington, DC: U.S. Government Printing Office.

U.S. Department of Health and Human Services. (1994). *Clinician's handbook of prevention services: Put prevention into practice.* Washington, DC: U.S. Government Printing Office.

Knowledge: Prescribed Activity

DEFINITION: Extent of understanding conveyed about prescribed activity and exercise

KNOWLEDGE: PRESCRIBED ACTIVITY	None 1	Limited 2	Moderate 3	Substantial 4	Extensive 5
INDICATORS:					
Description of prescribed activity	1	2	3	4	5
Explanation of purpose of activity	1	2	3	4	5
Description of expected effects of activity	1	2	3	4	5
Description of activity restrictions	1	2	3	4	5
Description of activity precautions	1	2	3	4	5
Description of factors that lower activity tolerance	1	2	3	4	5
Description of strategy for gradual activity increase	1	2	3	4	5
Description of how to monitor activity	1	2	3	4	5
Performance of self-monitoring activities	1	2	3	4	5
Description of obstacles to implementing routine	1	2	3	4	5
Description of realistic exercise plan	1	2	3	4	5
Description of proper performance of exercise	1	2	3	4	5
Proper performance of exercise	1	2	3	4	5
Other _____ Specify	1	2	3	4	5

BACKGROUND READINGS:

Bloomgarden, Z.T., Karmally, W., Metzger, J., Brothers, M., Nechemias, C., Bookman, J., Faierman, D., Ginsberg-Fellner, F., Rayfield, E., & Brown, W.V. (1987). Randomized controlled trial of diabetic patient education: Improved knowledge without improved metabolic status. *Diabetes Care, 10*(3), 263-272.

Bushnell, F. (1992, October). Self-care teaching for congestive heart failure patients. *Journal of Gerontological Nursing,* 27-32.

Devins, G.M., Binik, Y.M., Mandin, H., Litourneau, P.K., Hollomby, D.J., Barre, P.E., & Prichard, S. (1990). The kidney disease questionnaire: A test for measuring patient knowledge about end-stage renal disease. *Journal of Clinical Epidemiology, 43*(3), 297-307.

Garrard, J., Joynes, J.O., Mullen, L., McNeil, L., Mensing, C., Feste, C., & Etzwiler, D.D. (1987). Psychometric study of patient knowledge test. *Diabetes Care, 10*(4), 500-509.

Gilden, J.L., Hendryx, M., Casia, C., & Singh, S.P. (1989). The effectiveness of diabetes education programs for older patients and their spouses. *Journal of American Geriatrics Society, 37*(11), 1023-1030.

Mazzuca S.A., Moorman, N.H., Wheeler, M.L., Norton, J.A., Fineberg, N.S., Vinicor, F., Cohen, S.J., & Clark, C.M. (1986). The diabetes education study: A controlled trial of the effects of diabetes patient education. *Diabetes Care, 9*(1), 1-10.

Redman, B. (1993). Knowledge deficit (specify). In J.M. Thompson, G.K. McFarland, J.E. Hirsch, & S.M. Tucker (Eds.), *Mosby's clinical nursing* (pp. 1548-1552). St. Louis: Mosby.

Scherer, Y.K., Janelli, L.M., & Schmieder, L.E. (1992). A time-series perspective of effectiveness of a health teaching program on chronic obstructive pulmonary disease. *Journal of Healthcare Education and Training, 6*(3), 7-13.

Smith, M.M., Hicks, V.L., & Heyward, V.H. (1991). Coronary disease knowledge test: Developing a valid and reliable tool. *Nurse Practitioner, 16*(4), 28, 31, 35-38.

Knowledge: Substance Use Control

DEFINITION: Extent of understanding conveyed about managing substance use safely

KNOWLEDGE: SUBSTANCE USE CONTROL	None 1	Limited 2	Moderate 3	Substantial 4	Extensive 5
INDICATORS:					
Description of own risk for substance abuse	1	2	3	4	5
Description of health consequences of substance use	1	2	3	4	5
Description of benefits of eliminating substance use	1	2	3	4	5
Identification of dangers of substance use	1	2	3	4	5
Description of social consequences of substance use	1	2	3	4	5
Description of personal responsibility in managing substance use	1	2	3	4	5
Description of threats to substance use control	1	2	3	4	5
Description of support for substance use control	1	2	3	4	5
Description of actions to prevent substance use	1	2	3	4	5
Description of actions to manage substance use	1	2	3	4	5
Description of benefits of ongoing monitoring	1	2	3	4	5
Description of potential for relapse in efforts to control substance use	1	2	3	4	5
Description of actions to prevent and manage relapses in substance abuse	1	2	3	4	5
Description of signs of dependence during substance withdrawal	1	2	3	4	5
Other _____ Specify	1	2	3	4	5

Outcomes

BACKGROUND READINGS:

Eells, M.A.W. (1991). Strategies for promotion of avoiding harmful substances. *Nursing Clinics of North America, 26*(40), 915-927.

Simons-Morton, D.G., Mullen, P.D., Mains, D.A., Tabak, E.R., & Green, L.W. (1992). Characteristics of controlled studies of patient education and counseling for preventive health behaviors. *Patient Education and Counseling, 19,* 174-204.

Tanner, E.K. (1991). Assessment of a health-promotive lifestyle. *Nursing Clinics of North America, 26*(4), 845-854.

U.S. Department of Health and Human Services. (1990). *Healthy people 2000, National health promotion and disease prevention objectives.* Washington, DC: U.S. Government Printing Office.

U.S. Department of Health and Human Services. (1994). *Clinician's handbook of prevention services: Put prevention into practice.* Washington, DC: U.S. Government Printing Office.

Knowledge: Treatment Procedure(s)

DEFINITION: Extent of understanding conveyed about procedure(s) required as part of a treatment regimen

KNOWLEDGE: TREATMENT PROCEDURE(S)	None 1	Limited 2	Moderate 3	Substantial 4	Extensive 5
INDICATORS:					
Description of treatment procedure	1	2	3	4	5
Explanation of purpose of procedure	1	2	3	4	5
Description of steps in procedure	1	2	3	4	5
Description of how device works	1	2	3	4	5
Description of precautions related to procedure	1	2	3	4	5
Description of restrictions related to procedure	1	2	3	4	5
Description of proper care of equipment	1	2	3	4	5
Performance of treatment procedure	1	2	3	4	5
Description of appropriate action for complications	1	2	3	4	5
Description of potential side effects	1	2	3	4	5
Other _____ Specify	1	2	3	4	5

BACKGROUND READINGS:

Gronlund, N.E. (1978). *Stating objectives for classroom instruction* (2nd ed.). New York: Macmillan.

Redman, B.K. (1993). *The process of patient teaching* (7th ed.). St. Louis: Mosby.

Robinson, J., Gould, M.A., Burrows-Hudson, S., Baltz, P., Currier, H., Piwkiewicz, D., & Smith, L.J. (1991). A care plan for administration of epoetin alpha. *ANNA Journal, 18*(6), 573-580.

Sarisley, C. (1987). Designing a teaching program for outpatient antibiotic therapy. *Journal of Nursing Staff Development, Summer,* 128-135.

Smith, C.E. (1987). *Patient education: Nurses in partnership with other health professionals.* Orlando, FL: Gruen & Stratton.

Knowledge: Treatment Regimen

DEFINITION: Extent of understanding conveyed about a specific treatment regimen

KNOWLEDGE: TREATMENT REGIMEN	None 1	Limited 2	Moderate 3	Substantial 4	Extensive 5
INDICATORS:					
Description of rationale for treatment regimen	1	2	3	4	5
Description of self-care responsibilities for ongoing treatment	1	2	3	4	5
Description of self-care responsibilities for emergency situations	1	2	3	4	5
Description of expected effects of treatment	1	2	3	4	5
Description of prescribed diet	1	2	3	4	5
Description of prescribed medication	1	2	3	4	5
Description of prescribed activity	1	2	3	4	5
Description of prescribed exercise	1	2	3	4	5
Description of prescribed procedures	1	2	3	4	5
Performance of self-monitoring techniques	1	2	3	4	5
Performance of treatment procedure	1	2	3	4	5
Selection of foods recommended in diet	1	2	3	4	5
Other _____ Specify	1	2	3	4	5

Outcomes

BACKGROUND READINGS:

Bloomgarden, Z.T., Karmally, W., Metzger, J., Brothers, M., Nechemias, C., Bookman, J., Faierman, D., Ginsberg-Fellner, F., Rayfield, E., & Brown, W.V. (1987). Randomized controlled trial of diabetic patient education: Improved knowledge without improved metabolic status. *Diabetes Care, 10*(3), 263-272.

Bushnell, F. (1992, October). Self-care teaching for congestive heart failure patients. *Journal of Gerontological Nursing,* 27-32.

Devins, G.M., Binik, Y.M., Mandin, H., Litourneau, P.K., Hollomby, D.J., Barre, P.E., & Prichard, S. (1990). The kidney disease questionnaire: A test for measuring patient knowledge about end-stage renal disease. *Journal of Clinical Epidemiology, 43*(3), 297-307.

Garrard, J., Joynes, J.O., Mullen, L., McNeil, L., Mensing, C., Feste, C., & Etzwiler, D.D. (1987). Psychometric study of patient knowledge test. *Diabetes Care, 10*(4), 500-509.

Gilden, J.L., Hendryx, M., Casia, C., & Singh, S.P. (1989). The effectiveness of diabetes education programs for older patients and their spouses. *Journal of American Geriatrics Society, 37*(11), 1023-1030.

Mazzuca, S.A., Moorman, N.H., Wheeler, M.L., Norton, J.A., Fineberg, N.S., Vinicor, F., Cohen, S.J., & Clark, C.M. (1986). The diabetes education study: A controlled trial of the effects of diabetes patient education. *Diabetes Care, 9*(1), 1-10.

Redman, B. (1993). Knowledge deficit (specify). In J.M. Thompson, G.K. McFarland, J.E. Hirsch, & S.M. Tucker (Eds.), *Mosby's clinical nursing* (3rd ed., pp. 1548-1552). St. Louis: Mosby.

Continued.

Roe, B.H. (1990). Study of the effects of education on the management of urine drainage systems by patients and carers. *Journal of Advanced Nursing, 15,* 517-524.

Scherer, Y.K., Janelli, L.M., & Schmieder, L.E. (1992). A time-series perspective of effectiveness of a health teaching program on chronic obstructive pulmonary disease. *Journal of Healthcare Education & Training, 6*(3), 7-13.

Smith, M.M., Hicks, V.L., & Heyward, V.H. (1991). Coronary disease knowledge test: Developing a valid and reliable tool. *Nurse Practitioner, 16*(4), 28, 31, 35-38.

Outcomes

Leisure Participation

DEFINITION: Use of restful or relaxing activities as needed to promote well-being

LEISURE PARTICIPATION	Not adequate 1	Slightly adequate 2	Moderately adequate 3	Substantially adequate 4	Totally adequate 5
INDICATORS:					
Participation in activities other than regular work	1	2	3	4	5
Expression of satisfaction with leisure activities	1	2	3	4	5
Use of appropriate social and interactional skills	1	2	3	4	5
Reports of relaxation from leisure activities	1	2	3	4	5
Demonstration of creativity through leisure activities	1	2	3	4	5
Direction of own leisure	1	2	3	4	5
Identification of recreational options	1	2	3	4	5
Reports of restfulness of leisure activities	1	2	3	4	5
Other _____ Specify	1	2	3	4	5

BACKGROUND READINGS:

Ansello, E.F. (1985). *The activity coordinator as environmental press.* New York: The Haworth Press.

Godin, G., Jobin, J., & Bouillon, J. (1986). Assessment of leisure time exercise behavior by self-report: A concurrent validity study. *Canadian Journal of Public Health, 77*(5), 359-362.

Gordon, M.D. (1987). Pediatric recreational therapy after thermal injury. *Journal of Burn Rehabilitation, 8*(4), 336-340.

Johnson, S.W., McSweeney, M., & Webster, R.E. (1989). Leisure: How to promote inpatient motivation after discharge. *Journal of Psychosocial Nursing, 27*(9), 29-31.

Jongbloed, L., & Morgan, D. (1991). An investigation of involvement in leisure activities after a stroke. *The American Journal of Occupational Therapy, 45*(5), 420-427.

Klein, M.M. (1985). The therapeutics of recreation. *Physical Occupational Therapy Pediatrics, 4*(3): 9-11.

Peterson, C.A., & Gunn, S.L. (1984). *Therapeutic recreation program design: Principles and procedures.* Englewood Cliffs, NJ: Prentice-Hall.

Outcomes

Outcomes

Loneliness

DEFINITION: The extent of emotional, social, or existential isolation response					
LONELINESS	Extensive 1	Substantial 2	Moderate 3	Limited 4	None 5
INDICATORS:					
Expression of unfounded dread	1	2	3	4	5
Expression of desperation	1	2	3	4	5
Expression of extreme restlessness	1	2	3	4	5
Expression of hopelessness	1	2	3	4	5
Expression of lack of belonging	1	2	3	4	5
Expression of loss due to separation from another	1	2	3	4	5
Expression of social isolation	1	2	3	4	5
Expression of not being understood	1	2	3	4	5
Expression of being excluded	1	2	3	4	5
Complaints that time seems endless	1	2	3	4	5
Difficulty in planning	1	2	3	4	5
Difficulty in establishing contact with other people	1	2	3	4	5
Difficulty overcoming separateness	1	2	3	4	5
Difficulty in effecting a mutual relationship	1	2	3	4	5
Demonstration of mood fluctuations	1	2	3	4	5
Decrease in ability to concentrate	1	2	3	4	5
Demonstration of non-assertiveness	1	2	3	4	5
Difficulty making decisions	1	2	3	4	5
Eating disturbances	1	2	3	4	5
Sleep disturbances	1	2	3	4	5
Headaches	1	2	3	4	5
Nausea	1	2	3	4	5
Underactivity	1	2	3	4	5
Pain	1	2	3	4	5
Spiritual discomfort	1	2	3	4	5
Other _____ Specify	1	2	3	4	5

BACKGROUND READINGS:

Copel, L.C. (1988). Loneliness: A conceptual model. *Journal of Psychosocial Nursing, 26*(1), 14-19.

Ellison, C.W. (1978). Loneliness: A social-developmental analysis. *Journal of Psychology and Theology, 6*(1), 3-17.

Peplau, H.E. (1955). Loneliness. *American Journal of Nursing, 55*(12), 1476-1481.

Peplau, L.A., & Pearlman, D. (Eds.). (1982). *Loneliness: A sourcebook of current theory, research, and therapy.* New York: John Wiley.

Weiss, R.S. (Ed.). (1973). *Loneliness: The experience of emotional and social isolation.* Cambridge, MA: The MIT Press.

West, D.A., Kellner, R., & Moore-West, M. (1986). The effects of loneliness: A review of the literature. *Comparative Psychiatry, 27*(4), 351-363.

Outcomes

Memory

DEFINITION: Ability to cognitively retrieve and report previously stored information				
MEMORY	Never demonstrated 1	Rarely demonstrated 2	Sometimes demonstrated 3	Often demonstrated 4	Consistently demonstrated 5

INDICATORS:					
Recalls immediate information accurately	1	2	3	4	5
Recalls recent information accurately	1	2	3	4	5
Recalls remote information accurately	1	2	3	4	5
Other _____ Specify	1	2	3	4	5

BACKGROUND READINGS:

Abraham, I., & Reel, S. (1993). Cognitive nursing interventions with long-term residents: Effects on neurocognitive dimensions. *Archives of Psychiatric Nursing, VI*(6), 356-365.

Agostinelli, B., Demers, K., Garrigan, D., & Waszynski, C. (1994). Targeted interventions: Use of the mini-mental state exam. *Journal of Gerontological Nursing, 20*(8), 15-23.

Dellasega, C. (1992). Home health nurses' assessments of cognition. *Applied Nursing Research, 5*(3), 127-133.

Foreman, M., Theis, S., & Anderson, M.A. (1993). Adverse events in the hospitalized elderly. *Clinical Nursing Research, 2*(3) 360-370.

Foreman, M., Gilles, D., & Wagner, D. (1989). Impaired cognition in the critically ill elderly patient: Clinical implications. *Critical Care Nursing Quarterly, 12*(1), 61-73.

Inaba-Roland, K., & Maricle, R. (1992). Assessing delirium in the acute care setting. *Heart and Lung, 21*(1), 48-55.

Jubeck, M. (1992). Are you sensitive to the cognitive needs of the elderly? *Home Healthcare Nurse, 10*(5), 20-25.

Kupferer, S., Uebele, J., & Levin, D. (1988). Geriatric ambulatory surgery patients: Assessing cognitive functions. *AORN Journal, 47*(3), 752-766.

Mason, P. (1989). Cognitive assessment parameters and tools for the critically injured adult. *Critical Care Nursing Clinics of North America, 1*(1), 45-53.

Strub, R., & Black, W. (1993). *The mental status examination in neurology* (3rd ed.). Philadelphia: F.A. Davis.

Mobility Level

DEFINITION: Ability to move purposefully

MOBILITY LEVEL	Dependent, does not participate	Requires assistive person & device	Requires assistive person	Independent with assistive device	Completely independent
	1	**2**	**3**	**4**	**5**
INDICATORS:					
Balance performance	1	2	3	4	5
Body positioning performance	1	2	3	4	5
Muscle movement	1	2	3	4	5
Joint movement	1	2	3	4	5
Transfer performance	1	2	3	4	5
Ambulation: walking	1	2	3	4	5
Ambulation: wheelchair	1	2	3	4	5
Other _____ Specify	1	2	3	4	5

BACKGROUND READINGS:

Maas, M. (1991). Impaired physical mobility. In M. Maas, K. Buckwalter, & M. Hardy (Eds.), *Nursing diagnosis and interventions for the elderly* (pp. 263-284). Redwood City, CA: Addison-Wesley Nursing.

Outcomes

Mood Equilibrium

DEFINITION: Appropriate adjustment of prevailing emotional tone in response to circumstances

MOOD EQUILIBRIUM	Never demonstrated 1	Rarely demonstrated 2	Sometimes demonstrated 3	Often demonstrated 4	Consistently demonstrated 5
INDICATORS:					
Exhibits appropriate affect	1	2	3	4	5
Exhibits non-labile mood	1	2	3	4	5
Exhibits impulse control	1	2	3	4	5
Reports adequate sleep (at least 5 hr/24 hr)	1	2	3	4	5
Exhibits concentration	1	2	3	4	5
Speech at moderate pace	1	2	3	4	5
Exhibits absence of flight of ideas	1	2	3	4	5
Exhibits absence of grandiosity	1	2	3	4	5
Exhibits absence of euphoria	1	2	3	4	5
Exhibits appropriate grooming and hygiene	1	2	3	4	5
Wears appropriate clothing for situation and weather	1	2	3	4	5
Maintains stable weight	1	2	3	4	5
Reports normal appetite	1	2	3	4	5
Reports compliance with medication and therapeutic regimen	1	2	3	4	5
Shows interest in surroundings	1	2	3	4	5
Absence of suicide ideation	1	2	3	4	5
Reports appropriate energy level	1	2	3	4	5
Reports ability to accomplish daily tasks	1	2	3	4	5
Other _____ Specify	1	2	3	4	5

Outcomes

BACKGROUND READINGS:

George, L.K., Blazer, D.B., Hughes, D.C., & Fowler N. (1989). Social support and the outcome of major depression. *British Journal of Psychiatry 154,* 478-485.

Keitner, G.I., & Miller, I.W. (1990). Family functioning and major depression: An overview. *American Journal of Psychiatry, 147*(9), 1128-1137.

Maynard, C.K. (1993). Comparison of effectiveness of group interventions for depression in women. *Archives of Psychiatric Nursing, 7*(5), 277-283.

Maynard, C. (1993). Psychoeducational approach to depression in women. *Journal of Psychosocial Nursing and Mental Health Services, 31*(12), 9-14.

Stuart, G.W., & Sundeen, S.J. (1995). *Principles and practice of psychiatric nursing* (5th ed.). St. Louis: Mosby.

U.S. Department of Health and Human Services. (1993). *Depression in primary care: Vol. 2. Treatment of major depression* (AHCPR Publication No. 93-0551). Rockville, MD: Public Health Service Agency for Health Care Policy and Research.

U.S. Department of Health and Human Services. (1993). *Depression in primary care: Vol. 1. Detection and diagnosis* (AHCPR Publication No. 93-0550). Rockville, MD: Public Health Service Agency for Health Care Policy and Research.

Outcomes

Muscle Function

DEFINITION: Adequacy of muscle contraction needed for movement					
MUSCLE FUNCTION	Extremely compromised 1	Substantially compromised 2	Moderately compromised 3	Mildly compromised 4	Not compromised 5
INDICATORS:					
Strength of muscle contraction	1	2	3	4	5
Muscle tone	1	2	3	4	5
Sustained muscle movement	1	2	3	4	5
Muscle mass	1	2	3	4	5
Speed of movement	1	2	3	4	5
Steadiness of movement	1	2	3	4	5
Control of movement	1	2	3	4	5
Other _____ Specify	1	2	3	4	5

BACKGROUND READINGS:

Guyton, A.C. (1992). *Human physiology and mechanisms of disease*. Philadelphia: W.B. Saunders.

Matteson, M.A., & McConnell, E.S. (1988). *Gerontological nursing: Concepts and practice*. Philadelphia: W.B. Saunders.

Outcomes

Neglect Recovery

DEFINITION: Healing following the cessation of substandard care

NEGLECT RECOVERY	No evidence 1	Limited evidence 2	Moderate evidence 3	Substantial evidence 4	Extensive evidence 5
INDICATORS:					
Personal hygiene adequate	1	2	3	4	5
Absence of hunger	1	2	3	4	5
Nutrition adequate	1	2	3	4	5
Energy level adequate for daily activities	1	2	3	4	5
Dresses appropriately for weather	1	2	3	4	5
Living environment clean	1	2	3	4	5
Living environment safe	1	2	3	4	5
Skin intact	1	2	3	4	5
Supervision adequate	1	2	3	4	5
Demonstrates interest in life	1	2	3	4	5
Expresses pride in self	1	2	3	4	5
Expresses hope	1	2	3	4	5
Emotional needs met	1	2	3	4	5
Receives appropriate health care	1	2	3	4	5
Receives recommended diet	1	2	3	4	5
Receives recommended medication regimen	1	2	3	4	5
Receives appropriate equipment or appliance	1	2	3	4	5
Growth IER*	1	2	3	4	5
Cognitive learning IER	1	2	3	4	5
Development IER	1	2	3	4	5
Responsibilities appropriate for age	1	2	3	4	5
Seeks affection appropriately	1	2	3	4	5
Free of substance abuse	1	2	3	4	5
Behavior consistent w/social norms	1	2	3	4	5
Other _____ Specify	1	2	3	4	5

*IER = In expected range.

Continued.

Outcomes

BACKGROUND READINGS:

Aber, J.L., Allen, J.P., Carlson, V., & Cicchetti, D. (1990). The effects of maltreatment on development during early childhood: Recent studies and their theoretical, clinical, and policy implications. In D. Cicchetti & V. Carlson (Eds.), *Child maltreatment: Theory and research on the causes and consequences of child abuse and neglect* (pp. 579-619). New York: Cambridge University Press.

Campbell, J., & Humphreys, J. (1993). *Nursing care of survivors of family violence* (2nd ed.). St. Louis: Mosby.

Cicchetti, D., & Carlson, V. (Eds.). (1990). *Child maltreatment: Theory and research on the causes and consequences of child abuse and neglect.* New York: Cambridge University Press.

Fulmer, T., & Ashley, J. (1989). Clinical indicators of elder neglect. *Applied Nursing Research, 2*(4), 161-167.

Hudson, M.F., & Johnson, T.F. (1986). Elder neglect and abuse: A review of the literature [Monograph]. *Annual Review of Nursing Research, 6,* 81-134.

Lobo, M.L., Barnard, K.E., & Coombs, J.B. (1992). Failure to thrive: A parent-infant interaction perspective. *Journal of Pediatric Nursing, 7*(4), 251-261.

Olds, D.L., Henderson, C.R., Chamberlin, R., & Tatelbaum R. (1986). Preventing child abuse and neglect: A randomized trial of nurse home visitation. *Pediatrics, 78*(1), 65-78.

Polansky, N.A., Halley, C., & Polansky, N.F. (1977). Profile of neglect: A survey of the state of knowledge. Washington, DC: U.S. Department of Health, Education, and Welfare.

Rhodes, A.M. (1987). Identifying and reporting child abuse. *The American Journal of Maternal Child Nursing, 2*(3), 399.

Weinman, M.L., Schreiber, N.B., & Robinson, M. (1992). Adolescent mothers: Were there any gains in a parent education program? *Family and Community Health, 15*(3), 1-10.

Young, L. (1981). *Physical child neglect.* Chicago: The National Committee for Prevention of Child Abuse.

Neurological Status

DEFINITION: Extent to which the peripheral and central nervous systems receive, process, and respond to internal and external stimuli

NEUROLOGICAL STATUS	Extremely compromised 1	Substantially compromised 2	Moderately compromised 3	Mildly compromised 4	Not compromised 5
INDICATORS:					
Neurological status: consciousness	1	2	3	4	5
Neurological status: central motor control	1	2	3	4	5
Neurological status: cranial sensory/motor function	1	2	3	4	5
Neurological status: spinal sensory/motor function	1	2	3	4	5
Neurological status: autonomic	1	2	3	4	5
Intracranial pressure WNL*	1	2	3	4	5
Communication	1	2	3	4	5
Pupil size	1	2	3	4	5
Pupil reactivity	1	2	3	4	5
Eye movement pattern	1	2	3	4	5
Breathing pattern	1	2	3	4	5
Vital signs WNL	1	2	3	4	5
Rest-sleep pattern	1	2	3	4	5
Seizure activity not present	1	2	3	4	5
Headaches not present	1	2	3	4	5
Other _____ Specify	1	2	3	4	5

*WNL = Within normal limits.   *Continued.*

Outcomes

Outcomes

BACKGROUND READINGS:

American Nurses' Association Council on Medical-Surgical Nursing Practice and American Association of Neuroscience Nurses. (1985). *Neuroscience nursing practice: process and outcome criteria for selected diagnoses.* Washington, DC: U.S. Government Printing Office.

Hickey, J.V. (1992). *The clinical practice of neurological and neurosurgical nursing* (3rd ed.). Philadelphia: J.B. Lippincott.

Luckmann, J., & Sorensen, K. (1987). *Medical-surgical nursing: A psychophysiologic approach* (3rd ed.). Philadelphia: W.B. Saunders.

Mitchell, P.H., Hodges, L.C., Muwaswes, M., & Walleck, C.A. (Eds.). (1988). *AANN's neuroscience nursing: phenomena and practice.* Norwalk, CT: Appleton & Lange.

Riess, P.C. (1995). Validity and reliability of the Riess intracranial aneurysm assessment tool and the Glasgow coma scale in the aneurysm population. Master's thesis, The University of Iowa, Iowa City.

Neurological Status: Autonomic

DEFINITION: Extent to which the autonomic nervous system coordinates visceral function

NEUROLOGICAL STATUS: AUTO-NOMIC	Extremely compromised 1	Substantially compromised 2	Moderately compromised 3	Mildly compromised 4	Not compromised 5
INDICATORS:					
Heart rate WNL*	1	2	3	4	5
Systolic BP* WNL	1	2	3	4	5
Diastolic BP WNL	1	2	3	4	5
Cardiac pump effective-ness	1	2	3	4	5
Vasodilates appropriately	1	2	3	4	5
Vasoconstricts appropri-ately	1	2	3	4	5
Perspiration pattern	1	2	3	4	5
Goose bumps when appropriate	1	2	3	4	5
Bowel elimination pattern	1	2	3	4	5
Intestinal motility	1	2	3	4	5
Urinary elimination pat-tern	1	2	3	4	5
Pupil size	1	2	3	4	5
Thermoregulation	1	2	3	4	5
Peripheral tissue perfu-sion	1	2	3	4	5
Appropriate sexual organ response	1	2	3	4	5
Bronchospasms not present	1	2	3	4	5
Intestinal spasms not present	1	2	3	4	5
Bladder spasms not present	1	2	3	4	5
Other _____ Specify	1	2	3	4	5

*WNL = Within normal limits; *BP* = blood pressure.   *Continued.*

Outcomes

BACKGROUND READINGS:

Luckmann, J., & Sorensen, K. (1987). *Medical-surgical nursing: A psychophysiologic approach* (3rd ed.). Philadelphia: W.B. Saunders.

McCance, K.L., & Huether, S.E. (1994). *Pathophysiology: The biologic basis for disease in adults and children* (2nd ed.). St. Louis: Mosby.

NANDA. (1995-1996). *Nursing diagnoses: Definitions & classification.* Philadelphia: North American Nursing Diagnosis Association.

Neurological Status: Central Motor Control

DEFINITION: Extent to which skeletal muscle activity (body movement) is coordinated by the central nervous system

NEUROLOGICAL STATUS: CENTRAL MOTOR CONTROL	Extremely compromised 1	Substantially compromised 2	Moderately compromised 3	Mildly compromised 4	Not compromised 5
INDICATORS:					
Balance	1	2	3	4	5
Gait effectiveness	1	2	3	4	5
Maintenance of posture	1	2	3	4	5
Infantile reflexes (automatisms)	1	2	3	4	5
Babinski's reflex	1	2	3	4	5
Deep tendon reflexes	1	2	3	4	5
Spasticity not present	1	2	3	4	5
Involuntary movements not present	1	2	3	4	5
Nystagmus not present	1	2	3	4	5
Seizure activity not present	1	2	3	4	5
Other _____ Specify	1	2	3	4	5

BACKGROUND READINGS:

American Nurses' Association Council on Medical-Surgical Nursing Practice and American Association of Neuroscience Nurses. (1985). *Neuroscience nursing practice: process and outcome criteria for selected diagnoses.* Washington, DC: U.S. Government Printing Office.

Bates, B. (1987). *A guide to physical examination and history taking* (4th ed.). Philadelphia: J.B. Lippincott.

Hickey, J.V. (1992). *The clinical practice of neurological and neurosurgical nursing* (3rd ed.). Philadelphia: J.B. Lippincott.

Luckmann, J., & Sorensen, K. (1987). *Medical-surgical nursing: A psychophysiologic approach* (3rd ed.). Philadelphia: W.B. Saunders.

Mitchell, P.H., Hodges, L.C., Muwaswes, M., & Walleck, C.A. (Eds.). (1988). *AANN's neuroscience nursing: Phenomena and practice.* Norwalk, CT: Appleton & Lange.

Neurological Status: Consciousness

DEFINITION: Extent to which an individual arouses, orients, and attends to the environment

NEUROLOGICAL STATUS: CONSCIOUSNESS	Extremely compromised 1	Substantially compromised 2	Moderately compromised 3	Mildly compromised 4	Not compromised 5
INDICATORS:					
Opens eyes to external stimuli	1	2	3	4	5
Cognitive orientation	1	2	3	4	5
Communication appropriate to situation	1	2	3	4	5
Obeys commands	1	2	3	4	5
Motor responses to noxious stimuli	1	2	3	4	5
Attends to environmental stimuli	1	2	3	4	5
Seizure activity not present	1	2	3	4	5
Other _____ Specify	1	2	3	4	5

BACKGROUND READINGS:

American Nurses' Association Council on Medical-Surgical Nursing Practice and American Association of Neuroscience Nurses. (1985). *Neuroscience nursing practice: process and outcome criteria for selected diagnoses.* Washington, DC: U.S. Government Printing Office.

Hickey, J.V. (1992). *The clinical practice of neurological and neurosurgical nursing* (3rd ed.). Philadelphia: J.B. Lippincott.

Luckmann, J. & Sorensen, K. (1987). *Medical-surgical nursing: A psychophysiologic approach* (3rd ed.). Philadelphia: W.B. Saunders.

Mitchell, P.H., Hodges, L.C., Muwaswes, M., & Walleck, C.A. (Eds.), (1988). *AANN's neuroscience nursing: Phenomena and practice.* Norwalk, CT: Appleton & Lange.

Riess, P.C. (1995). Validity and reliability of the Riess intracranial aneurysm assessment tool and the Glasgow coma scale in the aneurysm population. Master's thesis, The University of Iowa: Iowa City.

Neurological Status: Cranial Sensory/Motor Function

DEFINITION: Extent to which cranial nerves convey sensory and motor information

NEUROLOGICAL STATUS: CRANIAL SENSORY/MOTOR FUNCTION	Extremely compromised 1	Substantially compromised 2	Moderately compromised 3	Mildly compromised 4	Not compromised 5
INDICATORS:					
Olfaction	1	2	3	4	5
Vision	1	2	3	4	5
Eye reflexes	1	2	3	4	5
Taste	1	2	3	4	5
Hearing	1	2	3	4	5
Facial sensation	1	2	3	4	5
Facial muscle movement	1	2	3	4	5
Swallowing	1	2	3	4	5
Gag reflex	1	2	3	4	5
Tongue movement	1	2	3	4	5
Head orientation	1	2	3	4	5
Head and shoulder movement	1	2	3	4	5
Autonomic function	1	2	3	4	5
Dizziness not present	1	2	3	4	5
Pronator drift not present	1	2	3	4	5
Other _____ Specify	1	2	3	4	5

BACKGROUND READINGS:

Bates, B. (1987). *A guide to physical examination and history taking* (4th ed.). Philadelphia: J.B. Lippincott.

Luckmann, J., & Sorensen, K. (1987). *Medical-surgical nursing: A psychophysiologic approach* (3rd ed.). Philadelphia: W.B. Saunders.

Riess, P.C. (1995). Validity and reliability of the Riess intracranial aneurysm assessment tool and the Glasgow coma scale in the aneurysm population. Master's thesis, The University of Iowa, Iowa City.

Outcomes

Neurological Status: Spinal Sensory/Motor Function

DEFINITION: Extent to which spinal nerves convey sensory and motor information

NEUROLOGICAL STATUS: SPINAL SENSORY/MOTOR FUNCTION	Extremely compromised 1	Substantially compromised 2	Moderately compromised 3	Mildly compromised 4	Not compromised 5
INDICATORS:					
Head and shoulder movement	1	2	3	4	5
Autonomic function	1	2	3	4	5
Deep tendon reflexes	1	2	3	4	5
Body skin sensation	1	2	3	4	5
Strength of extremity movement	1	2	3	4	5
Flaccidity not present	1	2	3	4	5
Pronator drift not present	1	2	3	4	5
Other _____ Specify	1	2	3	4	5

BACKGROUND READINGS:

Bates, B. (1987). *A guide to physical examination and history taking* (4th ed.). Philadelphia: J.B. Lippincott.

Luckmann, J., & Sorensen, K. (1987). *Medical-surgical nursing: A psychophysiologic approach* (3rd ed.). Philadelphia, W.B. Saunders.

Riess, P.C. (1995). Validity and reliability of the Riess intracranial aneurysm assessment tool and the Glasgow coma scale in the aneurysm population. Master's thesis, The University of Iowa, Iowa City.

Nutritional Status

DEFINITION: Extent to which nutrients are available to meet metabolic needs

NUTRITIONAL STATUS	Extremely compromised 1	Substantially compromised 2	Moderately compromised 3	Mildly compromised 4	Not compromised 5
INDICATORS:					
Nutrient intake	1	2	3	4	5
Food and fluid intake	1	2	3	4	5
Energy	1	2	3	4	5
Body mass	1	2	3	4	5
Weight	1	2	3	4	5
Biochemical measures	1	2	3	4	5
Other _____ Specify	1	2	3	4	5

Outcomes

BACKGROUND READINGS:

Chang, B.L., Uman, G.C., Linn, L.S., Ware, J.E., & Kane, R.L. (1985). Adherence to healthcare regimens among elderly women. *Nursing Research, 34*(1), 27-31.

Collinsworth, R., & Boyle, K. (1989). Nutritional assessment of the elderly. *Journal of Gerontological Nursing, 15*(12), 17-21.

Curtas, S., Chapman, G., & Meguid, M. (1989). Evaluation of nutritional status. *Nursing Clinics of North America, 24*(2), 301-313.

Folsom, A.R., Kaye, S.A., Sellers, T.A., Hang, C.P., Cerhan, J.R., Potter, J.D., Prineas, R.J. (1993). Body fat distribution and five year risk of death in older women. *Journal of the American Medical Association, 269*(4), 483-487.

Gianino, S., & St. John, R.E. (1993). Nutritional assessment of the patient in the intensive care unit. *Critical Care Nursing Clinics of North America, 5*(1), 1-16.

Nutritional Status: Biochemical Measures

DEFINITION: Body fluid components and chemical indices of nutritional status

NUTRITIONAL STATUS: BIOCHEMICAL MEASURES	Extreme deviation from expected range 1	Substantial deviation from expected range 2	Moderate deviation from expected range 3	Mild deviation from expected range 4	No deviation from expected range 5
INDICATORS:					
Serum albumin	1	2	3	4	5
Serum prealbumin	1	2	3	4	5
Hematocrit	1	2	3	4	5
Hemoglobin	1	2	3	4	5
Total iron binding capacity	1	2	3	4	5
Lymphocyte count	1	2	3	4	5
Blood glucose	1	2	3	4	5
Blood cholesterol	1	2	3	4	5
Blood triglycerides	1	2	3	4	5
Serum transferrin	1	2	3	4	5
24-hour urinary creatinine	1	2	3	4	5
Urinary urea nitrogen	1	2	3	4	5
Other _____ Specify	1	2	3	4	5

BACKGROUND READINGS:

Chang, B.L., Uman, G.C., Linn, L.S., Ware, J.E., & Kane, R.L. (1985). Adherence to healthcare regimens among elderly women. *Nursing Research, 34*(1), 27-31.

Collinsworth, R., & Boyle, K. (1989). Nutritional assessment of the elderly. *Journal of Gerontological Nursing, 15*(12), 17-21.

Curtas, S., Chapman, G., & Meguid, M. (1989). Evaluation of nutritional status. *Nursing Clinics of North America, 24*(2), 301-313.

Folsom, A.R., Kaye, S.A., Sellers, T.A., Hang, C.P., Cerhan, J.R., Potter, J.D., & Prineas, R.J. (1993). Body fat distribution and five year risk of death in older women. *Journal of American Medical Association, 269*(4), 483-487.

Gianino, S., & St. John, R.E. (1993). Nutritional assessment of the patient in the intensive care unit. *Critical Care Nursing Clinics of North America, 5*(1), 1-16.

Nutritional Status: Body Mass

DEFINITION: Congruence of body weight, muscle, and fat to height, frame, and gender

NUTRITIONAL STATUS: BODY MASS	Extreme deviation from expected range **1**	Substantial deviation from expected range **2**	Moderate deviation from expected range **3**	Mild deviation from expected range **4**	No deviation from expected range **5**
INDICATORS:					
Weight	1	2	3	4	5
Triceps skinfold thickness	1	2	3	4	5
Subscapular skinfold thickness	1	2	3	4	5
Waist/hip circumference ratio (women)	1	2	3	4	5
Neck/waist circumference ratio (men)	1	2	3	4	5
Body fat percentage	1	2	3	4	5
Head circumference percentile (child)	1	2	3	4	5
Height percentile (child)	1	2	3	4	5
Weight percentile (child)	1	2	3	4	5
Other _____ Specify	1	2	3	4	5

BACKGROUND READINGS:

Chang, B.L., Uman, G.C., Linn, L.S., Ware, J.E., & Kane, R.L. (1985). Adherence to healthcare regimens among elderly women. *Nursing Research, 34*(1), 27-31.

Collinsworth, R., & Boyle, K. (1989). Nutritional assessment of the elderly. *Journal of Gerontological Nursing, 15*(12), 17-21.

Curtas, S., Chapman, G., & Meguid, M. (1989). Evaluation of nutritional status. *Nursing Clinics of North America, 24*(2), 301-313.

Folsom, A.R., Kaye, S.A., Sellers, T.A., Hang, C.P., Cerhan, J.R., Potter, J.D., & Prineas, R.J. (1993). Body fat distribution and five year risk of death in older women. *Journal of the American Medical Association, 269*(4), 483-487.

Gianino, S., & St. John, R.E. (1993). Nutritional assessment of the patient in the intensive care unit. *Critical Care Nursing Clinics of North America, 5*(1), 1-16.

Nutritional Status: Energy

DEFINITION: Extent to which nutrients provide cellular energy

NUTRITIONAL STATUS: ENERGY	Extremely compromised 1	Substantially compromised 2	Moderately compromised 3	Mildly compromised 4	Not compromised 5
INDICATORS:					
Stamina	1	2	3	4	5
Endurance	1	2	3	4	5
Hand grip strength	1	2	3	4	5
Tissue healing	1	2	3	4	5
Infection resistance	1	2	3	4	5
Growth (children)	1	2	3	4	5
Other _____ Specify	1	2	3	4	5

BACKGROUND READINGS:

Chang, B.L., Uman, G.C., Linn, L.S., Ware, J.E., & Kane, R.L. (1985). Adherence to healthcare regimens among elderly women. *Nursing Research, 34*(1), 27-31.

Collinsworth, R., & Boyle, K. (1989). Nutritional assessment of the elderly. *Journal of Gerontological Nursing, 15*(12), 17-21.

Curtas, S., Chapman, G., & Meguid, M. (1989). Evaluation of nutritional status. *Nursing Clinics of North America, 24*(2), 301-313.

Folsom, A.R., Kaye, S.A., Sellers, T.A., Hang, C.P., Cerhan, J.R., Potter, J.D., Prineas, R.J. (1993). Body fat distribution and 5 year risk of death in older women. *Journal of American Medical Association, 269*(4), 483-487.

Gianino, S., & St. John, R.E. (1993). Nutritional assessment of the patient in the intensive care unit. *Critical Care Nursing Clinics of North America, 5*(1), 1-16.

Outcomes

Nutritional Status: Food & Fluid Intake

DEFINITION: Amount of food and fluid taken into the body over a 24 hour period

NUTRITIONAL STATUS: FOOD & FLUID INTAKE	Not adequate 1	Slightly adequate 2	Moderately adequate 3	Substantially adequate 4	Totally adequate 5
INDICATORS:					
Oral food intake	1	2	3	4	5
Tube feeding intake	1	2	3	4	5
Oral fluid intake	1	2	3	4	5
IV* fluid intake	1	2	3	4	5
TPN* intake	1	2	3	4	5
Other _____ Specify	1	2	3	4	5

*IV = Intravenous; TPN = total parenteral nutrition.

BACKGROUND READINGS:

Champagne, M.T., & Ashley, M.L. (1989). Nutritional support in the critically ill elderly patient. *Critical Care Nursing Quarterly, 12*(1), 15-25.

Gianino, S., & St. John, R.E. (1993). Nutritional assessment of the patient in the intensive care unit. *Critical Care Nursing Clinics of North America, 5*(1), 1-16.

Keithley, J.K., & Kohn, C.L. (1990). Managing nutritional problems in people with AIDS. *Oncology Nursing Forum, 17*(1), 23-27.

Outcomes

Nutritional Status: Nutrient Intake

DEFINITION: Adequacy of nutrients taken into the body

NUTRITIONAL STATUS: NUTRIENT INTAKE	Not adequate 1	Slightly adequate 2	Moderately adequate 3	Substantially adequate 4	Totally adequate 5
INDICATORS:					
Caloric intake	1	2	3	4	5
Protein intake	1	2	3	4	5
Fat intake	1	2	3	4	5
Carbohydrate intake	1	2	3	4	5
Vitamin intake	1	2	3	4	5
Mineral intake	1	2	3	4	5
Iron intake	1	2	3	4	5
Calcium intake	1	2	3	4	5
Other _____ Specify	1	2	3	4	5

BACKGROUND READINGS:

Champagne, M.T., & Ashley, M.L. (1989). Nutritional support in the critically ill elderly patient. *Critical Care Nursing Quarterly, 12*(1), 15-25.

Gianino, S., & St. John, R.E. (1993). Nutritional assessment of the patient in the intensive care unit. *Critical Care Nursing Clinics of North America, 5*(1), 1-16.

Keithley, J.K., & Kohn, C.L. (1990). Managing nutritional problems in people with AIDS. *Oncology Nursing Forum, 17*(1), 23-27.

Outcomes

Oral Health

DEFINITION: Condition of the mouth, teeth, gums, and tongue

ORAL HEALTH	Extremely compromised 1	Substantially compromised 2	Moderately compromised 3	Mildly compromised 4	Not compromised 5
INDICATORS:					
Cleanliness of mouth	1	2	3	4	5
Cleanliness of teeth	1	2	3	4	5
Cleanliness of gums	1	2	3	4	5
Cleanliness of tongue	1	2	3	4	5
Cleanliness of dentures	1	2	3	4	5
Cleanliness of dental appliances	1	2	3	4	5
Fit of dentures	1	2	3	4	5
Fit of dental appliances	1	2	3	4	5
Moistness of lips	1	2	3	4	5
Moisture of oral mucosa and tongue	1	2	3	4	5
Color of mucosa membranes	1	2	3	4	5
Oral mucosa integrity	1	2	3	4	5
Tongue integrity	1	2	3	4	5
Gum integrity	1	2	3	4	5
Tooth integrity	1	2	3	4	5
Breath odor	1	2	3	4	5
Breath free of halitosis	1	2	3	4	5
Other _____ Specify	1	2	3	4	5

Outcomes

BACKGROUND READINGS:

Fischman, S. (1993). Self-care: Practical periodontal care in today's practice. *International Dental Journal, 43,* 179-183.

Jones, J.A. (1989). Integrating the oral examination into clinical practice. *Hospital Practice, 24*(10A), 23-24, 26-27, 30.

Mattheson, M.A., & McConnell E.S. (1988). *Gerontological nursing: Concepts & practice.* Philadelphia: W.B. Saunders.

Raybould, T.P., Carpenter, A.D., Ferretti, G.A., Brown, A.T., Lillich, T.T., & Henslee, J. (1994). Emergence of gram-negative bacilli in the mouths of bone marrow transplant recipients using chlorhexidine mouth rinse. *Oncology Nursing Forum, 21*(4), 691-696.

Richardson, A. (1987). A process standard for oral care. *Nursing Times, 83,* 38-40.

Speedie, G. (1983). Nursology of mouth care: Preventing, comforting and seeking activities related to mouth care. *Journal of Advanced Nursing, 8*(1), 33-40.

Pain Control Behavior

DEFINITION: Personal actions to control pain

PAIN CONTROL BEHAVIOR	Never demonstrated 1	Rarely demonstrated 2	Sometimes demonstrated 3	Often demonstrated 4	Consistently demonstrated 5
INDICATORS:					
Recognizes causal factors	1	2	3	4	5
Recognizes pain onset	1	2	3	4	5
Uses preventive measures	1	2	3	4	5
Uses non-analgesic relief measures	1	2	3	4	5
Uses analgesics appropriately	1	2	3	4	5
Uses warning signs to seek care	1	2	3	4	5
Reports symptoms to health care professional	1	2	3	4	5
Uses available resources	1	2	3	4	5
Recognizes symptoms of pain	1	2	3	4	5
Uses pain diary	1	2	3	4	5
Reports pain controlled	1	2	3	4	5
Other _____ Specify	1	2	3	4	5

BACKGROUND READINGS:

Howe, C.J. (1993). A new standard of care for pediatric pain management. *MCN: American Journal of Maternal Child Nursing, 18*(6), 325-329.

Jacox, A., Carr, D.B., Payne, R. et al. (1994). *Management of cancer pain. Clinical practice guideline* No. 9 (AHCPR Publication No. 94-0592). Rockville, MD: Agency for Health Care Policy and Research, U.S. Department of Health and Human Services, Public Health Service.

Puntillo, K., & Weiss, S.J. (1994). Pain: Its mediators and associated morbidity in critically ill cardiovascular surgical patients. *Nursing Research, 43*(1), 31-36.

Sherbourne, C.D. (1992). Pain measures. In A.L. Stewart & J.E. Ware, Jr. (Eds.), *Measuring functioning and well-being* (pp. 220-234). Durham, NC: Duke University Press.

Acute Pain Management Guideline Panel. (1992). *Acute pain management: Operative or medical procedures and trauma. Clinical practice guideline* (AHCPR Publication No. 92-0032). Rockville, MD: Agency for Health Care Policy and Research, Public Health Service, U.S. Department of Health and Human Services.

Pain: Disruptive Effects

DEFINITION: Observed or reported disruptive effects of pain on emotions and behavior

PAIN: DISRUPTIVE EFFECTS	Severe 1	Substantial 2	Moderate 3	Slight 4	None 5
INDICATORS:					
Impaired interpersonal relationships	1	2	3	4	5
Impaired role performance	1	2	3	4	5
Compromised play	1	2	3	4	5
Compromised leisure activities	1	2	3	4	5
Compromised work	1	2	3	4	5
Compromised life enjoyment	1	2	3	4	5
Compromised sense of control	1	2	3	4	5
Impaired concentration	1	2	3	4	5
Compromised sense of hope	1	2	3	4	5
Impaired mood	1	2	3	4	5
Lack of patience	1	2	3	4	5
Disrupted sleep	1	2	3	4	5
Impaired physical mobility	1	2	3	4	5
Impaired self-care	1	2	3	4	5
Lack of appetite	1	2	3	4	5
Difficulty eating	1	2	3	4	5
Impaired elimination	1	2	3	4	5
Other _____ Specify	1	2	3	4	5

BACKGROUND READINGS:

Howe, C.J. (1993). A new standard of care for pediatric pain management. *MCN: American Journal of Maternal Child Nursing, 18,* 325-329.

Jacox, A., Carr, D.B., Payne, R. et al. (1994). *Management of cancer pain. Clinical practice guideline* No. 9 (AHCPR Publication No. 94-0592). Rockville, MD: Agency for Health Care Policy and Research, U.S. Department of Health and Human Services, Public Health Service.

Puntillo, K., & Weiss, S.J. (1994). Pain: Its mediators and associated mobility in critically ill cardiovascular surgical patients. *Nursing Research, 43*(1), 31-36.

Sherbourne, C.D. (1992). Pain measures. In A.L. Stewart & J.E. Ware, Jr. (Eds.), *Measuring functioning and well-being* (pp. 220-234). Durham, NC: Duke University Press.

Acute Pain Management Guideline Panel. (1992). *Acute pain management: Operative or medical procedures and trauma. Clinical practice guideline* (AHCPR Publication No. 92-0032). Rockville, MD: Agency for Health Care Policy and Research, Public Health Service, U.S. Department of Health and Human Services.

Pain Level

DEFINITION: Amount of reported or demonstrated pain

PAIN LEVEL	Severe 1	Substantial 2	Moderate 3	Slight 4	None 5
INDICATORS:					
Reported pain	1	2	3	4	5
Percent of body affected	1	2	3	4	5
Frequency of pain	1	2	3	4	5
Length of pain episodes	1	2	3	4	5
Oral expressions of pain	1	2	3	4	5
Facial expressions of pain	1	2	3	4	5
Protective body positions	1	2	3	4	5
Restlessness	1	2	3	4	5
Muscle tension	1	2	3	4	5
Change in respiratory rate	1	2	3	4	5
Change in heart rate	1	2	3	4	5
Change in BP*	1	2	3	4	5
Change in pupil size	1	2	3	4	5
Perspiration	1	2	3	4	5
Appetite loss	1	2	3	4	5
Other _____ Specify	1	2	3	4	5

*BP = Blood pressure.

BACKGROUND READINGS:

Howe, C.J. (1993). A new standard of care for pediatric pain management. *MCN: American Journal of Maternal Child Nursing, 18,* 325-329.

Jacox, A., Carr, D.B., Payne, R. et al. (1994). *Management of cancer pain. Clinical practice guideline* No. 9 (AHCPR Publication No. 94-0592). Rockville, MD: Agency for Health Care Policy and Research, U.S. Department of Health and Human Services, Public Health Service.

Puntillo, K., & Weiss, S.J. (1994). Pain: Its mediators and associated morbidity in critically ill cardiovascular surgical patients. *Nursing Research, 43*(1), 31-36.

Sherbourne, C.D. (1992). Pain measures. In A.L. Stewart, & J.E. Ware, Jr. (Eds.), *Measuring functioning and well-being* (pp. 220-234). Durham, NC: Duke University Press.

Acute Pain Management Guideline Panel. (1992). *Acute pain management: Operative or medical procedures and trauma. Clinical practice guideline* (AHCPR Publication No. 92-0032). Rockville, MD: Agency for Health Care Policy and Research, Public Health Service, U.S. Department of Health and Human Services.

Outcomes

Parent-Infant Attachment

PARENT-INFANT ATTACHMENT	Never demonstrated 1	Rarely demonstrated 2	Sometimes demonstrated 3	Often demonstrated 4	Consistently demonstrated 5

DEFINITION: Behaviors which demonstrate an enduring affectionate bond between a parent and infant

PARENT-INFANT ATTACHMENT	Never demonstrated 1	Rarely demonstrated 2	Sometimes demonstrated 3	Often demonstrated 4	Consistently demonstrated 5
INDICATORS:					
Parent(s) practice healthy behaviors during pregnancy	1	2	3	4	5
Parent(s) assign specific attributes to fetus	1	2	3	4	5
Parent(s) prepare for infant prior to birth	1	2	3	4	5
Parent(s) verbalize positive feelings toward infant	1	2	3	4	5
Parent(s) hold infant close	1	2	3	4	5
Parent(s) touch, stroke, pat infant	1	2	3	4	5
Parent(s) kiss infant	1	2	3	4	5
Parent(s) smile at infant	1	2	3	4	5
Parent(s) visit nursery	1	2	3	4	5
Parent(s) talk to infant	1	2	3	4	5
Parent(s) use en face position	1	2	3	4	5
Parent(s) use eye contact	1	2	3	4	5
Parent(s) smile and vocalize to infant	1	2	3	4	5
Parent(s) play with infant	1	2	3	4	5
Parent(s) respond to infant cues	1	2	3	4	5
Parent(s) console/soothe infant	1	2	3	4	5
Parent(s) feed infant	1	2	3	4	5
Parent(s) keep infant dry, clean, and warm	1	2	3	4	5
Infant looks at parent(s)	1	2	3	4	5
Infant responds to parent(s)' cues	1	2	3	4	5

Continued.

Outcomes

Outcomes

PARENT-INFANT ATTACHMENT— cont'd	Never demonstrated 1	Rarely demonstrated 2	Sometimes demonstrated 3	Often demonstrated 4	Consistently demonstrated 5
Infant seeks proximity with parent(s)	1	2	3	4	5
Infant explores environment	1	2	3	4	5
Other _____ Specify	1	2	3	4	5

BACKGROUND READINGS:

Ainsworth, M.S., & Wittig, B.A. (1969). Attachment and exploratory behavior of one-year olds in a strange situation. In B.M. Foss (Ed.), *Determinants of infant behavior* (pp. 111-133). London: Methuen.

Kennell, J., Jerauld, R., Wolfe, H., Chesler, D., Kreger, N.C., McAlpine, W., Steffa, M., & Klaus, M.H. (1974). Maternal behavior one year after early and extended post-partum contact. *Developmental Medicine and Child Neurology, 16,* 172-279.

Koniak-Griffin, D. (1988). The relationship between social support, self-esteem, and maternal-fetal attachment in adolescents. *Research in Nursing and Health, 11,* 269-278.

Norr, K.F., Roberts, J.E., & Freese, U. (1989). Early postpartum rooming-in and maternal attachment behaviors in a group of medically indigent primiparas. *Journal of Nurse-Midwifery, 34*(2), 85-91.

Parenting

DEFINITION: Provision of an environment that promotes optimum growth and development of dependent children

PARENTING	Not adequate 1	Slightly adequate 2	Moderately adequate 3	Substantially adequate 4	Totally adequate 5
INDICATORS:					
Provides for child's physical needs	1	2	3	4	5
Eliminates controllable environmental hazards	1	2	3	4	5
Provides regular preventative and episodic health care	1	2	3	4	5
Stimulates cognitive development	1	2	3	4	5
Stimulates social development	1	2	3	4	5
Stimulates emotional growth	1	2	3	4	5
Stimulates spiritual growth	1	2	3	4	5
Uses community and other resources as appropriate	1	2	3	4	5
Reports having a functional support system	1	2	3	4	5
Uses interactions appropriate for child's temperament	1	2	3	4	5
Uses behavior management if indicated	1	2	3	4	5
Uses appropriate discipline	1	2	3	4	5
Provides for child's special needs	1	2	3	4	5
Interacts positively with child	1	2	3	4	5
Demonstrates empathy toward child	1	2	3	4	5
Verbalizes positive attributes of child	1	2	3	4	5
Demonstrates a loving relationship with child	1	2	3	4	5
Has realistic expectations of parental role	1	2	3	4	5
Expresses satisfaction with parental role	1	2	3	4	5
Demonstrates positive self-esteem	1	2	3	4	5
Other _____ Specify	1	2	3	4	5

BACKGROUND READINGS:

Causby, V., Nixon, C., & Bright, J.M. (1991). Influences on adolescent mother-infant interactions. *Adolescence, 26*(103), 619-630.

Fulton, A.M., Murphy, K.R., & Anderson, S.L. (1991). Increasing adolescent mothers' knowledge of child development: An intervention program. *Adolescence, 26*(101), 73-81.

Greaves, P., Glik, D.C. Kronenfeld, J.J., & Jackson, K. (1994). Determinants of controllable in-home child safety hazards. *Health Education Research, 9*(3), 307-315.

Continued.

Mercer, R.T., & Ferketich, S.L. (1994). Predictors of maternal role competence by risk status. *Nursing Research, 43*(1), 38-43.

Ohashi, J.P. (1992). Maternal role satisfaction: A new approach to assessing parenting. *Scholarly Inquiry for Nursing Practice: An International Journal, 6*(2), 135-149.

Reece, S.M. (1995). Stress and maternal adaptation in first-time mothers more than 35 years old. *Applied Nursing Research, 8*(2), 61-66.

Thompson, P.J., Powell, M.J., Patterson, R.J., & Ellerbee, S.M. (1995). Adolescent parenting: Outcomes and maternal perceptions. *Journal of Obstetric, Gynecologic, and Neonatal Nursing, 24*(8), 713-718.

Parenting: Social Safety

Outcomes

DEFINITION: Parental actions to avoid social relationships that might cause harm or injury

PARENTING: SOCIAL SAFETY	Not adequate 1	Slightly adequate 2	Moderately adequate 3	Substantially adequate 4	Totally adequate 5
INDICATORS:					
Monitoring of playmates	1	2	3	4	5
Monitoring of social contacts	1	2	3	4	5
Monitoring of supplemental caregiver(s)	1	2	3	4	5
Selection of supplemental caregivers(s)	1	2	3	4	5
Recognition of risk of abuse	1	2	3	4	5
Intervention to eliminate risk(s) of abuse	1	2	3	4	5
Intervention to eliminate abuse	1	2	3	4	5
Provision of nurturing environment	1	2	3	4	5
Provision of supervision	1	2	3	4	5
Provision of age appropriate social opportunities	1	2	3	4	5
Initiation of agreement to prevent high-risk social behaviors	1	2	3	4	5
Intervention to prevent high-risk social behaviors	1	2	3	4	5
Intervention to prevent gang participation	1	2	3	4	5
Other _____ Specify	1	2	3	4	5

BACKGROUND READINGS:

Glick, D., Kronenfeld, J., & Jackson, K. (1993). Safety behaviors among parents of preschoolers. *Health Values, 17*(1), 18-27.

Jensen, L.R., Williams, S.D., Thurman, D.J., & Keller, P.A. (1992). Submersion injuries for children less than 5 years in urban Utah. *Western Journal of Medicine, 157*(6), 641-644.

Quan, L., Gore, E.J., Wentz, K., Allen, J., & Novack, A.H. (1989). Ten year study of pediatric drownings and near-drownings in King County, Washington: Lessons in injury prevention. *Pediatrics, 83*(6), 1035-1040.

Outcomes

Participation: Health Care Decisions

DEFINITION: Personal involvement in selecting and evaluating health care options

PARTICIPATION: HEALTH CARE DECISIONS	Never demonstrated 1	Rarely demonstrated 2	Sometimes demonstrated 3	Often demonstrated 4	Consistently demonstrated 5
INDICATORS:					
Claims decision making responsibility	1	2	3	4	5
Demonstrates self direction in decision making	1	2	3	4	5
Seeks information	1	2	3	4	5
Defines available options	1	2	3	4	5
Specifies health outcome preferences	1	2	3	4	5
Identifies health outcome priorities	1	2	3	4	5
Identifies barriers to desired outcome achievement	1	2	3	4	5
Uses problem solving techniques to achieve desired outcomes	1	2	3	4	5
States intent to act on decision	1	2	3	4	5
Identifies available support for achieving desired outcomes	1	2	3	4	5
Seeks services to meet desired outcomes	1	2	3	4	5
Negotiates for care preferences	1	2	3	4	5
Monitors barriers to outcome achievement	1	2	3	4	5
Identifies level of health care outcome achievement	1	2	3	4	5
Evaluates satisfaction with health care outcomes	1	2	3	4	5
Other _____ Specify	1	2	3	4	5

BACKGROUND READINGS:

Conn, V., Taylor S., & Casey, B. (1992). Cardiac rehabilitation program participation and outcomes after myocardial infarction. *Rehabilitation Nursing, 17*(2), 58-62.

Epstein, L., & Cluss (1982). A behavioral perspective on adherence for long-term medical regimens. *Journal of Consulting and Clinical Psychology, 50,* 950-971.

Hegyvary, S.T. (1993). Patient care outcomes related to management of symptoms. In J.J. Fitzpatrick & J.J. Stevenson (Eds.), *Annual review of nursing research.* (Vol. 11, pp. 145-168). New York: Springer.

Outcomes

Physical Aging Status

DEFINITION: Physical changes that commonly occur with adult aging

PHYSICAL AGING STATUS	Extreme deviation from expected range 1	Substantial deviation from expected range 2	Moderate deviation from expected range 3	Mild deviation from expected range 4	No deviation from expected range 5
INDICATORS:					
Mean body mass	1	2	3	4	5
Bone density	1	2	3	4	5
Cardiac output	1	2	3	4	5
Vital capacity	1	2	3	4	5
Blood pressure	1	2	3	4	5
Skin elasticity	1	2	3	4	5
Muscle strength	1	2	3	4	5
Hearing acuity	1	2	3	4	5
Visual acuity	1	2	3	4	5
Olfactory acuity	1	2	3	4	5
Taste acuity	1	2	3	4	5
Basal metabolic rate	1	2	3	4	5
Fat distribution pattern	1	2	3	4	5
Hair distribution pattern	1	2	3	4	5
Menstrual pattern	1	2	3	4	5
Sexual functioning	1	2	3	4	5
Other _____ Specify	1	2	3	4	5

BACKGROUND READINGS:

Frieberg, K. (1992). *Human development: A life span approach* (4th ed.). Boston: Jones and Bartlett.

Miller, B., & Keane, C. (1972). *Encyclopedia and dictionary of medicine and nursing.* Philadelphia: W.B. Saunders.

Schuster, C., & Ashburn, S. (1992). *The process of human development: A holistic approach* (3rd ed.). Philadelphia: J.B. Lippincott.

Whaley, L., & Wong, D. (1991). *Nursing care of infants and children* (4th ed.). St. Louis: Mosby.

Outcomes

Physical Maturation: Female

Outcomes

DEFINITION: Normal physical changes in the female that occur with the transition from childhood to adulthood

PHYSICAL MATURATION: FEMALE	Extreme deviation from expected range 1	Substantial deviation from expected range 2	Moderate deviation from expected range 3	Mild deviation from expected range 4	No deviation from expected range 5
INDICATORS:					
Growth spurt between 9.5-14.5 years of age	1	2	3	4	5
Bone closure	1	2	3	4	5
Voice changes	1	2	3	4	5
Adult hair distribution	1	2	3	4	5
Breast development	1	2	3	4	5
Menstruation onset	1	2	3	4	5
Increased muscle mass	1	2	3	4	5
Decreased body fat	1	2	3	4	5
Increase in sebaceous secretions	1	2	3	4	5
Increase in perspiration	1	2	3	4	5
Other _____ Specify	1	2	3	4	5

BACKGROUND READINGS:

Frieberg, K. (1992). *Human development: A life span approach* (4th ed.). Boston: Jones and Bartlett.

Miller, B., & Keane, C. (1972). *Encyclopedia and dictionary of medicine and nursing.* Philadelphia: W.B. Saunders.

Schuster, C., & Ashburn, S. (1992). *The process of human development: A holistic approach* (3rd ed.). Philadelphia: J.B. Lippincott.

Whaley, L., & Wong, D. (1991). *Nursing care of infants and children* (4th ed.). St. Louis: Mosby.

Physical Maturation: Male

DEFINITION: Normal physical changes in the male that occur with the transition from childhood to adulthood

PHYSICAL MATURATION: MALE	Extreme deviation from expected range 1	Substantial deviation from expected range 2	Moderate deviation from expected range 3	Mild deviation from expected range 4	No deviation from expected range 5
INDICATORS:					
Growth spurt between 10.5-16 years of age	1	2	3	4	5
Bone closure	1	2	3	4	5
Voice changes	1	2	3	4	5
Adult hair distribution	1	2	3	4	5
Testicular descent	1	2	3	4	5
Penis enlargement	1	2	3	4	5
First ejaculation of sperm (wet dream)	1	2	3	4	5
Increased muscle mass	1	2	3	4	5
Decreased body fat	1	2	3	4	5
Increase in sebaceous secretions	1	2	3	4	5
Increase in perspiration	1	2	3	4	5
Other _____ Specify	1	2	3	4	5

BACKGROUND READINGS:

Frieberg, K. (1992). *Human development: A life span approach* (4th ed.). Boston: Jones and Bartlett.

Miller, B., & Keane, C. (1972). *Encyclopedia and dictionary of medicine and nursing*. Philadelphia: W.B. Saunders.

Schuster, C., & Ashburn, S. (1992). *The process of human development: A holistic approach* (3rd ed.). Philadelphia: J.B. Lippincott.

Whaley, L., & Wong, D. (1991). *Nursing care of infants and children* (4th ed.). St. Louis: Mosby.

Outcomes

Play Participation

DEFINITION: Use of activities as needed for enjoyment, entertainment, and development by children

PLAY PARTICIPATION	Not adequate 1	Slightly adequate 2	Moderately adequate 3	Substantially adequate 4	Totally adequate 5
INDICATORS:					
Participation in play	1	2	3	4	5
Appropriateness of play	1	2	3	4	5
Expression of enjoyment in play	1	2	3	4	5
Use of social skills during play	1	2	3	4	5
Use of physical skills during play	1	2	3	4	5
Use of imagination during play	1	2	3	4	5
Expression of emotions during play	1	2	3	4	5
Use of role playing	1	2	3	4	5
Other _____ Specify	1	2	3	4	5

BACKGROUND READINGS:

Gillis, A.J. (1989). The effect of play on immobilized children in hospital. *International Journal of Nursing Studies, 26*(3), 261-269.

Gray, E. (1989). The emotional and play needs of the dying child. *Issues in Comprehensive Pediatric Nursing, 12*(2/3); 207-224.

Jack, L.W. (1987). Using play in psychiatric rehabilitation. *Journal of Psychosocial Nursing, 25*(7), 17-20.

Post, C. (1990). Play therapy with an abused child: A case study. *Journal of Child and Adolescent Psychiatric and Mental Health Nursing, 2*(2), 48-51.

Psychosocial Adjustment: Life Change

DEFINITION: Psychosocial adaptation of an individual to a life change

PSYCHOSOCIAL ADJUSTMENT: LIFE CHANGE	None 1	Limited 2	Moderate 3	Substantial 4	Extensive 5
INDICATORS:					
Realistic goal setting	1	2	3	4	5
Maintenance of self-esteem	1	2	3	4	5
Expressions of productivity	1	2	3	4	5
Expressions of usefulness	1	2	3	4	5
Expressions of optimism about present	1	2	3	4	5
Expressions of optimism about future	1	2	3	4	5
Expressions of feeling empowered	1	2	3	4	5
Identification of multiple coping strategies	1	2	3	4	5
Use of effective coping strategies	1	2	3	4	5
Effective financial management	1	2	3	4	5
Expressions of satisfaction with living arrangements	1	2	3	4	5
Expressions of feeling socially engaged	1	2	3	4	5
Expressions of adequate social support	1	2	3	4	5
Participation in leisure interests	1	2	3	4	5
Other _____ Specify	1	2	3	4	5

BACKGROUND READINGS:

Hernan, J.A. (1984). Exploding aging myths through retirement counseling. *Journal of Gerontological Nursing, 10*(4), 31-33.

Neuhs, H.P. (1991). Ready for retirement? *Geriatric Nursing, 12*(5), 240-241.

Rosenkoetter, M.M. (1985). Is your older client ready for a role change after retirement? *Journal of Gerontological Nursing, 11*(9), 21-24.

Tincher, B.J.V. (1992). Retirement: Perspectives and theory. *Physical & Occupational Therapy in Geriatrics, 11*(1), 55-62.

Quality of Life

DEFINITION: An individual's expressed satisfaction with current life circumstances

QUALITY OF LIFE	Extremely compromised 1	Substantially compromised 2	Moderately compromised 3	Mildly compromised 4	Not compromised 5
INDICATORS:					
Satisfaction with health status	1	2	3	4	5
Satisfaction with social circumstances	1	2	3	4	5
Satisfaction with environmental circumstances	1	2	3	4	5
Satisfaction with economic status	1	2	3	4	5
Satisfaction with education level	1	2	3	4	5
Satisfaction with occupation level	1	2	3	4	5
Satisfaction with close relationships	1	2	3	4	5
Satisfaction with achievement of life goals	1	2	3	4	5
Satisfaction with coping ability	1	2	3	4	5
Satisfaction with self-concept	1	2	3	4	5
Satisfaction with pervasive mood	1	2	3	4	5
Other _____ Specify	1	2	3	4	5

BACKGROUND READINGS:

Andrews, F., & Withey, S. (1976). *Social indicators of well-being: Americans' perceptions of life quality.* New York: Plenum Press.

Gill, L., & Flenstein, A.R. (1994). A critical appraisal of the quality of quality-of-life measurements. *Journal of the American Medical Association, 272*(8), 619-626.

Padilla, G., Ferrell, B., Grant, M., & Rhiner, M. (1990). Defining the content domain of quality of life for cancer patients with pain. *Cancer Nursing, 13*(2), 108-115.

Ragsdale, D., Kotarba, J., & Morrow, J. (1992). Quality of life of hospitalized persons with AIDS. *IMAGE-The Journal of Nursing Scholarship, 24*(4), 259-265.

Stewart, A., Ware, J., Sherbourne, C., & Wells, K. (1992). Psychological distress/well-being and cognitive functioning measures. In A. Stewart & J. Ware, Jr. (Eds.), *Measuring functioning and well-being: The medical outcomes study approach* (pp. 102-142). Durham, NC: Duke University Press.

Respiratory Status: Gas Exchange

DEFINITION: Alveolar exchange of CO_2 or O_2 to maintain arterial blood gas concentrations

RESPIRATORY STATUS: GAS EXCHANGE	Extremely compromised 1	Substantially compromised 2	Moderately compromised 3	Mildly compromised 4	Not compromised 5
INDICATORS:					
Neurological status IER*	1	2	3	4	5
Ease of breathing	1	2	3	4	5
Dyspnea at rest not present	1	2	3	4	5
Dyspnea with exertion not present	1	2	3	4	5
Restlessness not present	1	2	3	4	5
Cyanosis not present	1	2	3	4	5
Fatigue not present	1	2	3	4	5
Pao$_2$ WNL*	1	2	3	4	5
Paco$_2$ WNL	1	2	3	4	5
Arterial pH WNL	1	2	3	4	5
O$_2$ saturation WNL	1	2	3	4	5
End tidal (ET) CO$_2$ IER	1	2	3	4	5
Chest x-ray findings IER	1	2	3	4	5
Other _____ Specify	1	2	3	4	5

*IER = In expected range; WNL = within normal limits.

BACKGROUND READINGS:

Ahrens, T. (1993). Changing perspectives in the assessment of oxygenation. *Critical Care Nurse, 13*(4), 78-83.

Hayden, R. (1992). What keeps oxygenation on track? *American Journal of Nursing, 92*(12), 32-40.

Janson-Bjerklie, S. (1993). Predicting the outcomes of living with asthma. *Research in Nursing and Health, 16*(4), 241-249.

Morton, P. (1989). Respiratory systems. In *Health assessment in nursing* (pp. 243-281). Springhouse, PA: Springhouse.

Patrick, M. et al. (1991). *Medical-surgical nursing: Pathophysiological concepts* (2nd ed.). Philadelphia: J.B. Lippincott.

Potter, P., & Perry, A. (1991). *Oxygenation: Basic nursing theory and practice.* St. Louis: Mosby.

McCarty, K. & Wilkins, R. (1990). Synopsis of clinical findings in respiratory disorders. In R. Wilkins et al (Eds.), *Clinical assessment in respiratory care,* (2nd ed., pp. 294-302). St. Louis: Mosby.

Respiratory Status: Ventilation

DEFINITION: Movement of air in and out of the lungs

RESPIRATORY STATUS: VENTILATION	Extremely compromised 1	Substantially compromised 2	Moderately compromised 3	Mildly compromised 4	Not compromised 5
INDICATORS:					
Respiratory rate IER*	1	2	3	4	5
Respiratory rhythm IER	1	2	3	4	5
Depth of inspiration	1	2	3	4	5
Chest expansion symmetrical	1	2	3	4	5
Ease of breathing	1	2	3	4	5
Moves sputum out of airway	1	2	3	4	5
Vocalizes adequately	1	2	3	4	5
Expulsion of air	1	2	3	4	5
Accessory muscle use not present	1	2	3	4	5
Adventitious breath sounds not present	1	2	3	4	5
Chest retraction not present	1	2	3	4	5
Pursed lip breathing not present	1	2	3	4	5
Dyspnea at rest not present	1	2	3	4	5
Dyspnea with exertion not present	1	2	3	4	5
Orthopnea not present	1	2	3	4	5
SOB* not present	1	2	3	4	5
Tactile fremitus not present	1	2	3	4	5
Percussed sounds IER	1	2	3	4	5
Auscultated breath sounds IER	1	2	3	4	5
Auscultated vocalizations IER	1	2	3	4	5
Bronchophony IER	1	2	3	4	5
Egophony IER	1	2	3	4	5

*IER = In expected range; *SOB* = shortness of breath.   *Continued.*

Outcomes

RESPIRATORY STATUS: VENTILA-TION—cont'd	Extremely compromised 1	Substantially compromised 2	Moderately compromised 3	Mildly compromised 4	Not compromised 5
Whispered pectoriloquy IER	1	2	3	4	5
Tidal volume IER	1	2	3	4	5
Vital capacity IER	1	2	3	4	5
Chest x-ray findings IER	1	2	3	4	5
Pulmonary function tests IER	1	2	3	4	5
Other _____ Specify	1	2	3	4	5

BACKGROUND READINGS:

Ahrens, T. (1993). Changing perspectives in the assessment of oxygenation. *Critical Care Nurse, 13*(4), 78-83.

Hayden, R. (1992). What keeps oxygenation on track? *American Journal of Nursing, 92*(12), 32-40.

Janson-Bjerklie, S. (1993). Predicting the outcomes of living with asthma. *Research in Nursing and Health, 16*(4), 241-249.

Morton, P. (1989). Respiratory systems. In *Health Assessment in Nursing* (pp. 243-281). Springhouse, PA: Springhouse.

Potter, P., & Perry, A. (1990). *Oxygenation: Basic nursing theory and practice* (pp. 821-845). St. Louis: Mosby.

McCarty, K. & Wilkins, R. et al. (1990). Synopsis of clinical findings in respiratory disorders. In R. Wilkins et al (Eds.), *Clinical assessment in respiratory care* (2nd ed., pp. 294-302). St. Louis: Mosby.

Rest

DEFINITION: Extent and pattern of diminished activity for mental and physical rejuvenation

REST	Extremely compromised 1	Substantially compromised 2	Moderately compromised 3	Mildly compromised 4	Not compromised 5
INDICATORS:					
Amount of rest	1	2	3	4	5
Rest pattern	1	2	3	4	5
Rest quality	1	2	3	4	5
Physically rested	1	2	3	4	5
Mentally rested	1	2	3	4	5
Feelings of rejuvenation after rest	1	2	3	4	5
Other _____ Specify	1	2	3	4	5

BACKGROUND READINGS:

Brown, D.R., Morgan, W.P., & Raglin, J.S. (1993). Effects of exercise and rest on the state anxiety and blood pressure of physically challenged college students. *Journal of Sports Medicine and Physical Fitness, 33*(3), 300-305.

Ellis, J.R., & Nowlis, E.A. (1994). *Providing nursing care within the nursing process* (5th ed.). Philadelphia: J.B. Lippincott.

Luckman, J., & Sorensen, K.C. (1987). *Medical-surgical nursing: A psychophysiologic approach* (3rd ed.). Philadelphia: W.B. Saunders.

Potter, P.A., & Perry, A. (1989). *Fundamentals of nursing: Concepts, process, and practice* (2nd ed.). St. Louis: Mosby.

Outcomes

Risk Control

DEFINITION: Actions to eliminate or reduce actual, personal, and modifiable health threats

RISK CONTROL	Never demonstrated 1	Rarely demonstrated 2	Sometimes demonstrated 3	Often demonstrated 4	Consistently demonstrated 5
INDICATORS:					
Acknowledges risk	1	2	3	4	5
Monitors environmental risk factors	1	2	3	4	5
Monitors personal behavior risk factors	1	2	3	4	5
Develops effective risk control strategies	1	2	3	4	5
Adjusts risk control strategies as needed	1	2	3	4	5
Commits to risk control strategies	1	2	3	4	5
Follows selected risk control strategies.	1	2	3	4	5
Modifies lifestyle to reduce risk	1	2	3	4	5
Avoids exposure to health threats	1	2	3	4	5
Participates in screening for associated health problems	1	2	3	4	5
Participates in screening for identified risks	1	2	3	4	5
Obtains appropriate immunizations	1	2	3	4	5
Uses health care services congruent with need	1	2	3	4	5
Uses personal support systems to control risk	1	2	3	4	5
Uses community resources to control risk	1	2	3	4	5
Recognizes changes in health status	1	2	3	4	5
Monitors health status changes	1	2	3	4	5
Other _____ Specify	1	2	3	4	5

BACKGROUND READINGS:

Nease, R. (1994). Risk attitudes in gambles involving length of life: Aspirations, variations, and ruminations. *Medical Decision Making, 14*(2), 210-213.

Perez-Stable, E., Marin, G., & Marin, B. (1994). Behavioral risk factors: A comparison of Latinos and non-Latino whites in San Francisco. *American Journal of Public Health, 84*(6), 971-976.

Rost, K., Burnam, M., & Smith, G. (1993). Development of services for depressive disorders and substance abuse history. *Medical Care, 31*(3), 189-200.

Ryan, P. (1983). Altered health maintenance. In J.M. Thompston et al. (Eds.), *Mosby's clinical nursing.* (3rd ed., pp. 1425-1427). St. Louis: Mosby.

Simons-Morton, D.G., Mullen, P.D., Mains, D.A., Tabak, E.R., & Green, L.W. (1992). Characteristics of controlled studies of patient education and counseling for preventive health behaviors. *Patient Education and Counseling, 19,* 174-204.

U.S. Department of Health and Human Services. (1994). *Clinician's handbook of preventive services: Put prevention into practice.* Washington, DC: U.S. Government Printing Office.

Outcomes

Risk Control: Alcohol Use

DEFINITION: Actions to eliminate or reduce alcohol use that poses a threat to health

RISK CONTROL: ALCOHOL USE	Never demonstrated 1	Rarely demonstrated 2	Sometimes demonstrated 3	Often demonstrated 4	Consistently demonstrated 5
INDICATORS:					
Acknowledges risk for alcohol misuse	1	2	3	4	5
Acknowledges personal consequences associated with alcohol misuse	1	2	3	4	5
Monitors environment for factors encouraging alcohol abuse	1	2	3	4	5
Monitors personal alcohol use patterns	1	2	3	4	5
Develops effective alcohol use control strategies	1	2	3	4	5
Adjusts alcohol use control strategies as needed	1	2	3	4	5
Commits to alcohol use control strategies	1	2	3	4	5
Follows selected alcohol use control strategies	1	2	3	4	5
Participates in screening for associated health problems	1	2	3	4	5
Uses health care services congruent with need	1	2	3	4	5
Uses personal support systems to control alcohol misuse	1	2	3	4	5
Uses support groups to control alcohol misuse	1	2	3	4	5
Uses community resources to control alcohol misuse	1	2	3	4	5
Recognizes changes in health status	1	2	3	4	5
Monitors health status changes	1	2	3	4	5
Controls alcohol intake	1	2	3	4	5
Other _____ Specify	1	2	3	4	5

Outcomes

Outcomes

BACKGROUND READINGS:

McCuster, J., Stoddard, A.M., Zapka, J.G., & Lewis, B.F. (1993). Behavioral outcomes of AIDS educational interventions for drug users in short term treatment, *American Journal of Public Health, 83*(10), 1463-1466.

McDonald, B. (1994, January 18). Intake supervisor of MECCA-substance abuse services. Personal correspondence.

Simons-Morton, D.G., Mullen, P.D., Mains, D.A., Tabek, E.R., & Green, L.W. (1992). Characteristics of controlled studies of patient education and counseling for preventive health behaviors. *Patient Education and Counseling, 19,* 174-204.

Talashek, M.L., Gerace, L.M., & Starr, K.L. (1994). The substance abuse pandemic: Determinants to guide interventions. *Public Health Nursing, 11*(2), 131-139.

Risk Control: Drug Use

DEFINITION: Actions to eliminate or reduce drug use that poses a threat to health

RISK CONTROL: DRUG USE	Never demonstrated 1	Rarely demonstrated 2	Sometimes demonstrated 3	Often demonstrated 4	Consistently demonstrated 5
INDICATORS:					
Acknowledges risk for drug misuse	1	2	3	4	5
Acknowledges personal consequences associated with drug misuse	1	2	3	4	5
Monitors environment for factors encouraging drug misuse	1	2	3	4	5
Monitors personal drug use patterns	1	2	3	4	5
Develops effective drug use control strategies	1	2	3	4	5
Adjusts drug use control strategies as needed	1	2	3	4	5
Commits to drug use control strategies	1	2	3	4	5
Follows selected drug use control strategies	1	2	3	4	5
Participates in screening for associated health problems	1	2	3	4	5
Uses health care services congruent with need	1	2	3	4	5
Uses personal support systems to control drug misuse	1	2	3	4	5
Uses support groups to control drug misuse	1	2	3	4	5
Uses community resources to control drug misuse	1	2	3	4	5
Recognizes changes in health status	1	2	3	4	5
Monitor health status changes	1	2	3	4	5
Controls drug intake	1	2	3	4	5
Other _____ Specify	1	2	3	4	5

Outcomes

BACKGROUND READINGS:

McCuster, J., Stoddard, A.M., Zapka, J.G., & Lewis, B.F. (1993). Behavioral outcomes of AIDS educational interventions for drug users in short term treatment. *American Journal of Public Health, 83*(10), 1463-1466.

McDonald, B. (1994, January 18). Intake Supervisor of MECCA-Substance Abuse Services. Personal correspondence.

Simons-Morton, D.G., Mullen, P.D., Mains, D.A., Tabek, E.R., & Green, L.W. (1992). Characteristics of controlled studies of patient education and counseling for preventive health behaviors. *Patient Education and Counseling, 19,* 174-204.

Talashek, M.L., Gerace, L.M., & Starr, K.L. (1994). The substance abuse pandemic; Determinants to guide interventions. *Public Health Nursing, 11*(2), 131-139.

Outcomes

Risk Control: Sexually Transmitted Diseases (STD)

DEFINITION: Actions to eliminate or reduce behaviors associated with sexually transmitted disease

RISK CONTROL: SEXUALLY TRANS-MITTED DISEASES (STD)	Never demonstrated 1	Rarely demonstrated 2	Sometimes demonstrated 3	Often demonstrated 4	Consistently demonstrated 5
INDICATORS:					
Acknowledges individual risk for STD	1	2	3	4	5
Acknowledges personal consequences associated with STD	1	2	3	4	5
Monitors environment for STD exposure risks	1	2	3	4	5
Monitors personal behaviors for STD exposure risk	1	2	3	4	5
Develops effective strategies to reduce STD exposure	1	2	3	4	5
Adjusts exposure control strategies as needed	1	2	3	4	5
Commits to exposure control strategies	1	2	3	4	5
Follows selected exposure control strategies.	1	2	3	4	5
Inquires of partner(s)' STD status before sexual activity	1	2	3	4	5
Uses methods to control STD transmission	1	2	3	4	5
Recognizes STD signs and symptoms	1	2	3	4	5
Participates in screening for STD	1	2	3	4	5
Participates in screening for associated health problems	1	2	3	4	5
Uses community health services for STD treatment	1	2	3	4	5
Complies with recommended treatment for STDs	1	2	3	4	5

RISK CONTROL: SEXUALLY TRANSMITTED DISEASES (STD)	Never demonstrated 1	Rarely demonstrated 2	Sometimes demonstrated 3	Often demonstrated 4	Consistently demonstrated 5
Notifies sexual partner(s) in event of STD infection	1	2	3	4	5
Absence of STD	1	2	3	4	5
Other _____ Specify	1	2	3	4	5

Outcomes

BACKGROUND READINGS:

Rotheram, M.J., Reid, M.A., & Rosario, M. (1994). Factors mediating changes in sexual HIV risk behaviors among gay and bisexual male adolescents. *American Journal of Public Health, 84*(12), 1938-1946.

Simons-Morton, D.G., Mullen, P.D., Mains, D.A., Tabak, E.R., & Green, L.W. (1992). Characteristics of controlled studies of patient education and counseling for preventive health behaviors. *Patient Education and Counseling, 19*, 174-204.

U.S. Department of Health and Human Services. (1994). *Evaluation and management of early HIV infection* (AHCPR Publication No. 94-0572). Rockville, MD: Public Health Service Agency for Health Care Policy and Research.

Risk Control: Tobacco Use

DEFINITION: Actions to eliminate or reduce tobacco use

RISK CONTROL: TOBACCO USE	Never demonstrated 1	Rarely demonstrated 2	Sometimes demonstrated 3	Often demonstrated 4	Consistently demonstrated 5
INDICATORS:					
Acknowledges risk for tobacco use	1	2	3	4	5
Acknowledges personal consequences associated with tobacco use	1	2	3	4	5
Monitors environment for factors encouraging tobacco use	1	2	3	4	5
Monitors personal behaviors for tobacco use patterns	1	2	3	4	5
Develops effective strategies to eliminate tobacco use	1	2	3	4	5
Adjusts tobacco use control strategies as needed	1	2	3	4	5
Commits to tobacco use control strategies	1	2	3	4	5
Follows selected tobacco use control strategies	1	2	3	4	5
Participates in screening for associated health problems	1	2	3	4	5
Uses health services congruent with needs	1	2	3	4	5
Complies with recommended tobacco use monitoring	1	2	3	4	5
Uses personal support systems to eliminate tobacco use	1	2	3	4	5
Uses support group to eliminate tobacco use	1	2	3	4	5
Uses community resources to eliminate tobacco use	1	2	3	4	5

RISK CONTROL: TOBACCO USE	Never demonstrated 1	Rarely demonstrated 2	Sometimes demonstrated 3	Often demonstrated 4	Consistently demonstrated 5
Monitors health status changes	1	2	3	4	5
Eliminates tobacco use	1	2	3	4	5
Other _____ Specify	1	2	3	4	5

BACKGROUND READINGS:

Hirdes, J.P., & Maxwell, M.A. (1994). Smoking cessation and quality of life outcomes among older adults in the Campbell's survey on well-being. *Canadian Journal of Public Health, 85*(2), 99-102.

Simons-Morton, D.G., Mullen, P.D., Mains, D.A., Tabak, E.R., & Green, L.W. (1992). Characteristics of controlled studies of patient education and counseling for preventive health behaviors. *Patient Education and counseling, 19,* 174-204.

Sussman, S., Dent, C.W., Stacy, A.W., Sun, P., Craig, S., Simon, T.R., Burton, D., & Flay, B.R. (1993). Project towards no tobacco use: 1-year behavioral outcomes, *American Journal of Public Health, 83*(9), 1245-1250.

Talashek, M.L., Gerace, L.M., & Starr, K.L. (1994). The substance abuse pandemic: Determinants to guide interventions. *Public Health Nursing, 11*(2), 131-139.

Winsor, R.A., Lowe, J.B., Perkins, L.L., Smith-Yoder, D., Artz, L., Crawford, M., Amburgy, K., & Boyd, N.R. (1993). Health education for pregnant smokers: Its behavioral impact and cost benefit. *American Journal of Public Health, 83*(2), 201-206.

U.S. Department of Health and Human Services. (1996). *Smoking cessation* (AHCPR Publication No. 96-0692). Rockville, MD: Public Health Service Agency for Health Care Policy and Research.

Outcomes

Risk Control: Unintended Pregnancy

DEFINITION: Actions to reduce the possibility of unintended pregnancy

RISK CONTROL: UNINTENDED PREGNANCY	Never demonstrated 1	Rarely demonstrated 2	Sometimes demonstrated 3	Often demonstrated 4	Consistently demonstrated 5
INDICATORS:					
Acknowledges risk for unintended pregnancy	1	2	3	4	5
Describes signs and symptoms of pregnancy	1	2	3	4	5
Monitors personal consequences associated with unintended pregnancy	1	2	3	4	5
Monitors signs and symptoms of pregnancy	1	2	3	4	5
Understands physiological processes of conception	1	2	3	4	5
Develops effective pregnancy prevention strategies	1	2	3	4	5
Adjusts pregnancy prevention strategies as needed	1	2	3	4	5
Commits to pregnancy prevention strategies	1	2	3	4	5
Follows selected pregnancy prevention strategies	1	2	3	4	5
Uses support systems to enhance prevention strategy	1	2	3	4	5
Uses community resources for information/services	1	2	3	4	5
Identifies appropriate birth control method for self	1	2	3	4	5
Obtains contraceptive supplies and devices	1	2	3	4	5
Uses contraceptive methods correctly	1	2	3	4	5
Uses health care services congruent with need	1	2	3	4	5
Other _____ Specify	1	2	3	4	5

BACKGROUND READINGS:

Simons-Morton, D.G., Mullen, P.D., Mains, D.A., Tabak, E.R., & Green, L.W. (1992). Characteristics of controlled studies of patient education and counseling for preventive health behaviors. *Patient Education and Counseling, 19,* 174-204.

Risk Detection

DEFINITION: Actions taken to identify personal health threats

RISK DETECTION	Never demonstrated 1	Rarely demonstrated 2	Sometimes demonstrated 3	Often demonstrated 4	Consistently demonstrated 5
INDICATORS:					
Recognizes signs and symptoms that indicate risks	1	2	3	4	5
Identifies potential health risks	1	2	3	4	5
Seeks validation of perceived risks	1	2	3	4	5
Performs self-examinations at recommended intervals	1	2	3	4	5
Participates in screening at recommended intervals	1	2	3	4	5
Acquires knowledge of family history	1	2	3	4	5
Maintains updated knowledge of family history	1	2	3	4	5
Maintains updated knowledge of personal history	1	2	3	4	5
Uses resources to stay informed about potential risks	1	2	3	4	5
Uses health care services congruent with needs	1	2	3	4	5
Other _____ Specify	1	2	3	4	5

BACKGROUND READINGS:

Bamberg, R., Acton, R.T., Goodson, L., Go, R., Struempler, B., & Roseman, J.M. (1989). The effect of risk assessment in conjunction with health promotion education on compliance with preventive behaviors. *Journal of Allied Health, 18*(1), 271-281.

Simons-Morton, D.G., Mullen, P.D., Mains, D.A., Tabak, E.R., & Green, L.W. (1992). Characteristics of controlled studies of patient education and counseling for preventive health behaviors. *Patient Education and Counseling, 19*, 174-204.

Outcomes

Role Performance

DEFINITION: Congruence of an individual's role behavior with role expectations

ROLE PERFORMANCE	Not adequate 1	Slightly adequate 2	Moderately adequate 3	Substantially adequate 4	Totally adequate 5
INDICATORS:					
Ability to meet role expectations	1	2	3	4	5
Knowledge of role transition periods	1	2	3	4	5
Performance of family role behaviors	1	2	3	4	5
Performance of community role behaviors	1	2	3	4	5
Performance of work role behaviors	1	2	3	4	5
Performance of friendship role behaviors	1	2	3	4	5
Description of behavioral changes with illness or disability	1	2	3	4	5
Description of behavioral changes with elderly dependents	1	2	3	4	5
Description of behavioral changes with new family member	1	2	3	4	5
Description of behavioral changes when family member leaves home	1	2	3	4	5
Reported strategies for role change(s)	1	2	3	4	5
Reported comfort with role expectation	1	2	3	4	5
Performance of intimate role behaviors	1	2	3	4	5
Other _____ Specify	1	2	3	4	5

BACKGROUND READINGS:

Knutson, A.L. (1965). *The individual, society, and health behavior.* New York: Sage.

McCloskey, J.B., & Bulechek, G.M. (1992). *Nursing interventions classification.* St. Louis: Mosby.

Moorhead, S.A. (1985). Role supplementation. In G.M. Bulechek, & J.C. McCloskey (Eds.), *Nursing interventions: Treatments for nursing diagnoses.* Philadelphia: W.B. Saunders.

Outcomes

Safety Behavior: Fall Prevention

DEFINITION: Individual or caregiver actions to minimize risk factors that might precipitate falls

SAFETY BEHAVIOR: FALL PREVENTION	Not adequate 1	Slightly adequate 2	Moderately adequate 3	Substantially adequate 4	Totally adequate 5
INDICATORS:					
Correct use of assistive devices	1	2	3	4	5
Provision of personal assistance	1	2	3	4	5
Placement of barriers to prevent falls	1	2	3	4	5
Use of restraints as needed	1	2	3	4	5
Placement of handrailings as needed	1	2	3	4	5
Elimination of clutter, spills, glare from floors	1	2	3	4	5
Tacking down rugs	1	2	3	4	5
Arrangement for removal of snow and ice from walking surfaces	1	2	3	4	5
Appropriate use of stools/ladders	1	2	3	4	5
Use of well-fitting tied shoes	1	2	3	4	5
Adjustment of toilet height as needed	1	2	3	4	5
Adjustment of chair height as needed	1	2	3	4	5
Adjustment of bed height as needed	1	2	3	4	5
Use of rubber mats in tub/shower	1	2	3	4	5
Use of grab bars	1	2	3	4	5
Agitation and restlessness controlled	1	2	3	4	5
Use of precautions when taking medications that increase risk for falls	1	2	3	4	5
Use of vision-correcting devices	1	2	3	4	5
Use of safe transfer procedure	1	2	3	4	5
Compensation for physical limitations	1	2	3	4	5
Other _____ Specify	1	2	3	4	5

BACKGROUND READINGS:

Meller, J.L., & Shermeta, D.W. (1987). Falls in urban children. *American Journal of Diseases of Children, 14*(12), 1271-1275.

Moss, A.B. (1992). Are the elderly safe at home? *Journal of Community Health Nursing, 9*(1), 13-19.

O'Connor, M.S., Boyle, W.E., O'Connor, G.T., & Letellier, R. (1992). Self-reported safety practices in child care facilities. *American Journal of Preventative Medicine, 8*(1), 14-18.

Urton, M.M. (1991). A community home inspection approach to preventing falls among the elderly. *Public Health Reports, 106*(2), 192-196.

Outcomes

Safety Behavior: Home Physical Environment

DEFINITION: Individual or caregiver actions to minimize environmental factors that might cause physical harm or injury in the home

SAFETY BEHAVIOR: HOME PHYSICAL ENVIRONMENT	Not adequate 1	Slightly adequate 2	Moderately adequate 3	Substantially adequate 4	Totally adequate 5
INDICATORS:					
Provision of lighting	1	2	3	4	5
Placement of handrailings	1	2	3	4	5
Smoke detector maintenance	1	2	3	4	5
Use of personal alarm system	1	2	3	4	5
Provision of accessible telephone	1	2	3	4	5
Placement of appropriate hazard warning labels	1	2	3	4	5
Disposal of unused medicines	1	2	3	4	5
Provision of assistive devices in accessible location	1	2	3	4	5
Provision of equipment that meets safety standards	1	2	3	4	5
Storage of firearms to prevent accidents	1	2	3	4	5
Storage of hazardous materials to prevent injury	1	2	3	4	5
Safe disposal of hazardous materials	1	2	3	4	5
Arrangement of furniture to reduce risks	1	2	3	4	5
Provision of safe play area	1	2	3	4	5
Removal of unused refrigerator and freezer doors	1	2	3	4	5
Correction of lead hazard risks	1	2	3	4	5
Provision of age-appropriate toys	1	2	3	4	5
Use of electrical outlet covers	1	2	3	4	5
Room temperature regulation	1	2	3	4	5
Elimination of harmful noise levels	1	2	3	4	5
Placement of window guards as needed	1	2	3	4	5
Other _____ Specify	1	2	3	4	5

BACKGROUND READINGS:

Halperin, S.F., Bass, J.L., & Mehta, K.A., (1983). Knowledge of accident prevention among parents of young children in nine Massachusetts towns. *Public Health Reports, 98*(6), 548-552.

Mayhew, M.S. (1991). Strategies for promoting safety and preventing injury. *Nursing Clinics of North America, 26*(1), 885-893.

Wasserman, R.C., Dameron, D.O., Brozicevic, M.M., & Aronson, R.A. (1989). Injury hazards in home day care. *The Journal of Pediatrics, 114*(4), 591-593.

Outcomes

Safety Behavior: Personal

DEFINITION: Individual or caregiver efforts to control behaviors that might cause physical injury

SAFETY BEHAVIOR: PERSONAL	Not adequate 1	Slightly adequate 2	Moderately adequate 3	Substantially adequate 4	Totally adequate 5
INDICATORS:					
Balance of sleep and rest with activity	1	2	3	4	5
Storage of food to minimize illness	1	2	3	4	5
Preparation of food to minimize illness	1	2	3	4	5
Use of helmets as needed	1	2	3	4	5
Use of seatbelts or safety seats	1	2	3	4	5
Choice of appropriate clothing for activity	1	2	3	4	5
Correct use of assistive devices	1	2	3	4	5
Development of safe play and leisure habits	1	2	3	4	5
Practice of safe sexual behaviors	1	2	3	4	5
Correct use of tools	1	2	3	4	5
Correct use of machinery	1	2	3	4	5
Correct use of protective devices	1	2	3	4	5
Avoidance of recreational drugs	1	2	3	4	5
Arrangement for secure living environment	1	2	3	4	5
Use of precautions when taking mind altering drugs	1	2	3	4	5
Provision of secure living environment	1	2	3	4	5
Avoidance of tobacco products/by-products	1	2	3	4	5
Avoidance of alcohol misuse	1	2	3	4	5
Avoidance of high-risk behaviors	1	2	3	4	5
Observance of speed limits	1	2	3	4	5
Other _____ Specify	1	2	3	4	5

BACKGROUND READINGS:

Chang, A., Dillman, A.S., Leonard, E., & English, P. (1985). Teaching car passenger safety to preschool children. *Pediatrics, 76*(3), 425-428.

Greensher, J., & Mofenson, H.C. (1985). Injuries at play. *Pediatric Clinics of North America, 32*(1), 127-139.

Sorock, G.S. (1988). Falls among the elderly: Epidemiology and prevention. *Journal of Preventive Medicine, 4*(5), 252-255.

Outcomes

Safety Status: Falls Occurrence

DEFINITION: Number of falls in the past week					

SAFETY STATUS: FALLS OCCURRENCE	Over 9 **1**	7-9 **2**	4-6 **3**	1-3 **4**	None **5**
TOTAL NUMBER OF FALLS PER WEEK:					
Number of falls while standing	1	2	3	4	5
Number of falls while walking	1	2	3	4	5
Number of falls while sitting	1	2	3	4	5
Number of falls from bed	1	2	3	4	5
Number of falls while transferring	1	2	3	4	5
Number of falls climbing steps	1	2	3	4	5
Number of falls descending steps	1	2	3	4	5
Other _____ Specify	1	2	3	4	5

BACKGROUND READINGS:

Baker, L. (1992). Developing a safety plan that works for patients and nurses. *Rehabilitation Nursing, 17*(5), 264-266.

Nelson, R.C., & Amin, M.A. (1990). Falls in the elderly. *Emergency Care of the Elderly, 8*(2), 309-323.

Sorock, G.S. (1988). Falls among the elderly: Epidemiology and prevention. *American Journal of Preventive Medicine, 4*(5), 282-288.

Outcomes

Outcomes

Safety Status: Physical Injury

DEFINITION: Severity of injuries from accidents and trauma

SAFETY STATUS: PHYSICAL INJURY	Severe 1	Substantial 2	Moderate 3	Slight 4	None 5
INDICATORS:					
Skin abrasions	1	2	3	4	5
Bruises	1	2	3	4	5
Lacerations	1	2	3	4	5
Burns	1	2	3	4	5
Extremity sprains	1	2	3	4	5
Back sprains	1	2	3	4	5
Extremity fractures	1	2	3	4	5
Pelvic fractures	1	2	3	4	5
Hip fractures	1	2	3	4	5
Spinal fractures	1	2	3	4	5
Cranial fractures	1	2	3	4	5
Facial fractures	1	2	3	4	5
Dental injuries	1	2	3	4	5
Open head injuries	1	2	3	4	5
Closed head injuries	1	2	3	4	5
Impaired mobility	1	2	3	4	5
Impaired consciousness	1	2	3	4	5
Other _____ Specify	1	2	3	4	5

BACKGROUND READINGS:

Lawrence, J.I., & Maher, P.L. (1992). An interdisciplinary falls consult team: A collaborative approach to patient falls. *Journal of Nursing Care Quality, 6*(3), 21-29.

Llewellyn, J., Martin, B., Shekleton, M., & Firlit, S. (1988). Analysis of falls in the acute surgical and cardiovascular surgical patient. *Applied Nursing Research, 1*(3), 116-121.

Self-Care: Activities of Daily Living (ADL)

DEFINITION: Ability to perform the most basic physical tasks and personal care activities

SELF-CARE: ACTIVITIES OF DAILY LIVING (ADL)	Dependent, does not participate	Requires assistive person & device	Requires assistive person	Independent with assistive device	Completely independent
	1	2	3	4	5
INDICATORS:					
Eating	1	2	3	4	5
Dressing	1	2	3	4	5
Toileting	1	2	3	4	5
Bathing	1	2	3	4	5
Grooming	1	2	3	4	5
Hygiene	1	2	3	4	5
Oral hygiene	1	2	3	4	5
Ambulation: walking	1	2	3	4	5
Ambulation: wheelchair	1	2	3	4	5
Transfer performance	1	2	3	4	5
Other _____ Specify	1	2	3	4	5

BACKGROUND READINGS:

Katz, S., Ford, A.B., Moskowitz, R.W., Jackson, B.A., & Jaffe, M.W. (1963). Studies of illness in the aged. The index of ADL: A standardized measure of biological and psychosocial function. *Journal of the American Medical Association, 185*(12), 914-919.

Klein, R.M., & Bell, B. (1982). Self-care skills: Behavioral measurement with Klein-Bell ADL Scale. *Archives of Physical Medicine and Rehabilitation, 63*(7), 335-338.

Outcomes

Self-Care: Bathing

DEFINITION: Ability to cleanse own body

SELF-CARE: BATHING	Dependent, does not participate	Requires assistive person & device	Requires assistive person	Independent with assistive device	Completely independent
	1	2	3	4	5
INDICATORS:					
Gets in and out of bathroom	1	2	3	4	5
Gets bath supplies	1	2	3	4	5
Obtains water	1	2	3	4	5
Turns on water	1	2	3	4	5
Regulates water temperature	1	2	3	4	5
Regulates water flow	1	2	3	4	5
Bathes at sink	1	2	3	4	5
Bathes in tub	1	2	3	4	5
Bathes in shower	1	2	3	4	5
Washes body	1	2	3	4	5
Dries body	1	2	3	4	5
Other _____ Specify	1	2	3	4	5

BACKGROUND READINGS:

Gulick, E.E. (1990). The self-administered ADL scale for persons with multiple sclerosis. In C.F. Waltz, & O.L. Strickland (Eds.), *Measurement of nursing outcomes* (pp. 128-147). New York: Springer.

Klein, R.M., & Bell, B. (1982). Self-care skills: Behavioral measurement with Klein-Bell ADL scale. *Archives of Physical Medicine and Rehabilitation, 63,* 335-338.

McKeighten, R.J., Mehmert, P.A., & Dickel, C.A. (1990). Bathing/hygiene self-care deficit: Defining characteristics and related factors across age groups and diagnosis-related groups in an acute care setting. *Nursing Diagnosis, 1*(4), 155-161.

Shillam, L.L., & Beeman, C., & Loshin, P. (1983). Effect of occupational therapy intervention on bathing independence of disabled persons. *The American Journal of Occupational Therapy, 37*(11), 744-748.

Self-Care: Dressing

DEFINITION: Ability to dress self

SELF-CARE: DRESSING	Dependent, does not participate	Requires assistive person & device	Requires assistive person	Independent with assistive device	Completely independent
	1	**2**	**3**	**4**	**5**
INDICATORS:					
Chooses clothing	1	2	3	4	5
Gets clothes from drawer and closet	1	2	3	4	5
Picks up clothing	1	2	3	4	5
Puts clothing on upper body	1	2	3	4	5
Puts clothing on lower body	1	2	3	4	5
Buttons clothing	1	2	3	4	5
Uses fasteners	1	2	3	4	5
Uses zippers	1	2	3	4	5
Puts on socks	1	2	3	4	5
Puts on shoes	1	2	3	4	5
Removes clothes	1	2	3	4	5
Other _____ _Specify_	1	2	3	4	5

BACKGROUND READINGS:

Beck, C. (1988). Measurement of dressing performance in persons with dementia. *American Journal of Alzheimer's Care and Related Disorders and Research, 3*(3), 21-25.

Cole, S.L. (1992). Dress for success: A nurse's knowledge of simple clothing adaptations and dressing aids may make the difference between rehabilitation success and failure. *Geriatric Nursing, 13*(4), 217-221.

Cook, E.A., Luschen, L., & Sikes, S. (1991). Dressing training for an elderly woman with cognitive and perceptual impairments. *The American Journal of Occupational Therapy, 45,* 652-654.

Dudgeon, B.J., DeLisa, J.A., & Miller, R.M. (1984). Optokinetic nystagmus and upper extremity dressing independence after stroke. *Archives of Physical Medicine & Rehabilitation, 66,* 164-167.

Ford, L.J. (1975). Teaching dressing skills to a severely retarded child. *The American Journal of Occupational Therapy, 2*(29), 87-92.

Panikoff, L.B. (1983). Recovery trends of functional skills in the head injured adult. *The American Journal of Occupational Therapy, 37,* 735-743.

Runge, M. (1967). Self-dressing techniques for patients with spinal cord injury. *The American Journal of Occupational Therapy, 21,* 367-375.

Self-Care: Eating

DEFINITION: Ability to prepare and ingest food

SELF-CARE: EATING	Dependent, does not participate	Requires assistive person & device	Requires assistive person	Independent with assistive device	Completely independent
	1	2	3	4	5
INDICATORS:					
Prepares food for ingestion	1	2	3	4	5
Opens containers	1	2	3	4	5
Handles utensils	1	2	3	4	5
Gets food onto the utensil	1	2	3	4	5
Picks up cup or glass	1	2	3	4	5
Brings food to mouth with fingers	1	2	3	4	5
Brings food to mouth with container	1	2	3	4	5
Brings food to mouth with utensil	1	2	3	4	5
Drinks from a cup or glass	1	2	3	4	5
Places food in mouth	1	2	3	4	5
Manipulates food in mouth	1	2	3	4	5
Chews food	1	2	3	4	5
Swallows food	1	2	3	4	5
Completes a meal	1	2	3	4	5
Other _____ Specify	1	2	3	4	5

BACKGROUND READINGS:

Athlin, E., Norberg, A., Axelson, K., Moller, A., & Nordstrom, G. (1989). Aberrant eating behavior in elderly parkinsonian patients with and without dementia: Analysis of video-recorded meals. *Research in Nursing and Health, 12,* 41-51.

Luiselli, J.K. (1993). Training self-feeding skills in children who are deaf and blind. *Behavior Modification, 17,*(4), 457-473.

Piazza, C.C., Anderson, C., & Fisher, W. (1993). Teaching self-feeding skills to patients with Rett Syndrome. *Developmental Medicine and Child Neurology, 35,* 991-996.

Outcomes

Self-Care: Grooming

DEFINITION: Ability to maintain kempt appearance

SELF-CARE: GROOMING	Dependent, does not participate	Requires assistive person & device	Requires assistive person	Independent with assistive device	Completely independent
	1	2	3	4	5
INDICATORS:					
Shampoos hair	1	2	3	4	5
Combs or brushes hair	1	2	3	4	5
Shaves	1	2	3	4	5
Applies makeup	1	2	3	4	5
Cares for nails	1	2	3	4	5
Maintains neat appearance	1	2	3	4	5
Uses a mirror	1	2	3	4	5
Other _____ Specify	1	2	3	4	5

BACKGROUND READINGS:

Cole, G. (1991). Hygiene and care of the patient's environment. In G. Cole (Ed.), *Basic nursing skills and concepts* (pp. 261-290). St. Louis: Mosby.

Hallstrom, R., & Beck, S.L. (1993). Implementation of the AORN skin shaving standard: Evaluation of a planned change. *AORN Journal, 58*(3), 498-506.

Wong, S.E., Flanagan, S.G., Kuehnel, T.G., Liberman, R.P., Hunnicut, R., & Adams-Badgett, J. (1988). Training chronic mental patients to independently practice personal grooming skills, *Hospital and Community Psychiatry, 39*(8), 874-879.

Self-Care: Hygiene

DEFINITION: Ability to maintain own hygiene

SELF-CARE: HYGIENE	Dependent, does not participate	Requires assistive person & device	Requires assistive person	Independent with assistive device	Completely independent
	1	2	3	4	5
INDICATORS:					
Washes hands	1	2	3	4	5
Applies deodorant	1	2	3	4	5
Cleans perineal area	1	2	3	4	5
Cleans ears	1	2	3	4	5
Keeps nose blown and clean	1	2	3	4	5
Maintains oral hygiene	1	2	3	4	5
Other _____ Specify	1	2	3	4	5

BACKGROUND READINGS:

Cole, G. (1991). Hygiene and care of the patient's environment. In G. Cole (Ed.), *Basic nursing skills and concepts* (pp. 261-290). St. Louis: Mosby.

Hylen, A.M., Karlsson, E., Svanberg, L., & Walder, M. (1983). Hygiene for the newborn—To bathe or to wash? *Journal of Hygiene, 91*(3), 529-534.

McKeighten, R.J., Mehmert, P.A., & Dickel, C.A. (1990). Bathing/hygiene self-care deficit: Defining characteristics and related factors across age groups and diagnosis-related groups in an acute care setting. *Nursing Diagnosis, 1*(4), 155-161.

Ney, D.F. (1993). Cerumen impaction, ear hygiene practices, and hearing acuity. *Geriatric Nursing—American Journal of Care for the Aging, 14*(2), 70-73.

Outcomes

Self-Care: Instrumental Activities of Daily Living (IADL)

DEFINITION: Ability to perform activities needed to function in the home or community

SELF-CARE: INSTRUMENTAL ACTIVITIES OF DAILY LIVING (IADL)	Dependent, does not participate 1	Requires assistive person & device 2	Requires assistive person 3	Independent with assistive device 4	Completely independent 5
INDICATORS:					
Shops for groceries	1	2	3	4	5
Shops for clothing	1	2	3	4	5
Shops for household needs	1	2	3	4	5
Prepares meals	1	2	3	4	5
Serves meals	1	2	3	4	5
Uses telephone	1	2	3	4	5
Handles written communication	1	2	3	4	5
Opens containers	1	2	3	4	5
Performs housework	1	2	3	4	5
Performs household repairs	1	2	3	4	5
Does yard work	1	2	3	4	5
Manages money	1	2	3	4	5
Manages business affairs	1	2	3	4	5
Travels on public transportation	1	2	3	4	5
Drives own car	1	2	3	4	5
Does own laundry	1	2	3	4	5
Manages medications	1	2	3	4	5
Other _____ Specify	1	2	3	4	5

BACKGROUND READINGS:

Fillenbaum, G.G., Smyer, M.A. (1981). The development, validity, and reliability of the OARS multidimensional functional assessment questionnaire. *Journal of Gerontology, 36,* 428.

Jette, A.M. (1980). Functional status index: Reliability of a chronic disease evaluation instrument. *Archives of Physical Medicine & Rehabilitation, 61,* 395-401.

Lawton, M.P. (1983). Assessment of behaviors required to maintain residence in the community. In T. Crook, S. Ferris, & R. Bartus (Eds.), *Assessment in geriatric psychopharmacology* (pp. 119-135). New Canaan, CT: Mark Powley Associates.

Lawton, M.P., & Brody, E.M. (1969). Assessment of older people: Self-maintaining and instrumental activities of daily living. *Gerontologist, 9,* 179-186.

Linn, M.W., & Linn, B.W. (1982). The rapid disability rating scale-2. *Journal of the American Geriatric Society, 30,* 378-382.

Continued.

Outcomes

Meenan, R.F., Gertman, P.M., & Mason, J.H. (1980). Measuring health status in arthritis: The arthritis impact measurement scales. *Arthritis Rheumatism, 23*(2), 146-152.

Pearlman, R. (1987). Development of a functional assessment questionnaire for geriatric patients: The comprehensive older persons' evaluation (COPE). *Journal of Chronic Disease, 40*(56), 85S-94S.

Shanas, E., Townsend, P., Wedderburn, D., Friis, H., Milhoj, P., & Stehouwer, J. (1968). *Old people in three industrial societies.* New York: Atherton Press.

Self-Care: Non-Parenteral Medication

DEFINITION: Ability to administer oral and topical medications to meet therapeutic goals

SELF-CARE: NON-PARENTERAL MEDICATION	Dependent, does not participate	Requires assistive person & device	Requires assistive person	Independent with assistive device	Completely independent
	1	**2**	**3**	**4**	**5**
INDICATORS:					
Identifies medication	1	2	3	4	5
States correct dose	1	2	3	4	5
Describes action of medication	1	2	3	4	5
Adjusts dose appropriately	1	2	3	4	5
Describes medication precautions	1	2	3	4	5
Describes side effects of medication	1	2	3	4	5
Uses memory aids	1	2	3	4	5
Performs self-monitoring activities	1	2	3	4	5
Uses monitoring equipment accurately	1	2	3	4	5
Maintains needed supplies	1	2	3	4	5
Administers medication correctly	1	2	3	4	5
Stores medication properly	1	2	3	4	5
Disposes of medication appropriately	1	2	3	4	5
Seeks needed laboratory tests	1	2	3	4	5
Other _____ Specify	1	2	3	4	5

BACKGROUND READINGS:

Barry, K. (1993). Patient self-medication: An innovative approach to medication teaching. *Journal of Nursing Care Quality, 8,* 75-82.

Felsenthal, G., Glomski, N., & Jones, D. (1986, January). Medication education program in an inpatient geriatric rehabilitation unit. *Archives of Physical Medication and Rehabilitation, 67,* 27-29.

Lorish, D.D., Richards, B., & Brown, S. (1990). Perspective of the patient with rheumatoid arthritis on issues related to missed medication. *Arthritis Care and Research, 3*(2), 78-84.

Outcomes

Self-Care: Oral Hygiene

DEFINITION: Ability to care for own mouth and teeth

SELF-CARE: ORAL HYGIENE	Dependent, does not participate	Requires assistive person & device	Requires assistive person	Independent with assistive device	Completely independent
	1	2	3	4	5
INDICATORS:					
Brushes teeth	1	2	3	4	5
Flosses teeth	1	2	3	4	5
Cleans mouth, gums, and tongue	1	2	3	4	5
Cleans dentures or dental appliances	1	2	3	4	5
Handles necessary equipment	1	2	3	4	5
Uses fluoridation	1	2	3	4	5
Obtains regular dental care	1	2	3	4	5
Maintains low risk for caries diet	1	2	3	4	5
Other _____ Specify	1	2	3	4	5

BACKGROUND READINGS:

Fischman, S. (1993). Self-care: Practical periodontal care in today's practice. *International Dental Journal, 43,* 179-183.

Horowitz, L.G. (1990). Dental patient education: Self-care to healthy human development. *Patient Education and Counseling, 15*(1), 65-71.

Rayant, G.A., & Sheiham, A. (1980). An analysis of factors affecting compliance with tooth-cleaning recommendations. *Journal of Clinical Periodontology, 7,* 289-299.

Richardson, A. (1987). A process standard for oral care. *Nursing Times, 83,* 38-40.

Outcomes

Self-Care: Parenteral Medication

DEFINITION: Ability to administer parenteral medications to meet therapeutic goals

SELF-CARE: PARENTERAL MEDICATION	Dependent, does not participate	Requires assistive person & device	Requires assistive person	Independent with assistive device	Completely independent
	1	2	3	4	5
INDICATORS:					
Identifies medication	1	2	3	4	5
States correct dose	1	2	3	4	5
Describes action of medication	1	2	3	4	5
Adjusts dose appropriately	1	2	3	4	5
Describes medication precautions	1	2	3	4	5
Describes side effects of medication	1	2	3	4	5
Uses memory aids	1	2	3	4	5
Performs self-monitoring activities	1	2	3	4	5
Uses monitoring equipment accurately	1	2	3	4	5
Maintains needed supplies	1	2	3	4	5
Administers medication correctly	1	2	3	4	5
Stores medication properly	1	2	3	4	5
Disposes of medication appropriately	1	2	3	4	5
Maintains asepsis	1	2	3	4	5
Monitors injection sites	1	2	3	4	5
Seeks needed laboratory tests	1	2	3	4	5
Other _____ Specify	1	2	3	4	5

BACKGROUND READINGS:

Robinson, J., Gould, M.A., Burrows-Hudson, S., Baltz, P., Currier, H., Piwkiewicz, D., & Smith, L.J. (1991). A care plan for self-administration of epoetin alpha. *ANNA Journal, 18*(6), 573-580.

Sarisley, C. (1987). Designing a teaching program for outpatient antibiotic therapy. *Journal of Nursing Staff Development, 3*(3), 128-135.

Outcomes

Self-Care: Toileting

DEFINITION: Ability to toilet self

SELF-CARE: TOILETING	Dependent, does not participate	Requires assistive person & device	Requires assistive person	Independent with assistive device	Completely independent
	1	2	3	4	5
INDICATORS:					
Recognizes and responds to full bladder	1	2	3	4	5
Recognizes and responds to urge to have a bowel movement	1	2	3	4	5
Gets to and from toilet	1	2	3	4	5
Removes clothing	1	2	3	4	5
Positions self on toilet or commode	1	2	3	4	5
Empties bladder or bowel	1	2	3	4	5
Wipes self after urinating or bowel movement	1	2	3	4	5
Gets up from toilet	1	2	3	4	5
Adjusts clothing after toileting	1	2	3	4	5
Other _____ Specify	1	2	3	4	5

BACKGROUND READINGS:

Burgio, K.L., Burgio, L.D., McCormick, K.A., & Engel, B.T. (1991). Assessing toileting skills and habits in an adult day care center. *Journal of Gerontological Nursing, 17*(12), 32-35.

Okamoto, G.A., Sousa, J., Telzrow, R.W., Holm, R.A., McCartin, R., & Shurtleff, D.B. (1984). Toileting skills in children with myelomeningocele: Rates of learning. *Archives of Physical Medicine and Rehabilitation, 65,* 182-185.

Seim, H.C. (1989). Toilet training in first children. *The Journal of Family Practice, 29*(6), 633-636.

Outcomes

Self-Esteem

DEFINITION: Personal judgment of self-worth

SELF-ESTEEM	Never positive 1	Rarely positive 2	Sometimes positive 3	Often positive 4	Consistently positive 5
INDICATORS:					
Verbalizations of self-acceptance	1	2	3	4	5
Acceptance of self-limitations	1	2	3	4	5
Maintenance of erect posture	1	2	3	4	5
Maintenance of eye contact	1	2	3	4	5
Description of self	1	2	3	4	5
Regard for others	1	2	3	4	5
Open communication	1	2	3	4	5
Fulfillment of personally significant roles	1	2	3	4	5
Maintenance of grooming/hygiene	1	2	3	4	5
Balance of participation and listening in groups	1	2	3	4	5
Confidence level	1	2	3	4	5
Acceptance of compliments from others	1	2	3	4	5
Expected response from others	1	2	3	4	5
Acceptance of constructive criticism	1	2	3	4	5
Willingness to confront others	1	2	3	4	5
Description of success in work or school	1	2	3	4	5
Description of success in social groups	1	2	3	4	5
Description of pride in self	1	2	3	4	5
Feelings about self-worth	1	2	3	4	5
Other _____ Specify	1	2	3	4	5

BACKGROUND READINGS:

Bonham, P., & Cheney, A. (1982). *Concept of self: A framework for nursing assessment.* In P.L. Chinn (Ed.), *Advances in nursing theory development* (pp. 173-189). Rockville, MD: Aspen.

Carroll-Johnson, R. (1989). *Classification of nursing diagnoses: Proceedings of the eighth conference (North American Nursing Diagnosis Association).* Philadelphia: J.B. Lippincott.

Coopersmith, S. (1967). *The antecedents of self-esteem.* San Francisco: W.H. Freeman.

Crandall, R. (1973). The measurement of self-esteem and related constructs. In J.P. Robinson & P.R. Shaver (Eds.), *Measures of social psychological attitudes.* Institute for Social Research, University of Michigan. Ann Arbor.

Driever, M. (1984). Self-esteem. In C. Roy (Ed.), *Introduction to nursing: An adaptation model* (pp. 394-404). Englewood Cliffs, NJ: Prentice-Hall.

Fitts, W. (1965). *Manual for the Tennessee self-concept scale.* Nashville, TN: Counselor Recordings & Tests.

Continued.

Norris, J., & Kunes-Connell, M. (1985). Self-esteem disturbance. *Nursing Clinics of North America, 20*(4), 745-761.

Norris, J. (1992). Nursing intervention for self-esteem disturbances. *Nursing Diagnosis, 3*(2), 48-53.

Roid, G., & Fitts, W. (1988). *Tennessee self-concept scale: Revised manual.* Los Angeles: Western Psychological Services.

Rosenberg, M. (1965). *Society & adolescent self image.* Princeton, NJ: Princeton University Press.

Soukup, B. (1991). *Self-esteem and job satisfaction among hospital staff nurses.* Master's thesis, University of Iowa: Iowa City.

Stanwyck, D. (1983). Self-esteem through the life span. *Family & Community Health, 6,* 11-28.

Townsend, M. (1988). *Nursing diagnoses in psychiatric nursing: Pocket guide for care plan construction.* Philadelphia: F.A. Davis.

Outcomes

Self-Mutilation Restraint

DEFINITION: Ability to refrain from intentional self-inflicted injury (non-lethal)

SELF-MUTILATION RESTRAINT	Never demonstrated 1	Rarely demonstrated 2	Sometimes demonstrated 3	Often demonstrated 4	Consistently demonstrated 5
INDICATORS:					
Refrains from gathering means for self-injury	1	2	3	4	5
Seeks help when feeling urge to injure self	1	2	3	4	5
Requires no treatment for self-injuries	1	2	3	4	5
Upholds contract to not harm self	1	2	3	4	5
Maintains self-control without supervision	1	2	3	4	5
Does not injure self	1	2	3	4	5
Other _____ Specify	1	2	3	4	5

BACKGROUND READINGS:

Burrow, S. (1994). Nursing management of self-mutilation. *British Journal of Nursing, 3*(8), 382-386.

Coler, M.S., & Vincent, K.G. (1995). Psychiatric mental health nursing. In K.V. Gettrust (Series Ed.), *Plans of care for specialty practice.* Albany, NY: Delmar Publishers.

Faye, P. (1995). Addictive characteristics of the behavior of self-mutilation. *Journal of Psychosocial Nursing and Mental Health Services, 33*(2), 19-22.

Stuart, G.W., & Sundeen, S.J. (1995). *Principles and practice of psychiatric nursing* (5th ed.). St. Louis: Mosby.

Valente, S.M. (1991). Deliberate self-injury management in a psychiatric setting. *Journal of Psychosocial Nursing and Mental Health Services, 29*(12), 19-25.

Winchel, R.M. (1991). Self-injurious behavior. A review of the behavior and biology of self-mutilation. *American Journal of Psychiatry, 148*(3), 306-17.

Outcomes

Sleep

DEFINITION: Extent and pattern of sleep for mental and physical rejuvenation

SLEEP	Extremely compromised 1	Substantially compromised 2	Moderately compromised 3	Mildly compromised 4	Not compromised 5
INDICATORS:					
Hours of sleep	1	2	3	4	5
Observed hours of sleep	1	2	3	4	5
Sleep pattern	1	2	3	4	5
Sleep quality	1	2	3	4	5
Sleep efficiency (ratio of sleep time/total time trying)	1	2	3	4	5
Uninterrupted sleep	1	2	3	4	5
Sleep routine	1	2	3	4	5
Feelings of rejuvenation after sleep	1	2	3	4	5
Napping appropriate for age	1	2	3	4	5
Wakeful at appropriate times	1	2	3	4	5
EEG IER*	1	2	3	4	5
EMG* IER	1	2	3	4	5
EOG* IER	1	2	3	4	5
Vital signs IER	1	2	3	4	5
Other _____ Specify	1	2	3	4	5

*EEG = Electroencephalogram; *IER* = in expected range; *EMG* = electromyogram; *EOG* = electro-olfactogram.

BACKGROUND READINGS:

Ellis, J.R., & Nowlis, E.A. (1994). *Providing nursing care within the nursing process* (5th ed.). Philadelphia: J.B. Lippincott.

Hoch, C.C., Reynolds, C.F., Houck, P. (1988). Sleep patterns in Alzheimer, depressed, and healthy elderly. *Western Journal of Nursing Research, 10*(3), 239-256.

Mead-Bennet, E. (1989). The relationship of primigravid sleep experience and select moods on the first postpartum day. *Journal of Obstetic, Gynecologic, & Neonatal Nursing, 19*(2), 146-152.

Paulsen, V.M., & Shaver, J.L. (1991). Stress, support, psychological states and sleep. *Social Science and Medicine, 32*(11), 1237-1243.

Potter, P.A., & Perry, A. (1989). *Fundamentals of nursing: Concepts, process, and practice* (2nd ed.). St. Louis: Mosby.

Topf, M. (1992). Effects of personal control over hospital noise on sleep. *Research in Nursing and Health, 15*, 19-22.

Topf, M., & Davis, J.E. (1993). Critical care unit noise and rapid eye movement sleep. *Heart and Lung, 22*(3), 252-258.

Williams, P.D., White, M.A., Powell, G.M., Alexander, D.J., & Conlon, M. (1988). Activity level in hospitalized children during sleep onset latency. *Computers in Nursing, 6*(2), 70-76.

Outcomes

Social Interaction Skills

DEFINITION: An individual's use of effective interaction behaviors

SOCIAL INTERACTION SKILLS	None 1	Limited 2	Moderate 3	Substantial 4	Extensive 5
INDICATORS:					
Disclosure	1	2	3	4	5
Receptiveness	1	2	3	4	5
Cooperation	1	2	3	4	5
Sensitivity	1	2	3	4	5
Assertiveness	1	2	3	4	5
Confrontation	1	2	3	4	5
Consideration	1	2	3	4	5
Genuineness	1	2	3	4	5
Warmth	1	2	3	4	5
Poise	1	2	3	4	5
Relaxation	1	2	3	4	5
Engagement	1	2	3	4	5
Trust	1	2	3	4	5
Compromise	1	2	3	4	5
Other _____ Specify	1	2	3	4	5

BACKGROUND READINGS:

Erickson, D.H., Beiser, M., Iacono, W.G., Fleming, J.A.E., & Lin, T. (1989). The role of social relationships in the course of first-episode schizophrenia and affective psychosis. *American Journal of Psychiatry, 146*(11), 1456-1461.

Gotcher, J.M. (1992). Interpersonal communication and psychosocial adjustment. *Journal of Psychosocial Oncology, 10*(3), 21-39.

Heltsley, M.E., & Powers, R.C. (1975). Social interaction and perceived adequacy of interaction of the rural aged. *The Gerontologist, 15*(6), 533-536.

Levin, J., & Levin, W.C. (1981). Willingness to interact with an old person. *Research on Aging, 3*(2), 211-217.

Nussbaum, J.F. (1983). Relational closeness of elderly interaction: Implications for life satisfaction. *Western Journal of Speech Communication, 47*, 229-243.

Richter, G., & Richter, J. (1989). Social relationships reflected by depressive inpatients. *Acta Psychiatrica Scandinavica, 80*, 573-578.

Sheppard, M. (1993). Client satisfaction, extended intervention and interpersonal skills in community mental health. *Journal of Advanced Nursing, 18*, 246-259.

Webb, L., Delaney, J.J., & Young, L.R. (1989). Age, interpersonal attraction, and social interaction. *Research on Aging, 11*(1), 107-123.

Social Involvement

DEFINITION: Frequency of an individual's social interactions with persons, groups, or organizations

SOCIAL INVOLVEMENT	None 1	Limited 2	Moderate 3	Substantial 4	Extensive 5
INDICATORS:					
Interaction with close friends	1	2	3	4	5
Interaction with neighbors	1	2	3	4	5
Interaction with family members	1	2	3	4	5
Interaction with members of work group(s)	1	2	3	4	5
Participation as member of church	1	2	3	4	5
Participation in active church work	1	2	3	4	5
Participation as club member	1	2	3	4	5
Participation as club officer	1	2	3	4	5
Participation as a volunteer group member	1	2	3	4	5
Performance of volunteer activities	1	2	3	4	5
Participation in leisure activities	1	2	3	4	5
Other _____ Specify	1	2	3	4	5

BACKGROUND READINGS:

Erickson, D.H., Beiser, M., Iacono, W.G., Fleming, J.A.E., & Lin, T. (1989). The role of social relationships in the course of first-episode schizophrenia and affective psychosis. *American Journal of Psychiatry, 146*(11), 1456-1461.

Gotcher, J.M. (1992). Interpersonal communication and psychosocial adjustment. *Journal of Psychosocial Oncology, 10*(3), 21-39.

Heltsley, M.E., & Powers, R.C. (1975). Social interaction and perceived adequacy of interaction of the rural aged. *The Gerontologist, 15*(6), 533-536.

Levin, J., & Levin, W.C. (1981). Willingness to interact with an old person. *Research on Aging, 3*(2), 211-217.

Nussbaum, J.F. (1983). Relational closeness of elderly interaction: Implications for life satisfaction. *Western Journal of Speech Communication, 47,* 229-243.

Richter, G., & Richter, J. (1989). Social relationships reflected by depressive inpatients. *Acta Psychiatrica Scandinavica, 80,* 573-578.

Sheppard, M. (1993). Client satisfaction, extended intervention and interpersonal skills in community mental health. *Journal of Advanced Nursing, 18,* 246-259.

Webb, L., Delaney, J.J., & Young, L.R. (1989). Age, interpersonal attraction, and social interaction. *Research on Aging, 11*(1), 107-123.

Outcomes

Outcomes

Social Support

DEFINITION: Perceived availability and actual provision of reliable assistance from other persons

SOCIAL SUPPORT	None 1	Limited 2	Moderate 3	Substantial 4	Extensive 5
INDICATORS:					
Reports of money provided by others	1	2	3	4	5
Reports of time provided by others	1	2	3	4	5
Reports of labor provided by others	1	2	3	4	5
Reports of information provided by others	1	2	3	4	5
Reports of emotional assistance provided by others	1	2	3	4	5
Reports of confidant relationship(s)	1	2	3	4	5
Reports of persons who can help when needed	1	2	3	4	5
Evidence of willingness to call on others for help	1	2	3	4	5
Reports of assistive social network	1	2	3	4	5
Reports of adequate supportive social contacts	1	2	3	4	5
Reports of stable social network	1	2	3	4	5
Reports of help offered by others	1	2	3	4	5
Other _____ Specify	1	2	3	4	5

BACKGROUND READINGS:

Dimond, M., & Jones, S.L. (1983). Social support: A review and theoretical integration. In P.L. Chinn (Ed.), *Advances in nursing theory development* (pp. 235-249). Rockville, MD: Aspen.

Norbeck, J.S. (1981). Social support: A model for clinical research and application. *Advances in Nursing Science, 3*(4): 43-59.

Tilden, V.P. (1985). Issues of conceptualization and measurement of social support in the construction of nursing theory. *Research in Nursing and Health, 8,* 199-206.

Spiritual Well-Being

DEFINITION: Personal expressions of connectedness with self, others, higher power, all life, nature, and the universe that transcend and empower the self

SPIRITUAL WELL-BEING	Extremely compromised 1	Substantially compromised 2	Moderately compromised 3	Mildly compromised 4	Not compromised 5
INDICATORS:					
Expression of faith	1	2	3	4	5
Expression of hope	1	2	3	4	5
Expression of meaning and purpose in life	1	2	3	4	5
Expression of spiritual world view	1	2	3	4	5
Expression of serenity	1	2	3	4	5
Expression of love	1	2	3	4	5
Expression of forgiveness	1	2	3	4	5
Mystical experiences	1	2	3	4	5
Prayer	1	2	3	4	5
Worship	1	2	3	4	5
Participation in spiritual rites and passages	1	2	3	4	5
Interaction with spiritual leaders	1	2	3	4	5
Meditation	1	2	3	4	5
Expression through song	1	2	3	4	5
Spiritual reading	1	2	3	4	5
Connectedness with inner-self	1	2	3	4	5
Connectedness with others to share thoughts, feelings, and belief	1	2	3	4	5
Other _____ Specify	1	2	3	4	5

Outcomes

Outcomes

BACKGROUND READINGS:

Burkhardt, M.A. (1989). Spirituality: An analysis of the concept. *Holistic Nursing Practice, 3*(3), 69-77.

Emblen, J.D. (1992). Religion and spirituality defined according to current use in nursing literature. *Journal of Professional Nursing, 8*(1), 41-47.

Haase, J.E. et al. (1992). Simultaneous concept analysis of spiritual perspective, hope, acceptance and self-transcendence. *IMAGE-The Journal of Nursing Scholarship, 24*(2), 141-146.

Labun, E. (1988). Spiritual care: An element in nursing care planning. *Journal of Advanced Nursing, 13*(3), 314-320.

Pender, N. (1996). *Health promotion in nursing practice* (3rd ed.). Stanford, CT: Appleton & Lange.

Reed, P.G. (1992). An emerging paradigm for the investigation of spirituality in nursing. *Research in Nursing and Health, 15*(5), 349-357.

Substance Addiction Consequences

DEFINITION: Compromise in health status and social functioning due to substance addiction

SUBSTANCE ADDICTION CONSEQUENCES	Severe 1	Substantial 2	Moderate 3	Slight 4	None 5
INDICATORS:					
Sustained decrease in physical activity	1	2	3	4	5
Chronic impaired motor function	1	2	3	4	5
Chronic decreased endurance	1	2	3	4	5
Chronic fatigue	1	2	3	4	5
Chronic impaired cognitive function	1	2	3	4	5
Chronic impaired breathing	1	2	3	4	5
Prolonged recovery from illnesses	1	2	3	4	5
Absenteeism from work or school	1	2	3	4	5
Difficulty maintaining employment	1	2	3	4	5
Difficulty maintaining adequate housing	1	2	3	4	5
Difficulty supporting self financially	1	2	3	4	5
Repeated traffic accidents within the last year	1	2	3	4	5
Habitual arrests within the last year	1	2	3	4	5
Repeated ER* visits within the last year	1	2	3	4	5
Repeated hospitalizations within the last year	1	2	3	4	5
Other _____ Specify	1	2	3	4	5

*ER = Emergency room.

BACKGROUND READINGS:

McCuster, J., Stoddard, A.M., Zapka, J.G., & Lewis, B.F. (1993). Behavioral outcomes of AIDS educational interventions for drug users in short term treatment. *American Journal of Public Health, 83*(10), 1463-1466.

McDonald, B. (1994, January 18). Intake Supervisor of MECCA-Substance Abuse Services. Personal correspondence.

Simons-Morton, D.G., Mullen, P.D., Mains, D.A., Tabak, E.R., & Green, L.W. (1992). Characteristics of controlled studies of patient education and counseling for preventive health behaviors. *Patient Education and Counseling, 19,* 174-204.

Talashek, M.L., Gerace, L.M., & Starr, K.L. (1994). The substance abuse pandemic: Determinants to guide interventions. *Public Health Nursing, 11*(2), 131-139.

Outcomes

Suicide Self-Restraint

DEFINITION: Ability to refrain from gestures and attempts at killing self

SUICIDE SELF-RESTRAINT	Never demonstrated 1	Rarely demonstrated 2	Sometimes demonstrated 3	Often demonstrated 4	Consistently demonstrated 5
INDICATORS:					
Expresses feelings	1	2	3	4	5
Maintains connectedness in relationships	1	2	3	4	5
Seeks help when feeling self-destructive	1	2	3	4	5
Verbalizes suicidal ideas	1	2	3	4	5
Verbalizes control of impulses	1	2	3	4	5
Refrains from gathering means for suicide	1	2	3	4	5
Does not give away possessions	1	2	3	4	5
Does not require treatment for suicide gestures or attempts	1	2	3	4	5
Refrains from using mood altering substance(s)	1	2	3	4	5
Discloses plan for suicide	1	2	3	4	5
Upholds suicide contract	1	2	3	4	5
Maintains self-control without supervision	1	2	3	4	5
Does not attempt suicide	1	2	3	4	5
Other _____ Specify	1	2	3	4	5

BACKGROUND READINGS:

Beck, A.T., Steer, R.A., & Brown, G. (1993). Dysfunctional attitudes and suicidal ideation in psychiatric outpatients. *Suicide and Life-Threatening Behavior, 23*(1), 11-20.

Cugino, A., Markovich, E.I., Rosenblatt, S., Jarjoura, D., Blend, D., & Whittier, F.C. (1992). Searching for a pattern: Repeat suicide attempts. *Journal of Psychosocial Nursing, 30,* 23-25.

Forrester, P. (1994). Accurate assessment of short-term suicide risk in a crisis. *Psychiatric Annals, 24,* 603-609.

Josepho, S.A., & Plutchek, R. (1994). Stress, coping, and suicide risk in psychiatric inpatients. *Suicide and Life-Threatening Behavior, 24*(1), 48-57.

Lipshitz, A. (1995). Suicide prevention in young adults (age 18-30). *Suicide and Life-Threatening Behavior, 25*(1), 155-169.

Mellick, E., Buckwalter, K.C., & Stolley, J.M. (1992). Suicide among elderly white men: Development of a profile. *Journal of Psychosocial Nursing, 30,* 29-34.

Continued.

Muczkowski, T.A., Sweeney, J.A., Haas, G.L., Junker, B.W., Brown, R.P., & Mann, J.J. (1993). Factor composition of the suicide intent scale. *Suicide and Life-Threatening Behavior, 23*(1), 48-57.

Steer, R.A., Rismiller, D.J., Ranieri, W.F., & Beck, A.T. (1993). Dimensions of suicidal ideation in psychiatric inpatients. *Behavior Research Therapy, 31*(2), 229-236.

Stuart, G.W., & Sundeen, S.J. (1995). *Principles and practices of psychiatric nursing* (5th ed.). St. Louis: Mosby.

Symptom Control Behavior

SYMPTOM CONTROL BEHAVIOR	Never demonstrated 1	Rarely demonstrated 2	Sometimes demonstrated 3	Often demonstrated 4	Consistently demonstrated 5

DEFINITION: Personal actions to minimize perceived adverse changes in physical and emotional functioning

INDICATORS:					
Recognizes symptom onset	1	2	3	4	5
Recognizes symptom persistence	1	2	3	4	5
Recognizes symptom severity	1	2	3	4	5
Recognizes symptom frequency	1	2	3	4	5
Recognizes symptom variation	1	2	3	4	5
Uses preventive measures	1	2	3	4	5
Uses relief measures	1	2	3	4	5
Uses warning signs to seek health care	1	2	3	4	5
Uses available resources	1	2	3	4	5
Uses symptom diary	1	2	3	4	5
Reports controlling symptoms	1	2	3	4	5
Other _____ Specify	1	2	3	4	5

Outcomes

BACKGROUND READINGS:

Epstein, L., & Cluss (1982). A behavioral perspective on adherence for long-term medical regimens. *Journal of Consulting and Clinical Psychology, 50,* 950-971.

Hartford, M., Karlson, B.W., Sjolin, M., Holmber, S. & Herlitz, J. (1993). Symptoms, thoughts, and environmental factors in suspected acute myocardial infarction. *Heart and Lung, 22*(1), 64-70.

Hegyvary, S.T. (1993). Patient care outcomes related to management of symptoms. In J.J. Fitzpatrick & J.S. Stevenson (Eds.), *Annual Review of Nursing Research, 11,* 145-168.

McCorkle, R., & Young, K. (1978). Development of a symptom distress scale. *Cancer Nursing, 10,* 373-378.

Sherbourne, C.D., Allen, H.M., Kamberg, C.J., & Wells, K.B. (1992). Physical/psychophysiological symptoms measure. In A.L. Stewart & J.E. Ware, Jr. (Eds.), *Measuring functioning and well-being* (pp. 261-272): Durham, NC: Duke University Press.

Strauss, A.L., Corbin, J., Fagerhaugh, S., Glaser, B.G., Maines, D., Suczek, B., & Wiener, C.L. (1984). Symptom control. In *Chronic illness and the quality of life.* (2nd ed., pp. 49-59). St. Louis: Mosby.

Symptom Severity

DEFINITION: Extent of perceived adverse changes in physical, emotional, and social functioning

SYMPTOM SEVERITY	Severe 1	Substantial 2	Moderate 3	Slight 4	None 5
INDICATORS:					
Symptom intensity	1	2	3	4	5
Symptom frequency	1	2	3	4	5
Symptom persistence	1	2	3	4	5
Associated discomfort	1	2	3	4	5
Associated restlessness	1	2	3	4	5
Associated fear	1	2	3	4	5
Associated anxiety	1	2	3	4	5
Impaired physical mobility	1	2	3	4	5
Impaired role performance	1	2	3	4	5
Impaired interpersonal relationship	1	2	3	4	5
Impaired mood	1	2	3	4	5
Compromised life enjoyment	1	2	3	4	5
Disrupted sleep	1	2	3	4	5
Lack of appetite	1	2	3	4	5
Other _____ Specify	1	2	3	4	5

BACKGROUND READINGS:

Hartford, M., Karlson, B.W., Sjolin, M., Homberg, S., & Herlitz, J. (1993). Symptoms, thoughts, and environmental factors in suspected acute myocardial infarction. *Heart and Lung, 22*(1), 64-70.

Hegyvary, S.T. (1993). Patient care outcomes related to management of symptoms. In J.J. Fitzpatrick & J.S. Stevenson (Eds.), *Annual Review of Nursing Research, 11,* 145-168.

McCorkle, R., & Young, K. (1978). Development of a symptom distress scale. *Cancer Nursing, 10,* 373-378.

Sherbourne, C.D., Allen, H.M., Kamberg, C.J., & Wells, K.B. (1992). Physical/psychophysiologic symptoms measure. In A.L. Stewart & J.E. Ware, Jr. (Eds.), *Measure functioning and well-being* (pp. 261-272). Durham, NC: Duke University Press.

Strauss, A.L., Corbin, J., Fagerhaugh, S., Glaser, B.G., Maines, D., Suczek, B., & Wiener, C.L. (1984). Symptom control. In *Chronic illness and the quality of life* (2nd ed., pp. 49-59). St. Louis: Mosby.

Outcomes

Thermoregulation

DEFINITION: Balance among heat production, heat gain, and heat loss

THERMOREGU-LATION	Extremely compromised 1	Substantially compromised 2	Moderately compromised 3	Mildly compromised 4	Not compromised 5
INDICATORS:					
Skin temperature IER*	1	2	3	4	5
Body temperature WNL*	1	2	3	4	5
Headache not present	1	2	3	4	5
Muscle aches not present	1	2	3	4	5
Irritability not present	1	2	3	4	5
Drowsiness not present	1	2	3	4	5
Skin color changes not present	1	2	3	4	5
Muscle twitching not present	1	2	3	4	5
Presence of goose bumps when cold	1	2	3	4	5
Sweating when hot	1	2	3	4	5
Shivering when cold	1	2	3	4	5
Pulse rate IER	1	2	3	4	5
Respiratory rate IER	1	2	3	4	5
Hydration adequate	1	2	3	4	5
Reported thermal comfort	1	2	3	4	5
Other _____ Specify	1	2	3	4	5

*IER = In expected range; WNL = within normal limits.

BACKGROUND READINGS:

Caruso, C., Hadley, B., Shuklou, R., & Frame, P. (1992). Cooling effects and comfort of four cooling blanket temperatures in humans with fever. *Nursing Research, 41*(2), 68-72.

Erickson, R., & Kerklin, S. (1992). Comparison of methods for core temperature measurement. *Heart and Lung, 21*(3), 297.

Finke, C. (1991). Measurement of the thermoregulatory response: A review. *Focus on Critical Care, 18*(5), 408-412.

Franceschl, V. (1991). Accuracy and feasibility of measuring oral temperature in critically ill adults. *Focus on Critical Care, 18*(3), 221-228.

Hollander, H. (1993). Neurological and febrile syndromes in HIV. *Emergency Medicine, 25*(4), 26-40.

Holtzclaw, B.J. (1992). The febrile response in critical care: State of the science. *Heart and Lung, 21*(5), 482-501.

Kluger, M. (1978). Fever versus hyperthermia. *New England Journal of Medicine, 299*(10), 555.

Continued.

Murphy, K. (1992). Acetaminophen and ibuprofen: Finer control and overdose. *Pediatric Nursing, 18*(4), 428-431.

Segatore, M. (1992). Fever after traumatic brain injury. *American Association of Neuroscience Nurse, 24*(2), 104-109.

Stewart, G., & Webster, D. (1992). Re-evaluation of the tympanic thermometer in the emergency department. *Annals of Emergency Medicine, 21*(2), 158-161.

Summers, S., Dudgeon, N., Byram, K., & Zingsheim, K. (1990). The effects of two warming methods on core and surface temperatures, hemoglobin oxygen saturation, blood pressure, and perceived comfort of hypothermic postanesthesia patients. *Journal of Post Anesthesia Nursing, 5*(5), 354-364.

Thermoregulation: Neonate

DEFINITION: Balance among heat production, heat gain, and heat loss during the neonatal period

THERMOREGULA-TION: NEONATE	Extremely compromised 1	Substantially compromised 2	Moderately compromised 3	Mildly compromised 4	Not compromised 5
INDICATORS:					
Body temperature WNL*	1	2	3	4	5
Respiratory distress not present	1	2	3	4	5
Restlessness not present	1	2	3	4	5
Lethargy not present	1	2	3	4	5
Skin color changes IER*	1	2	3	4	5
Weight gain IER	1	2	3	4	5
Non-shivering thermogenesis	1	2	3	4	5
Use of heat retention posture	1	2	3	4	5
Use of heat dissipation posture	1	2	3	4	5
Weaning to crib from Isolette	1	2	3	4	5
Hydration adequate	1	2	3	4	5
Blood glucose WNL	1	2	3	4	5
Acid-base balance WNL	1	2	3	4	5
Bilirubin WNL	1	2	3	4	5
Other _____ Specify	1	2	3	4	5

*IER = In expected range; WNL = within normal limits.

BACKGROUND READINGS:

Bliss-Holtz, J. (1992). Temperature relationships in cold-stressed infants. *Neonatal network, 11*(2), 72.

Greer, P. (1988). Head coverings for newborns under radiant warmers. *Journal of Obstetric, Gynecologic, and Neonatal Nursing, 17*(4), 265-270.

Keeling, E. (1992). Thermoregulation and axillary temperature measurements in neonates: A review of the literature. *Maternal-Child Nursing Journal, 20*(3,4), 124-140.

Konrad, C. (1980). *Nursing interventions to assess and control fever in infants and small children.* Unpublished master's thesis, The University of Iowa, Iowa City.

Outcomes

Tissue Integrity: Skin & Mucous Membranes

DEFINITION: Structural intactness and normal physiological function of skin and mucous membranes

TISSUE INTEGRITY: SKIN & MUCOUS MEMBRANES	Extremely compromised 1	Substantially compromised 2	Moderately compromised 3	Mildly compromised 4	Not compromised 5
INDICATORS:					
Tissue temperature IER*	1	2	3	4	5
Sensation IER	1	2	3	4	5
Elasticity IER	1	2	3	4	5
Hydration IER	1	2	3	4	5
Pigmentation IER	1	2	3	4	5
Perspiration IER	1	2	3	4	5
Color IER	1	2	3	4	5
Texture IER	1	2	3	4	5
Thickness IER	1	2	3	4	5
Tissue lesion free	1	2	3	4	5
Tissue perfusion	1	2	3	4	5
Hair growth on skin IER	1	2	3	4	5
Skin intactness	1	2	3	4	5
Other _____ Specify	1	2	3	4	5

*IER = In expected range.

BACKGROUND READINGS:

Cohen, R.K., Diegelmann, R.F., & Lindblad, W.L. (1992). *Wound healing: biochemical and clinical aspects.* Philadelphia: W.B. Saunders.

Lazarus, G.S., Cooper, D.M., Knighton, D.R., Margohs, D.J., Pecoraro, R.E., Rodeheaver, G., & Robson, M.C. (1994). Definitions and guidelines for assessment of wounds and evaluation of healing. *Archives of Dermatology, 130,* 489-493.

Potter, P.A., & Perry, A.G. (1993). *Fundamentals of nursing: Concepts, process, and practice* (3rd ed.). St. Louis: Mosby.

Rijswijk, L et al. (1993). Full-thickness leg ulcers: Patient demographics and predictors of healing. *The Journal of Family Practice, 36*(6), 625-632.

Sieggreen, M., & Maklebust, J. (1991). *Pressure ulcers: Guidelines for prevention and nursing management.* Springhouse, PA: Springhouse.

U.S. Department of Health and Human Services. (1992). *Pressure ulcers in adults: Prediction and prevention* (AHCPR Publication No. 92-0047). Rockville, MD: Public Health Service Agency for Health Care Policy and Research.

U.S. Department of Health and Human Services. (1994). *Treatment of pressure ulcers* (AHCPR Publication No. 95-0652). Rockville, MD: Public Health Service Agency for Health Care Policy and Research.

Tissue Perfusion: Abdominal Organs

DEFINITION: Extent to which blood flows through the small vessels of the abdominal viscera and maintains organ function

TISSUE PERFUSION: ABDOMINAL ORGANS	Extremely compromised 1	Substantially compromised 2	Moderately compromised 3	Mildly compromised 4	Not compromised 5
INDICATORS:					
Vital signs	1	2	3	4	5
Urine output	1	2	3	4	5
Electrolyte and acid/base balance	1	2	3	4	5
Fluid balance	1	2	3	4	5
Bowel sounds	1	2	3	4	5
Appetite	1	2	3	4	5
Abnormal thirst not present	1	2	3	4	5
Abdominal pain not present	1	2	3	4	5
Nausea not present	1	2	3	4	5
Vomiting not present	1	2	3	4	5
Malabsorption deficiencies not present	1	2	3	4	5
Chronic gastritis not present	1	2	3	4	5
Abdominal distention not present	1	2	3	4	5
Ascites not present	1	2	3	4	5
Gastrointestinal varices not present	1	2	3	4	5
Constipation not present	1	2	3	4	5
Diarrhea not present	1	2	3	4	5
Urine specific gravity WNL*	1	2	3	4	5
BUN* WNL	1	2	3	4	5
Plasma creatinine WNL	1	2	3	4	5
Liver function tests WNL	1	2	3	4	5
Pancreatic enzymes WNL	1	2	3	4	5
Other _____ Specify	1	2	3	4	5

*WNL = Within normal limits; BUN = blood urea nitrogen.   *Continued.*

BACKGROUND READINGS:

Lewis, S.M., & Collier, I.C. (1992). *Medical-surgical nursing: Assessment & management of clinical problems* (3rd ed.). St. Louis: Mosby.

McCance, K.L., & Huether, S.E. (1994). *Pathophysiology: The biologic basis for disease in adults and children* (2nd ed.). St. Louis: Mosby.

Outcomes

Tissue Perfusion: Cardiac

DEFINITION: Extent to which blood flows through the coronary vasculature and maintains heart function

TISSUE PERFUSION: CARDIAC	Extremely compromised 1	Substantially compromised 2	Moderately compromised 3	Mildly compromised 4	Not compromised 5
INDICATORS:					
Cardiac pump effectiveness	1	2	3	4	5
Angina not present	1	2	3	4	5
Profuse diaphoresis not present	1	2	3	4	5
Nausea not present	1	2	3	4	5
Vomiting not present	1	2	3	4	5
Vital signs WNL*	1	2	3	4	5
ECG* WNL	1	2	3	4	5
Cardiac enzymes WNL	1	2	3	4	5
Coronary angiogram WNL	1	2	3	4	5
Thallium scan WNL	1	2	3	4	5
Other _____ Specify	1	2	3	4	5

*WNL = Within normal limits; ECG = electrocardiogram.

BACKGROUND READINGS:

Lewis, S.M., & Collier, I.C. (1992). *Medical-surgical nursing: Assessment & management of clinical problems* (3rd ed.). St. Louis: Mosby.

McCance, K.L., & Huether, S.E. (1994). *Pathophysiology: The biologic basis for disease in adults and children* (2nd ed.). St. Louis: Mosby.

Tissue Perfusion: Cerebral

DEFINITION: Extent to which blood flows through the cerebral vasculature and maintains brain function

TISSUE PERFUSION: CEREBRAL	Extremely compromised 1	Substantially compromised 2	Moderately compromised 3	Mildly compromised 4	Not compromised 5
INDICATORS:					
Neurological status	1	2	3	4	5
Intracranial pressure WNL*	1	2	3	4	5
Headache not present	1	2	3	4	5
Carotid bruit not present	1	2	3	4	5
Restlessness not present	1	2	3	4	5
Listlessness not present	1	2	3	4	5
Unexplained anxiety not present	1	2	3	4	5
Agitation not present	1	2	3	4	5
Vomiting not present	1	2	3	4	5
Hiccoughs not present	1	2	3	4	5
Syncope not present	1	2	3	4	5
Other _____ Specify	1	2	3	4	5

*WNL = Within normal limits.

BACKGROUND READINGS:

Lewis, S.M., & Collier, I.C. (1992). *Medical-surgical nursing: Assessment & management of clinical problems* (3rd ed.). St. Louis: Mosby.

McCance, K.L., & Huether, S.E. (1994). *Pathophysiology: The biologic basis for disease in adults and children* (2nd ed.). St. Louis: Mosby.

Tissue Perfusion: Peripheral

DEFINITION: Extent to which blood flows through the small vessels of the extremities and maintains tissue function

TISSUE PERFUSION: PERIPHERAL	Extremely compromised 1	Substantially compromised 2	Moderately compromised 3	Mildly compromised 4	Not compromised 5
INDICATORS:					
Capillary refill brisk	1	2	3	4	5
Distal peripheral pulses strong	1	2	3	4	5
Proximal peripheral pulses strong	1	2	3	4	5
Distal peripheral pulses symmetrical	1	2	3	4	5
Proximal peripheral pulses symmetrical	1	2	3	4	5
Sensation level normal	1	2	3	4	5
Skin color normal	1	2	3	4	5
Muscle function intact	1	2	3	4	5
Skin intact	1	2	3	4	5
Extremity temperature warm	1	2	3	4	5
Extremity bruits not present	1	2	3	4	5
Peripheral edema not present	1	2	3	4	5
Localized extremity pain not present	1	2	3	4	5
Other _____ Specify	1	2	3	4	5

BACKGROUND READINGS:

Cohen, R.K., Diegelmann, R.F., & Lindblad, W.L. (1992). *Wound healing: Biochemical and clinical aspects*. Philadelphia: W.B. Saunders.

Lazarus, G.S., Cooper, D.M., Knighton, D.R., Margohs, D.J., Pecoraro, R.E., Rodeheaver, G., & Robson, M.C. (1994). Definitions and guidelines for assessment of wounds and evaluation of healing. *Archives of Dermatology, 130,* 489-493.

Potter, P.A., & Perry, A.G. (1993). *Fundamentals of nursing: Concepts, process, and practice* (3rd ed.). St. Louis: Mosby.

Rijswijk, L. et al. (1993). Full-thickness leg ulcers: Patient demographics and predictors of healing. *The Journal of Family Practice, 36*(6), 625-632.

Sieggreen, M., & Maklebust, J. (1991). *Pressure ulcers: Guidelines for prevention and nursing management*. Springhouse, PA: Springhouse.

Outcomes

Tissue Perfusion: Pulmonary

DEFINITION: Extent to which blood flows through intact pulmonary vasculature with appropriate pressure and volume, perfusing alveoli/capillary unit

TISSUE PERFUSION: PULMONARY	Extremely compromised 1	Substantially compromised 2	Moderately compromised 3	Mildly compromised 4	Not compromised 5
INDICATORS:					
Respiratory status: gas exchange	1	2	3	4	5
Respiratory status: ventilation	1	2	3	4	5
Cardiac pump effectiveness	1	2	3	4	5
Vital signs	1	2	3	4	5
Chest pain not present	1	2	3	4	5
Pleural friction rub not present	1	2	3	4	5
Hemoptysis not present	1	2	3	4	5
Unexplained anxiety not present	1	2	3	4	5
Arterial blood gases WNL*	1	2	3	4	5
Ventilation-perfusion scan WNL	1	2	3	4	5
Pulmonary artery pressure (PAP) WNL	1	2	3	4	5
ECG* WNL	1	2	3	4	5
Other _____ Specify	1	2	3	4	5

*WNL = Within normal limits; ECG = electrocardiogram.

BACKGROUND READINGS:

Lewis, S.M., & Collier, I.C. (1992). *Medical-surgical nursing: Assessment & management of clinical problems* (3rd ed.). St. Louis: Mosby.

McCance, K.L., & Huether, S.E. (1994). *Pathophysiology: The biologic basis for disease in adults and children* (2nd ed.). St. Louis: Mosby.

Transfer Performance

DEFINITION: Ability to change body locations

TRANSFER PERFORMANCE	Dependent, does not participate	Requires assistive person & device	Requires assistive person	Independent with assistive device	Completely independent
	1	**2**	**3**	**4**	**5**
INDICATORS:					
Transfers from bed to chair	1	2	3	4	5
Transfers from chair to bed	1	2	3	4	5
Transfers from chair to chair	1	2	3	4	5
Transfers from wheel-chair to vehicle	1	2	3	4	5
Transfers from vehicle to wheelchair	1	2	3	4	5
Other _____ Specify	1	2	3	4	5

BACKGROUND READINGS:

Kane, R.L, & Kane, R.A. (1981). *Assessing the elderly: A practical guide to measurement.* Lexington, MA: Lexington Books.

Mikulic, M.A., Griffith, E.R., & Jebsen, R.H. (1976). Clinical application of a standardized mobility test. *Archives of Physical Medicine and Rehabilitation, 57*(3), 143-146.

Outcomes

Treatment Behavior: Illness or Injury

DEFINITION: Personal actions to palliate or eliminate pathology

TREATMENT BEHAVIOR: ILLNESS OR INJURY	Never demonstrated 1	Rarely demonstrated 2	Sometimes demonstrated 3	Often demonstrated 4	Consistently demonstrated 5
INDICATORS:					
Complies with recommended precautions	1	2	3	4	5
Complies with recommended treatment regimen	1	2	3	4	5
Complies with prescribed treatments	1	2	3	4	5
Complies with prescribed activities	1	2	3	4	5
Complies with medication regimen	1	2	3	4	5
Avoids behaviors that potentiate pathology	1	2	3	4	5
Performs self-care consistent with ability	1	2	3	4	5
Monitors for treatment effects	1	2	3	4	5
Monitors for treatment side effects	1	2	3	4	5
Monitors for disease side effects	1	2	3	4	5
Monitors changes in disease status	1	2	3	4	5
Uses devices correctly	1	2	3	4	5
Alters role functions to meet treatment requirements	1	2	3	4	5
Balances treatment, exercise, work, leisure, rest, and nutrition	1	2	3	4	5
Seeks advice from health provider as needed	1	2	3	4	5
Arranges personal visit with health care provider as needed	1	2	3	4	5
Other _____ Specify	1	2	3	4	5

BACKGROUND READINGS:

Conn, V., Taylor, S., & Casey, B. (1992). Cardiac rehabilitation program participation and outcomes after myocardial infarction. *Rehabilitation Nursing, 17*(2), 58-62.

Woods, N. (1989). Conceptualizations of self-care: Toward health-oriented models. *Advances in Nursing Science, 12*(1), 1-13.

Outcomes

Urinary Continence

DEFINITION: Control of the elimination of urine

URINARY CONTINENCE	Never demonstrated 1	Rarely demonstrated 2	Sometimes demonstrated 3	Often demonstrated 4	Consistently demonstrated 5
INDICATORS:					
Recognizes urge to void	1	2	3	4	5
Predictable pattern to passage of urine	1	2	3	4	5
Responds in timely manner to urge	1	2	3	4	5
Voids in appropriate receptacle	1	2	3	4	5
Adequate time to reach toilet between urge and evacuation of urine	1	2	3	4	5
Voids >150 cc each time	1	2	3	4	5
Free of urine leakage between voidings	1	2	3	4	5
Able to start and stop stream	1	2	3	4	5
Empties bladder completely	1	2	3	4	5
Absence of post void residual >100-200 cc	1	2	3	4	5
No urine leakage with increased abdominal pressure (e.g., sneezing, laughing, lifting)	1	2	3	4	5
Underclothing dry during day	1	2	3	4	5
Underclothing or bedding dry during night	1	2	3	4	5
Absence of urinary tract infection (<100,000 WBC)*	1	2	3	4	5
Fluid intake IER*	1	2	3	4	5
Able to manage clothing independently	1	2	3	4	5
Able to toilet independently	1	2	3	4	5

URINARY CONTINENCE	Never demonstrated 1	Rarely demonstrated 2	Sometimes demonstrated 3	Often demonstrated 4	Consistently demonstrated 5
Maintains environment barrier-free to independent toileting	1	2	3	4	5
Free of medications that interfere with urinary control	1	2	3	4	5
Other _____ Specify	1	2	3	4	5

*WBC = White blood (cell) count; IER = in expected range.

BACKGROUND READINGS:

Palmer, M.H., McCormick, K.A., Langford, A., Langlais, J., & Alvaran, M. (1992). Continence outcomes: Documentation on medical records in the nursing home environment. *Journal of Nursing Care Quality, 6*(3), 36-43.

Specht, J., Tunink, P., Maas, M., & Bulechek, G. (1991). Urinary incontinence. In M. Maas, K. Buckwalter, & M. Hardy (Eds.), *Nursing diagnoses and interventions for the elderly.* Redwood City, CA: Addison-Wesley Nursing.

Urinary Incontinence Guideline Panel. (1992). *Urinary incontinence in adults: Clinical practice guideline* (AHCPR Publication No. 92-0038). Rockville, MD: Agency for Health Care Policy and Research, Public Health Service, U.S. Department of Health and Human Services.

Outcomes

Urinary Elimination

DEFINITION: Ability of the urinary system to filter wastes, conserve solutes, and to collect and discharge urine in a healthy pattern

URINARY ELIMINATION	Extremely compromised 1	Substantially compromised 2	Moderately compromised 3	Mildly compromised 4	Not compromised 5
INDICATORS:					
Elimination pattern IER*	1	2	3	4	5
Urine odor IER	1	2	3	4	5
Urine amount IER	1	2	3	4	5
Urine color IER	1	2	3	4	5
Urine free of particles	1	2	3	4	5
Urine clarity	1	2	3	4	5
Digestion of adequate fluids	1	2	3	4	5
24-hour intake and output balanced	1	2	3	4	5
Urine passes without pain	1	2	3	4	5
Urine passes without hesitancy	1	2	3	4	5
Urine passes without urgency	1	2	3	4	5
Urinary continence	1	2	3	4	5
Empties bladder completely	1	2	3	4	5
Recognition of urge	1	2	3	4	5
BUN WNL*	1	2	3	4	5
Serum creatinine WNL	1	2	3	4	5
Urine specific gravity WNL	1	2	3	4	5
Urine proteins WNL	1	2	3	4	5
Urine glucose WNL	1	2	3	4	5
Urine free of blood	1	2	3	4	5
Urine ketones WNL	1	2	3	4	5
Urine pH WNL	1	2	3	4	5
Urine microscopic findings WNL	1	2	3	4	5
Urine electrolytes WNL	1	2	3	4	5
Arterial P_{CO_2} WNL	1	2	3	4	5

*IER = In expected range; BUN = blood urea nitrogen; WNL = within normal limits.

URINARY ELIMINATION	Extremely compromised 1	Substantially compromised 2	Moderately compromised 3	Mildly compromised 4	Not compromised 5
Arterial pH WNL	1	2	3	4	5
Serum electrolytes WNL	1	2	3	4	5
Other _____ Specify	1	2	3	4	5

BACKGROUND READINGS:

Brundage, D.J. & Linton, A.D. (1997). Age related changes in the genitourinary system. In M.A. Matteson, E.S. McConnell, & A.D. Linton (Eds.), *Gerontological nursing: Concepts in practice* (2nd ed.). Philadelphia, W.B. Saunders.

Fantl J.A., Newman, D.K., Colling, J. et al. (1996). *Urinary incontinence in adults: Acute and chronic management.* Clinical practice guideline, No. 2, 1996 update. (AHCPR Publication No. 96-0682). Rockville, MD: U.S. Department of Health and Human Services. Public Health Service, Agency for Health Care and Policy Research.

McConnell, J.D., Barry, M.J., Brusketwitz, R.C. et al. (1994). *Benign prostatic hyperplasia: Diagnosis and treatment. Clinical practice guideline,* No. 8. (AHCPR Publication No. 94-0582). Rockville, MD: Agency for Health Care Policy and Research, Public Health Service, U.S. Department of Health and Human Services.

Morton, P.G. (1989). *Health assessment in nursing.* Springhouse, PA: Springhouse.

Palmer, M.H., McCormick, K.A., Langford, A., Langlais, J., & Alvaran, M. (1992). Continence outcomes: Documentation on medical records in the nursing home environment. *Journal of Nursing Care Quality, 6*(3), 36-43.

Potter, P., & Potter, A. (1993). *Fundamentals of nursing: Concepts, process, and practice* (3rd ed.). St. Louis: Mosby.

Specht, J., Tunink, P., Maas, M., & Bulechek, G. (1991). Urinary incontinence. In M. Maas, K. Buckwalter & M. Hardy (Eds.), *Nursing diagnoses and interventions for the elderly.* Redwood City, CA: Addison-Wesley.

Urinary Incontinence Guideline Panel. (1992). *Urinary incontinence in adults: clinical practice guidelines* (AHCPR Publication No. 92-0038). Rockville, MD: Agency for Health Care Policy and Research, Public Health Service, U.S. Department of Health and Human Services.

Outcomes

Vital Signs Status

DEFINITION: Temperature, pulse, respiration, and blood pressure within expected range for the individual

VITAL SIGNS STATUS	Extreme deviation from expected range	Substantial deviation from expected range	Moderate deviation from expected range	Mild deviation from expected range	No deviation from expected range
	1	2	3	4	5
INDICATORS:					
Temperature	1	2	3	4	5
Apical pulse rate	1	2	3	4	5
Radial pulse rate	1	2	3	4	5
Respiration rate	1	2	3	4	5
Systolic BP*	1	2	3	4	5
Diastolic BP	1	2	3	4	5
Other _____ Specify	1	2	3	4	5

*BP = Blood pressure.

BACKGROUND READINGS:

Caruso, C., Hadley, B., Shukla, R., & Frame, P. (1992). Cooling effects and comfort of four cooling blanket temperatures in humans with fever. *Nursing Research, 41*(2), 68-72.

Finke, C. (1991). Measurement of the thermoregulatory response: A review. *Focus on Critical Care, 18*(5), 408-412.

Summers, S., Dudgeon, N., Byram, K., & Zingsheim, K. (1990). The effects of two warming methods on core and surface temperatures, hemoglobin oxygen saturation, blood pressure, and perceived comfort of hypothermic postanesthesia patients. *Journal of Post Anesthesia Nursing, 5*(5), 354-364.

Outcomes

Well-Being

DEFINITION: An individual's expressed satisfaction with health status

WELL-BEING	Extremely compromised 1	Substantially compromised 2	Moderately compromised 3	Mildly compromised 4	Not compromised 5
INDICATORS:					
Satisfaction with ADL* performance	1	2	3	4	5
Satisfaction with psycho-logical functioning	1	2	3	4	5
Satisfaction with social interaction	1	2	3	4	5
Satisfaction with spiritual life	1	2	3	4	5
Satisfaction with physio-logical functioning	1	2	3	4	5
Satisfaction with cognitive functioning	1	2	3	4	5
Satisfaction with ability to cope	1	2	3	4	5
Satisfaction with ability to relax	1	2	3	4	5
Satisfaction with level of happiness	1	2	3	4	5
Satisfaction with ability to express emotions	1	2	3	4	5
Other _____ Specify	1	2	3	4	5

*ADL = Activities of daily living.

BACKGROUND READINGS:

Brook, J.R., Davies, A. et al. (1980). *Conceptualization and measurement of health for adults in the health Insurance Study.* (Publication No. R-1987/HEW). Santa Monica, CA: Rand Corporation.

Ferrell, B.R., Dow, K.H., Leigh, S., Ly, J., & Gulasekaram, P. (1995). Quality of life in long-term cancer survivors. *Oncology Nursing Forum, 22*(6), 915-922.

Ferrell, B., Grant, M., Schmidt, G.M., Rhiner, M., Whitehead, C.P., & Forman, S.J. (1992). The meaning of quality of life for bone marrow transplant survivors. Part 1. *Cancer Nursing, 15*(3), 153-160.

Kozier, B., Erb, G., & Blais, K. (1992). *Concepts and issues in nursing practice* (2nd ed.). Redwood City, CA: Addison-Wesley Nursing.

Stewart, A., Ware, J., Jr., Sherbourne, C., & Wells, K. (1992). Psychological distress/well-being and cognitive functioning measures. In A. Stewart & J. Ware, Jr. (Eds.), *Measuring functioning and well-being: The medical outcomes study approach* (pp. 102-142). Durham, NC: Duke University Press.

Whedon, M., & Ferrell, B.R. (1994). Quality of life in adult bone marrow transplant patients: Beyond the first year. *Seminars in Oncology Nursing, 10*(1), 42-57.

Outcomes

Will to Live

DEFINITION: Desire, determination, and effort to survive					
WILL TO LIVE	**Extremely compromised** **1**	**Substantially compromised** **2**	**Moderately compromised** **3**	**Mildly compromised** **4**	**Not compromised** **5**
INDICATORS:					
Expression of determination to live	1	2	3	4	5
Expression of hope	1	2	3	4	5
Expression of optimism	1	2	3	4	5
Expression of sense of control	1	2	3	4	5
Expression of feelings	1	2	3	4	5
Inquires about one's illness/treatment	1	2	3	4	5
Seeks information about one's illness/treatment	1	2	3	4	5
Use of strategies to compensate for problems associated with disease	1	2	3	4	5
Use of strategies to enhance health	1	2	3	4	5
Use of strategies to lengthen life	1	2	3	4	5
Other _____ Specify	1	2	3	4	5

BACKGROUND READINGS:

Gaskins, S., & Brown, K. (1992). Psychosocial responses among individuals with human immunodeficiency virus infection. *Applied Nursing Research, 5*(3), 111-121.

Greer, S., Morris, T., & Pettingale, K. (1979). Psychological response to breast cancer: Effect on outcome. *The Lancet, 10,* 785-787.

Hagopian, G. (1993). Cognitive strategies used in adapting to a cancer diagnosis. *Oncology Nursing Forum, 20*(5), 759-763.

Katz, R., & Lowe, L. (1989). The "will to live" as perceived by nurses and physicians. *Issues in Mental Health Nursing, 10,* 15-22.

Weisman, A. (1972). *On death and denying: A psychiatric study of terminality.* New York: Behavioral Publications.

Outcomes

Wound Healing: Primary Intention

DEFINITION: The extent to which cells and tissues have regenerated following intentional closure

WOUND HEALING: PRIMARY INTENTION	None 1	Slight 2	Moderate 3	Substantial 4	Complete 5
INDICATORS:					
Skin approximation	1	2	3	4	5
Resolution of purulent drainage	1	2	3	4	5
Resolution of serous drainage from wound	1	2	3	4	5
Resolution of sanguineous drainage from wound	1	2	3	4	5
Resolution of serosanguineous drainage from wound	1	2	3	4	5
Resolution of sanguineous drainage from drain	1	2	3	4	5
Resolution of serosanguineous drainage from drain	1	2	3	4	5
Resolution of surrounding skin erythema	1	2	3	4	5
Resolution of periwound edema	1	2	3	4	5
Resolution of skin temperature elevation	1	2	3	4	5
Resolution of wound odor	1	2	3	4	5
Other _____ Specify	1	2	3	4	5

BACKGROUND READINGS:

Bergstrom, N., Bennett, M.A., Carlson, C.E. et al. (1994). *Treatment of pressure ulcers.* Clinical practice guideline, No. 15 (AHCPR Publication No. 95-0652). Rockville, MD: U.S. Department of Health and Human Services, Agency for Health Care Policy and Research.

Cohen, R.K., Diegelmann, R.F., Lindblad, W.L. (1992). *Wound healing: Biochemical and clinical aspects.* Philadelphia: W.B. Saunders.

Lazarus, G.S., Cooper, D.M., Knighton, D.R., Margohs, D.J., Pecoraro, R.E., Rodeheaver, G., & Robson, M.C. (1994). Definitions and guidelines for assessment of wounds and evaluation of healing. *Archives of Dermatology, 130,* 489-493.

Potter, P.A., Perry, A.G. (1993). *Fundamentals of nursing: Concepts, process, and practice* (3rd ed.). St. Louis: Mosby.

Outcomes

Wound Healing: Secondary Intention

DEFINITION: The extent to which cells and tissues in an open wound have regenerated

WOUND HEALING: SECONDARY INTENTION	None 1	Slight 2	Moderate 3	Substantial 4	Complete 5
INDICATORS:					
Granulation	1	2	3	4	5
Epithelialization	1	2	3	4	5
Resolution of purulent drainage	1	2	3	4	5
Resolution of serous drainage	1	2	3	4	5
Resolution of sanguineous drainage	1	2	3	4	5
Resolution of serosanguineous drainage	1	2	3	4	5
Resolution of surrounding skin erythema	1	2	3	4	5
Resolution of periwound edema	1	2	3	4	5
Resolution of abnormal surrounding skin	1	2	3	4	5
Resolution of blistered skin	1	2	3	4	5
Resolution of macerated skin	1	2	3	4	5
Resolution of necrosis	1	2	3	4	5
Resolution of sloughing	1	2	3	4	5
Resolution of tunneling	1	2	3	4	5
Resolution of undermining	1	2	3	4	5
Resolution of sinus tract formation	1	2	3	4	5
Resolution of wound odor	1	2	3	4	5
Resolution of wound size	1	2	3	4	5
Other _____ Specify	1	2	3	4	5

Decreased area (length × width) of wound _____ (cm)

Decreased depth of wound _____ (cm)

BACKGROUND READINGS:

Bergstrom, N., Bennett, M.A., Carlson, C.E. et al. (1994). *Treatment of pressure ulcers.* Clinical practice guideline, No. 15 (AHCPR Publication No. 95-0652). Rockville, MD: U.S. Department of Health and Human Services, Agency for Health Care Policy and Research.

Cohen, R.K., Diegelmann, R.F., Lindblad, W.L. (1992). *Wound healing: Biochemical and clinical aspects.* Philadelphia: W.B. Saunders.

Flanagan, M. (1994). Assessment criteria. *Nursing Times, 90*(35), 76-88.

Frantz, R.A., & Gardner S. (1994). Elderly skin care: Principles of chronic wound care. *Journal of Gerontological Nursing, 20*(9), 35-44.

Lazarus, G.S., Cooper, D.M., Knighton, D.R., Margohs, D.J., Pecoraro, R.E., Rodeheaver, G., & Robson, M.C. (1994). Definitions and guidelines for assessment of wounds and evaluation of healing. *Archives of Dermatology, 130,* 489-493.

Outcomes

Potter, P.A., & Perry, A.G. (1993). *Fundamentals of nursing: Concepts, process, and practice* (3rd ed.). St. Louis: Mosby.

Rijswijk, L. et al. (1993). Full-thickness leg ulcers: Patient demographics and predictors of healing. *The Journal of Family Practice, 36*(6), 625-632.

Sieggreen, M., & Maklebust, J. (1991). *Pressure ulcers: Guidelines for prevention and nursing management*. Springhouse, PA: Springhouse.

Outcomes

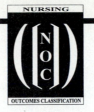

PART THREE

APPENDICES

NANDA-NOC Linkages

Gail Keenan

Appendix A provides linkages between the North American Nursing Diagnosis Association's nursing diagnoses[1] and the Nursing-sensitive Outcomes Classification (NOC) outcomes. A *linkage* is defined as a set of individual **NOC** outcomes that singly or in combination **may be** influenced by the nursing care provided to a patient with a specific NANDA diagnosis. The linkages are not prescriptive; rather they are suggested linkages that require validation through clinical research.[2]

Linkages are needed for the following reasons:

1. To identify specific outcomes that nurses may want to monitor in patients with a specific nursing diagnosis
2. To facilitate diagnostic reasoning relative to achieving desired nursing outcomes
3. To help familiarize nurses with the NOC language and facilitate its use in practice, education, and research
4. To provide initial direction for clinical-nursing–information-system data base structures
5. To facilitate field testing and validation of the linkages

The linkages should assist nurses in using the NOC. Although the NOC labels include familiar terminology, nurses are relatively unaccustomed to thinking in terms of variable outcomes. A linkage provides a list of outcomes from which the nurse may choose to monitor in a patient with a specific NANDA diagnosis. Eventually, ongoing use of the NOC is expected to facilitate knowledge development and result in the creation of more outcomes in the classification.

The list of NOC outcomes linked to a NANDA diagnosis is a representative set and is not intended to be exhaustive of all of the possible outcomes the nurse might consider monitoring for a patient with a particular diagnosis. The outcomes selected will ultimately depend on the nurse's judgment relative to the patient care situation. Each list includes outcomes that nurses may want to monitor for most patients with a particular diagnosis and other outcomes that are important but more specific to the related factors in NANDA diagnoses. Finally, the linkages are identified as NOC outcomes that have been developed to date. Additional linkages will be identified as more outcomes are added to the NOC.

METHODOLOGY USED TO DEVELOP LINKAGES

Several methodologies were initially tested to develop the linkages. In an effort to provide a practical and useful set of outcomes for each diagnosis, the following methodology was used to link NANDA diagnoses with NOC outcomes:

1. The process used to identify linkages was established:
   a. All diagnoses appearing in the *Nursing Diagnoses: Definitions & Classification 1995-1996*[1] were linked to NOC outcomes, if possible
   b. All NOC outcomes that were developed at the time of this text's publication were reviewed for appropriateness for each linkage list
   c. For each NANDA diagnosis:
      (1) The **definition, defining characteristics, related factors,** and **related risk factors** were reviewed
      (2) The definitions of the NOC outcomes were reviewed
      (3) Those outcomes expected to be influenced by nursing care provided to patients with the diagnosis were identified
      (4) Information related to each NANDA diagnosis was considered to identify linkages for a syndrome or set of nursing diagnoses that occur together
      (5) Outcomes for the linkage list that were inclusive of all ages appropriate to the diagnosis were selected
2. A research assistant familiar with the NOC outcomes compiled a preliminary list of outcomes for each NANDA diagnosis according to the established process.*
3. A small group composed of NOC team members with diverse clinical backgrounds and varying levels of knowledge of NANDA carefully evaluated the preliminary lists. The group met regularly and used the established process as a guide to evaluate the appropriateness of outcomes contained in the preliminary lists. The original lists were revised and outcomes were added and dropped through group discussion and consensus.
4. The small group arranged each revised list of outcomes linked to a NANDA diagnosis into the following two categories: (1) *Suggested Outcomes,* those most likely to be monitored in patients with the diagnosis, and (2) *Additional Associated Outcomes,* those more dependent on the etiologic factors of the diagnosis. In general the outcomes appearing in the *Suggested Outcomes* list were matched to the **definition** and **defining characteristics** of a diagnosis, and the outcomes included in *Additional Associated Outcomes* list were matched to **related factors** or **risk factors.** The outcomes are listed alphabetically in each category.

HOW TO USE THE LINKAGES

The following steps are suggested when using the linkages to assist with the identification of outcomes that may be important to monitor in patients with a particular diagnosis:
   1. Review the *Suggested Outcomes* for consideration first
   2. Review the *Additional Associated Outcomes*

---

*There are nine NANDA diagnoses for which there are no applicable **NOC** outcomes currently developed. All of these are community or family diagnoses: Community Coping, Ineffective; Community Coping, Potential for Enhanced; Community Management of Therapeutic Regimen, Ineffective; Family Coping: Compromised, Ineffective; Family Coping: Disabling, Ineffective; Family Coping: Potential for Growth; Family, Management of Therapeutic Regimen, Ineffective; Family Processes, Altered; and Family Processes, Altered: Alcoholism. As was stated earlier, the **NOC** outcomes currently are directed at individuals (patients or family caregivers) and not at groups of patients, families, or communities. In addition, two NANDA diagnoses—Health Seeking Behaviors and Individual Management of Therapeutic Regimen, Effective—are included in the linkages but reflect outcomes (desired states) rather than diagnoses.

3. Finally, if all of the outcomes that need to be monitored are not in the lists, review the general NOC list for other outcomes that may be more applicable to the patient care situation

4. Rate the selected outcomes at baseline and at subsequent intervals determined by the nurse

References

1. NANDA. (1994). Nursing Diagnoses: Definitions and Classification (1995-1996). Philadelphia: North American Nursing Diagnosis Association.

2. Iowa Outcomes Project (1996). NANDA-NOC Linkages. Iowa City, IA: University of Iowa, College of Nursing.

NANDA-NOC Linkages

Activity Intolerance

DEFINITION: A state in which an individual has insufficient physiological or psychological energy to endure or complete required or desired daily activities.

SUGGESTED OUTCOMES:

Endurance

Energy Conservation

Self-Care: Instrumental Activities of Daily Living (IADL)

Self-Care: Activities of Daily Living (ADL)

ADDITIONAL ASSOCIATED OUTCOMES:

Ambulation: Walking
Ambulation: Wheelchair
Cardiac Pump Effectiveness
Circulation Status
Health Beliefs: Perceived Ability to Perform
Immobility Consequences: Physiological
Mobility Level

Mood Equilibrium
Nutritional Status: Energy
Pain: Disruptive Effects
Respiratory Status: Gas Exchange
Respiratory Status: Ventilation
Symptom Severity

Activity Intolerance, Risk for

DEFINITION: A state in which an individual is at risk of experiencing insufficient physiological or psychological energy to endure or complete required or desired daily activities.

SUGGESTED OUTCOMES:

Cardiac Pump Effectiveness

Circulation Status

Coping

Energy Conservation

Respiratory Status: Gas Exchange

Respiratory Status: Ventilation

ADDITIONAL ASSOCIATED OUTCOMES:

Health Beliefs: Perceived Control
Immobility Consequences: Physiological
Immobility Consequences: Psycho-Cognitive
Knowledge: Diet
Knowledge: Disease Process
Knowledge: Prescribed Activity
Mood Equilibrium

Nutritional Status: Body Mass
Nutritional Status: Energy
Pain: Disruptive Effects
Pain Level
Symptom Severity
Symptom Control Behavior

Adjustment, Impaired

DEFINITION: The state in which the individual is unable to modify his/her lifestyle/behavior in a manner consistent with a change in health status.

SUGGESTED OUTCOMES:

Acceptance: Health Status

Coping

Grief Resolution

Health Seeking Behavior

Participation: Health Care Decisions

Psychosocial Adjustment: Life Change

Treatment Behavior: Illness or Injury

ADDITIONAL ASSOCIATED OUTCOMES:

Cognitive Ability   Impulse Control
Health Beliefs: Perceived Ability to Perform   Self-Esteem
Health Beliefs: Perceived Control   Social Support

Airway Clearance, Ineffective

DEFINITION: A state in which an individual is unable to clear secretions or obstructions from the respiratory tract to maintain airway patency.

SUGGESTED OUTCOMES:

Respiratory Status: Gas Exchange

Respiratory Status: Ventilation

Symptom Control Behavior

Treatment Behavior: Illness or Injury

ADDITIONAL ASSOCIATED OUTCOMES:

Cognitive Ability   Infection Status
Comfort Level   Knowledge: Treatment Regimen
Endurance

Anxiety

DEFINITION: A vague uneasy feeling whose source is often nonspecific or unknown to the individual.

SUGGESTED OUTCOMES:

Aggression Control

Anxiety Control

Coping

Impulse Control

Self-Mutilation Restraint

Social Interaction Skills

ADDITIONAL ASSOCIATED OUTCOMES:

Acceptance: Health Status   Psychosocial Adjustment: Life Change
Grief Resolution   Symptom Control Behavior
Parent-Infant Attachment

Aspiration, Risk for

DEFINITION: The state in which an individual is at risk for entry of gastrointestinal secretions, oropharyngeal secretions, or solids or fluids into tracheobronchial passages.

SUGGESTED OUTCOMES:

Cognitive Ability

Immobility Consequences: Physiological

Neurological Status

ADDITIONAL ASSOCIATED OUTCOMES:

Endurance   Respiratory Status: Ventilation
Infection Status   Self-Care: Non-Parenteral Medication
Knowledge: Treatment Procedure(s)   Self-Care: Oral Hygiene
Respiratory Status: Gas Exchange

Body Image Disturbance

DEFINITION: Disruption in the way one perceives one's body image.

SUGGESTED OUTCOMES:

Body Image

Child Development: 2 Years

Child Development: 3 Years

Child Development: 4 Years

Child Development: 5 Years

Child Development: Middle Childhood (6-11 Years)

Child Development: Adolescence (12-17 Years)

Distorted Thought Control

Grief Resolution

Psychosocial Adjustment: Life Change

Self-Esteem

ADDITIONAL ASSOCIATED OUTCOMES:

Acceptance: Health Status
Self-Mutilation Restraint
Social Involvement

Body Temperature, Risk for Altered

DEFINITION: The state in which the individual is at risk for failure to maintain body temperature within normal range.

SUGGESTED OUTCOMES:

Hydration

Infection Status

ADDITIONAL ASSOCIATED OUTCOMES:

Adherence Behavior
Compliance Behavior
Immune Status

Neglect Recovery
Risk Control

Breastfeeding, Effective

DEFINITION: The state in which a mother/infant dyad/family exhibits adequate proficiency and satisfaction with breastfeeding process.

SUGGESTED OUTCOMES:

Breastfeeding Establishment: Infant

Breastfeeding Establishment: Maternal

Breastfeeding Maintenance

Breastfeeding Weaning

ADDITIONAL ASSOCIATED OUTCOMES:

Anxiety Control

Cognitive Ability

Hydration

Knowledge: Breastfeeding

Nutritional Status: Food & Fluid Intake

Parent-Infant Attachment

Social Support

Breastfeeding, Ineffective

DEFINITION: The state in which a mother, infant, or child experiences dissatisfaction or difficulty with the breastfeeding process.

SUGGESTED OUTCOMES:

Breastfeeding Establishment: Infant

Breastfeeding Establishment: Maternal

Breastfeeding Maintenance

Breastfeeding Weaning

Knowledge: Breastfeeding

ADDITIONAL ASSOCIATED OUTCOMES:

Anxiety Control

Cognitive Ability

Hydration

Nutritional Status: Food & Fluid Intake

Parent-Infant Attachment

Social Support

Breastfeeding, Interrupted

DEFINITION: A break in the continuity of the breastfeeding process as a result of inability or inadvisability to put baby to breast for feeding.

SUGGESTED OUTCOMES:

Breastfeeding Establishment: Infant

Breastfeeding Establishment: Maternal

Breastfeeding Maintenance

Knowledge: Breastfeeding

Parent-Infant Attachment

ADDITIONAL ASSOCIATED OUTCOMES:

Breastfeeding Weaning

Caregiver Adaptation to Patient Institutionalization

Parenting

Risk Control: Alcohol Use

Risk Control: Drug Use

Role Performance

Breathing Pattern, Ineffective

DEFINITION: The state in which an individual's inhalation and/or exhalation pattern does not enable adequate pulmonary inflation or emptying.

SUGGESTED OUTCOMES:

Respiratory Status: Ventilation

Vital Signs Status

ADDITIONAL ASSOCIATED OUTCOMES:

Anxiety Control

Electrolyte & Acid/Base Balance

Energy Conservation

Muscle Function

Neurological Status

Pain Level

Cardiac Output, Decreased

DEFINITION: A state in which the blood pumped by an individual's heart is sufficiently reduced that it is inadequate to meet the needs of the body's tissues.

SUGGESTED OUTCOMES:

Cardiac Pump Effectiveness

Circulatory Status

Tissue Perfusion: Abdominal Organs

Tissue Perfusion: Peripheral

Vital Signs Status

ADDITIONAL ASSOCIATED OUTCOMES:

Cognitive Ability	Hydration
Electrolyte & Acid/Base Balance	Neurological Status: Autonomic
Endurance	Respiratory Status: Gas Exchange
Energy Conservation	Respiratory Status: Ventilation
Fluid Balance	Urinary Elimination

Caregiver Role Strain

DEFINITION: A caregiver's felt difficulty in performing the family caregiver role.

SUGGESTED OUTCOMES:

Caregiver Stressors

Caregiver Well-Being

ADDITIONAL ASSOCIATED OUTCOMES:

Caregiver Emotional Health	Caregiver Physical Health
Caregiver Lifestyle Disruption	Role Performance
Caregiver-Patient Relationship	

Caregiver Role Strain, Risk for

DEFINITION: A caregiver is vulnerable for felt difficulty in performing the family caregiver role.

SUGGESTED OUTCOMES:

Caregiver Emotional Health

Caregiver Home Care Readiness

Caregiver Lifestyle Disruption

Caregiver-Patient Relationship

Caregiver Performance: Direct Care

Caregiver Performance: Indirect Care

Caregiver Physical Health

Caregiver Stressors

Caregiving Endurance Potential

Risk Control

Role Performance

ADDITIONAL ASSOCIATED OUTCOMES:

Knowledge: Energy Conservation

Knowledge: Health Behaviors

Knowledge: Health Resources

Rest

Communication, Impaired Verbal

DEFINITION: The state in which an individual experiences a decreased or absent ability to use or understand language in human interaction.

SUGGESTED OUTCOMES:

Communication Ability

Communication: Expressive Ability

Communication: Receptive Ability

ADDITIONAL ASSOCIATED OUTCOMES:

Cognitive Ability

Cognitive Orientation

Distorted Thought Control

Information Processing

Muscle Function

Neurological Status

NANDA-NOC Linkages

Confusion, Acute

DEFINITION: The abrupt onset of a cluster of global, transient changes and disturbances in attention, cognition, psychomotor activity level of consciousness, and/or sleep/wake cycle.

SUGGESTED OUTCOMES:

Cognitive Ability

Distorted Thought Control

Information Processing

Memory

Neurological Status: Consciousness

Safety Behavior: Personal

Sleep

ADDITIONAL ASSOCIATED OUTCOMES:

Cognitive Orientation   Risk Control: Alcohol Use
Concentration   Risk Control: Drug Use
Electrolyte & Acid/Base Balance   Safety Behavior: Fall Prevention
Fluid Balance   Thermoregulation
Respiratory Status: Gas Exchange

Confusion, Chronic

DEFINITION: An irreversible, long-standing and/or progressive deterioration of intellect and personality characterized by decreased ability to interpret environmental stimuli, decreased capacity for intellectual thought processes and manifested by disturbances of memory, orientation, and behavior.

SUGGESTED OUTCOMES:

Cognitive Ability

Cognitive Orientation

Concentration

Decision Making

Distorted Thought Control

Identity

Information Processing

Memory

Neurological Status: Consciousness

ADDITIONAL ASSOCIATED OUTCOMES:

Communication Ability   Safety Behavior: Fall Prevention
Parenting: Social Safety   Safety Behavior: Home Physical Environment
Risk Control: Alcohol Use   Safety Behavior: Personal
Risk Control: Drug Use   Social Interaction Skills

Constipation

DEFINITION: A state in which an individual experiences a change in normal bowel habits characterized by a decrease in frequency and/or passage of hard dry stools.

SUGGESTED OUTCOMES:
Bowel Elimination

ADDITIONAL ASSOCIATED OUTCOMES:

Hydration
Mobility Level

Nutritional Status: Food & Fluid Intake
Treatment Behavior: Illness or Injury

Constipation, Colonic

DEFINITION: The state in which an individual's pattern of elimination is characterized by hard, dry stool which results from a delay in passage of food residue.

SUGGESTED OUTCOMES:
Bowel Elimination

ADDITIONAL ASSOCIATED OUTCOMES:

Hydration
Mobility Level

Nutritional Status: Food & Fluid Intake
Treatment Behavior: Illness or Injury

Constipation, Perceived

DEFINITION: The state in which an individual makes a self-diagnosis of constipation and ensures a daily bowel movement through abuse of laxatives, enemas, and suppositories.

SUGGESTED OUTCOMES:
Bowel Elimination

Health Beliefs

Health Beliefs: Perceived Threat

ADDITIONAL ASSOCIATED OUTCOMES:

Adherence Behavior
Hydration
Knowledge: Health Behaviors

Mobility Level
Nutritional Status: Food & Fluid Intake
Treatment Behavior: Illness or Injury

NANDA-NOC Linkages

Decisional Conflict (Specify)

DEFINITION: The state of uncertainty about course of action to be taken when choice among competing actions involves risk, loss, or challenge to personal life values.

SUGGESTED OUTCOMES:

Decision Making

Information Processing

Participation: Health Care Decisions

ADDITIONAL ASSOCIATED OUTCOMES:

Coping	Knowledge: Treatment Regimen
Health Beliefs	Psychosocial Adjustment: Life Change
Health Orientation	Social Support
Knowledge: Disease Process	

Defensive Coping

DEFINITION: The state in which an individual repeatedly projects falsely positive self evaluation based on a self-protective pattern which defends against underlying perceived threats to positive self regard.

SUGGESTED OUTCOMES:

Acceptance: Health Status

Child Development: Adolescence (12-17 Years)

Coping

Self-Esteem

Social Interaction Skills

ADDITIONAL ASSOCIATED OUTCOMES:

Grief Resolution	Risk Control: Drug Use
Impulse Control	Risk Control: Tobacco Use
Psychosocial Adjustment: Life Change	Social Involvement
Risk Control: Alcohol Use	Social Support

Denial, Ineffective

DEFINITION: The state of conscious or unconscious attempt to disavow the knowledge or meaning of an event to reduce anxiety/fear to the detriment of health.

SUGGESTED OUTCOMES:

Acceptance: Health Status

Anxiety Control

Health Beliefs: Perceived Threat

Symptom Control Behavior

ADDITIONAL ASSOCIATED OUTCOMES:

Coping

Health Beliefs

Health Seeking Behavior

Mood Equilibrium

Psychosocial Adjustment: Life Change

Diarrhea

DEFINITION: A state in which an individual experiences a change in normal bowel habits characterized by the frequent passage of loose, fluid, unformed stools.

SUGGESTED OUTCOMES:

Bowel Elimination

Electrolyte & Acid/Base Balance

Fluid Balance

Hydration

Treatment Behavior: Illness or Injury

ADDITIONAL ASSOCIATED OUTCOMES:

Infection Status

Nutritional Status: Biochemical Measures

Nutritional Status: Food & Fluid Intake

NANDA-NOC Linkages

Disuse Syndrome, Risk for

DEFINITION: A state in which an individual is at risk for deterioration of body systems as the result of prescribed or unavoidable musculoskeletal inactivity.

SUGGESTED OUTCOMES:

Endurance

Immobility Consequences: Physiological

Mobility Level

Neurological Status: Consciousness

Pain Level

ADDITIONAL ASSOCIATED OUTCOMES:

Energy Conservation   Joint Movement: Passive

Joint Movement: Active   Muscle Function

Diversional Activity Deficit

DEFINITION: The state in which an individual experiences a decreased stimulation from (or interest or engagement in) recreational or leisure activities.

SUGGESTED OUTCOMES:

Leisure Participation

Play Participation

Social Involvement

ADDITIONAL ASSOCIATED OUTCOMES:

Child Development: 2 Years   Child Development: Adolescence (12-17 Years)

Child Development: 3 Years   Health Promoting Behavior

Child Development: 4 Years   Rest

Child Development: 5 Years   Social Interaction Skills

Child Development: Middle Childhood (6-11 Years) Well-Being

Dysreflexia

DEFINITION: The state in which an individual with a spinal cord injury at T7 or above experiences a life-threatening uninhibited sympathetic response of the nervous system to a noxious stimulus.

SUGGESTED OUTCOMES:

Neurological Status

Vital Signs Status

ADDITIONAL ASSOCIATED OUTCOMES:

Symptom Severity
Tissue Integrity: Skin & Mucous Membranes
Treatment Behavior: Illness or Injury

Energy Field Disturbance

DEFINITION: A disruption of the flow of energy surrounding a person's being which results in disharmony of the body, mind, and/or spirit.

SUGGESTED OUTCOMES:

Spiritual Well-Being

Well-Being

ADDITIONAL ASSOCIATED OUTCOMES:

Comfort Level
Coping
Pain Level

Environmental Interpretation Syndrome, Impaired

DEFINITION: Consistent lack of orientation to person, place, time or circumstances over more than three to six months necessitating a protective environment.

SUGGESTED OUTCOMES:

Cognitive Orientation

Information Processing

Memory

Neurological Status: Consciousness

ADDITIONAL ASSOCIATED OUTCOMES:

Cognitive Ability   Safety Behavior: Fall Prevention
Concentration   Safety Behavior: Home Physical Environment
Decision Making   Safety Behavior: Personal
Parenting: Social Safety

Fatigue

DEFINITION: An overwhelming sustained feeling of exhaustion and decreased capacity for physical and mental work.

SUGGESTED OUTCOMES:

Concentration

Endurance

Energy Conservation

Nutritional Status: Energy

ADDITIONAL ASSOCIATED OUTCOMES:

Comfort Level	Rest
Mobility Level	Self-Care: Activities of Daily Living (ADL)
Mood Equilibrium	Self-Care: Non-Parenteral Medication
Pain Level	Self-Care: Parenteral Medication
Quality of Life	

Fear

DEFINITION: Feeling of dread related to an identifiable source which the person validates.

SUGGESTED OUTCOMES:

Fear Control

ADDITIONAL ASSOCIATED OUTCOMES:

Anxiety Control
Comfort Level
Coping

Fluid Volume Deficit

DEFINITION: The state in which an individual experiences vascular, cellular, or intracellular dehydration.

SUGGESTED OUTCOMES:

Electrolyte & Acid/Base Balance

Fluid Balance

Hydration

Nutritional Status: Flood & Fluid Intake

ADDITIONAL ASSOCIATED OUTCOMES:

Bowel Elimination	Thermoregulation: Neonate
Knowledge: Medication	Urinary Elimination
Thermoregulation	

Fluid Volume Deficit, Risk for

DEFINITION: The state in which an individual is at risk of experiencing vascular, cellular, or intra-cellular dehydration.

SUGGESTED OUTCOMES:

Electrolyte & Acid/Base Balance

Fluid Balance

Hydration

Nutritional Status: Food & Fluid Intake

ADDITIONAL ASSOCIATED OUTCOMES:

Bowel Elimination   Knowledge: Treatment Regimen
Knowledge: Disease Process   Thermoregulation
Knowledge: Health Behaviors   Thermoregulation: Neonate
Knowledge: Medication   Urinary Elimination

Fluid Volume Excess

DEFINITION: The state in which an individual experiences increased fluid retention and edema.

SUGGESTED OUTCOMES:

Electrolyte & Acid/Base Balance

Fluid Balance

Hydration

ADDITIONAL ASSOCIATED OUTCOMES:

Cardiac Pump Effectiveness   Respiratory Status: Ventilation
Knowledge: Disease Process   Self-Care: Parenteral Medication
Knowledge: Treatment Regimen   Urinary Elimination
Nutritional Status: Food & Fluid Intake

Gas Exchange, Impaired

DEFINITION: The state in which the individual experiences a decreased passage of oxygen and/or carbon dioxide between the aveoli of the lungs and the vascular system.

SUGGESTED OUTCOMES:

Respiratory Status: Gas Exchange

Respiratory Status: Ventilation

ADDITIONAL ASSOCIATED OUTCOMES:

Cognitive Ability   Tissue Perfusion: Abdominal Organs
Electrolyte & Acid/Base Balance   Tissue Perfusion: Peripheral

NANDA-NOC Linkages

Grieving, Anticipatory

DEFINITION: Intellectual and emotional responses and behaviors by which individuals work through the process of modifying self-concept based on the perception of potential loss.

SUGGESTED OUTCOMES:

Coping

Grief Resolution

Psychosocial Adjustment: Life Change

ADDITIONAL ASSOCIATED OUTCOMES:

Aggression Control
Communication Ability
Sleep

Grieving, Dysfunctional

DEFINITION: Extended, unsuccessful use of intellectual and emotional responses by which individuals attempt to work through the process of modifying self-concept based upon the perception of loss.

SUGGESTED OUTCOMES:

Coping

Grief Resolution

Psychosocial Adjustment: Life Change

ADDITIONAL ASSOCIATED OUTCOMES:

Aggression Control
Child Development: 3 Years
Child Development: 4 Years
Child Development: 5 Years
Child Development: Middle Childhood (6-11 Years)

Child Development: Adolescence (12-17 Years)
Communication Ability
Mood Equilibrium
Self-Esteem
Sleep

Growth and Development, Altered

DEFINITION: The state in which an individual demonstrates deviations in norms from his/her age group.

SUGGESTED OUTCOMES:

Child Development: 2 Months

Child Development: 4 Months

Child Development: 6 Months

Child Development: 12 Months

Child Development: 2 Years

Child Development: 3 Years

Child Development: 4 Years

Child Development: 5 Years

Child Development: Middle Childhood (6-11 Years)

Child Development: Adolescence (12-17 Years)

Growth

Physical Aging Status

Physical Maturation: Female

Physical Maturation: Male

ADDITIONAL ASSOCIATED OUTCOMES:

Abuse Recovery: Emotional

Abuse Recovery: Physical

Caregiver-Patient Relationship

Caregiver Performance: Direct Care

Caregiver Performance: Indirect Care

Neglect Recovery

Nutritional Status: Body Mass

Parenting

Parenting: Social Safety

Psychosocial Adjustment: Life Change

NANDA-NOC Linkages

Health Maintenance, Altered

DEFINITION: Inability to identify, manage, and/or seek out help to maintain health.

SUGGESTED OUTCOMES:

Health Beliefs: Perceived Resources

Health Promoting Behavior

Health Seeking Behavior

Knowledge: Health Behaviors

Knowledge: Health Resources

Knowledge: Treatment Regimen

Participation: Health Care Decisions

Psychosocial Adjustment: Life Change

Risk Detection

Social Support

Treatment Behavior: Illness or Injury

ADDITIONAL ASSOCIATED OUTCOMES:

Anxiety Control	Grief Resolution
Cognitive Ability	Information Processing
Communication Ability	Risk Control
Coping	Spiritual Well-Being
Decision Making	Symptom Control Behavior

Health Seeking Behaviors (Specify)

DEFINITION: A state in which an individual in stable health is actively seeking ways to alter personal health habits and/or the environment in order to move toward a higher level of health.

SUGGESTED OUTCOMES:

Adherence Behavior

Health Beliefs

Health Orientation

Health Promoting Behavior

Health Seeking Behavior

ADDITIONAL ASSOCIATED OUTCOMES:

Energy Conservation	Risk Control
Participation: Health Care Decisions	Safety Behavior: Home Physical Environment
Psychosocial Adjustment: Life Change	Safety Behavior: Personal
Quality of Life	Well-Being

Home Maintenance Management, Impaired

DEFINITION: Inability to independently maintain a safe growth-promoting immediate environment.

SUGGESTED OUTCOMES:

Parenting

Parenting: Social Safety

Role Performance

Self-Care: Instrumental Activities of Daily Living (IADL)

ADDITIONAL ASSOCIATED OUTCOMES:

Caregiver Emotional Health	Mobility Level
Caregiver Physical Health	Physical Aging Status
Cognitive Ability	Safety Behavior: Home Physical Environment
Coping	Social Support
Decision Making	

Hopelessness

DEFINITION: A subjective state in which an individual sees limited or no alternatives or personal choices available and is unable to mobilize energy on own behalf.

SUGGESTED OUTCOMES:

Decision Making

Hope

Mood Equilibrium

Nutritional States: Food & Fluid Intake

Quality of Life

Sleep

ADDITIONAL ASSOCIATED OUTCOMES:

Comfort Level	Pain: Disruptive Effects
Endurance	Pain Level
Grief Resolution	Spiritual Well-Being
Immobility Consequences: Physiological	Symptom Severity

Hyperthermia

DEFINITION: A state in which an individual's body temperature is elevated above his/her normal range.

SUGGESTED OUTCOMES:

Thermoregulation

Thermoregulation: Neonate

ADDITIONAL ASSOCIATED OUTCOMES:

Blood Transfusion Reaction Control	Neurological Status
Hydration	Safety Behavior: Personal
Immune Status	Vital Signs Status
Infection Status	

Hypothermia

DEFINITION: The state in which an individual's body temperature is reduced below normal range.

SUGGESTED OUTCOMES:

Thermoregulation

Thermoregulation: Neonate

ADDITIONAL ASSOCIATED OUTCOMES:

Neurological Status
Vital Signs Status

Incontinence, Bowel

DEFINITION: A state in which an individual experiences a change in normal bowel habits characterized by involuntary passage of stool.

SUGGESTED OUTCOMES:

Bowel Continence

Bowel Elimination

ADDITIONAL ASSOCIATED OUTCOMES:

Cognitive Ability	Nutritional Status: Food & Fluid Intake
Hydration	Self-Care: Toileting
Knowledge: Disease Process	Symptom Control Behavior
Muscle Function	Symptom Severity
Neurological Status	Treatment Behavior: Illness or Injury

Incontinence, Functional

DEFINITION: The state in which an individual experiences an involuntary, unpredictable passage of urine.

SUGGESTED OUTCOMES:

Urinary Continence

Urinary Elimination

ADDITIONAL ASSOCIATED OUTCOMES:

Cognitive Ability
Knowledge: Disease Process
Knowledge: Medication
Knowledge: Treatment Regimen
Mobility Level
Muscle Function
Self-Care: Hygiene

Self-Care: Toileting
Self-Esteem
Social Involvement
Symptom Control Behavior
Symptom Severity
Tissue Integrity: Skin & Mucous Membranes
Treatment Behavior: Illness or Injury

Incontinence, Reflex

DEFINITION: The state in which an individual experiences an involuntary loss of urine, occurring at somewhat predictable intervals when a specific bladder volume is reached.

SUGGESTED OUTCOMES:

Urinary Continence

Urinary Elimination

ADDITIONAL ASSOCIATED OUTCOMES:

Cognitive Ability
Knowledge: Disease Process
Knowledge: Treatment Regimen
Muscle Function
Neurological Status
Self-Care: Hygiene
Self-Care: Toileting

Self-Esteem
Social Involvement
Symptom Control Behavior
Symptom Severity
Tissue Integrity: Skin & Mucous Membranes
Treatment Behavior: Illness or Injury

NANDA-NOC Linkages

Incontinence, Stress

DEFINITION: The state in which an individual experiences a loss of urine of less than 50 ml occurring with increased abdominal pressure.

SUGGESTED OUTCOMES:

Urinary Continence

Urinary Elimination

ADDITIONAL ASSOCIATED OUTCOMES:

Knowledge: Treatment Regimen
Muscle Function
Self-Care: Hygiene
Self-Care: Toileting
Self-Esteem

Social Development
Symptom Control Behavior
Symptom Severity
Tissue Integrity: Skin & Mucous Membranes
Treatment Behavior: Illness or Injury

Incontinence, Total

DEFINITION: The state in which an individual experiences a continuous and unpredictable loss of urine.

SUGGESTED OUTCOMES:

Urinary Continence

Urinary Elimination

ADDITIONAL ASSOCIATED OUTCOMES:

Knowledge: Treatment Procedure(s)
Neurological Status
Self-Care: Hygiene
Self-Care: Toileting
Self-Esteem

Social Involvement
Symptom Control Behavior
Symptom Severity
Tissue Integrity: Skin & Mucous Membranes
Treatment Behavior: Illness or Injury

NANDA-NOC Linkages

Incontinence, Urge

DEFINITION: The state in which an individual experiences involuntary passage of urine occurring soon after a strong sense of urgency to void.

SUGGESTED OUTCOMES:

Urinary Continence

Urinary Elimination

ADDITIONAL ASSOCIATED OUTCOMES:

Cognitive Ability

Knowledge: Disease Process

Knowledge: Treatment Regimen

Mobility Level

Muscle Function

Self-Care: Hygiene

Self-Care: Toileting

Self-Esteem

Social Involvement

Symptom Control Behavior

Tissue Integrity: Skin & Mucous Membranes

Treatment Behavior: Illness or Injury

Individual Coping, Ineffective

DEFINITION: Impairment of adaptive behaviors and problem-solving abilities of a person in meeting life's demands and roles.

SUGGESTED OUTCOMES:

Coping

Decision Making

Impulse Control

Information Processing

ADDITIONAL ASSOCIATED OUTCOMES:

Abusive Behavior Self-Control

Aggression Control

Anxiety Control

Caregiver Stressors

Grief Resolution

Psychosocial Adjustment: Life Change

Quality of Life

Risk Control: Alcohol Use

Risk Control: Drug Use

Risk Control: Tobacco Use

Role Performance

Self-Mutilation Restraint

Social Interaction Skills

Suicide Self-Restraint

Well-Being

NANDA-NOC Linkages

Individual, Management of Therapeutic Regimen, Effective

DEFINITION: A pattern of regulating and integrating into daily living a program for treatment of illness and its sequelae that are satisfactory for meeting specific health goals.

SUGGESTED OUTCOMES:

Adherence Behavior

Compliance Behavior

Knowledge: Treatment Regimen

Participation: Health Care Decisions

Risk Control

Symptom Control Behavior

ADDITIONAL ASSOCIATED OUTCOMES:

Decision Making

Energy Conservation

Health Beliefs: Perceived Ability to Perform

Health Promoting Behavior

Knowledge: Diet

Knowledge: Disease Process

Knowledge: Energy Conservation

Knowledge: Medication

Knowledge: Prescribed Activity

Knowledge: Treatment Procedure(s)

Self-Care: Non-Parenteral Medication

Self-Care: Parenteral Medication

Individual, Management of Therapeutic Regimen, Ineffective

DEFINITION: A pattern of regulating and integrating into daily living a program for treatment of illness and the sequelae of illness that are unsatisfactory for meeting specific health goals.

SUGGESTED OUTCOMES:

Knowledge: Treatment Regimen

Participation: Health Care Decisions

Treatment Behavior: Illness or Injury

ADDITIONAL ASSOCIATED OUTCOMES:

Adherence Behavior

Compliance Behavior

Health Beliefs

Health Beliefs: Perceived Ability to Perform

Health Beliefs: Perceived Control

Health Beliefs: Perceived Resources

Health Beliefs: Perceived Threat

Health Orientation

Knowledge: Disease Process

Infant Behavior, Disorganized

DEFINITION: Alteration in integration and modulation of the physiological and behavioral systems of functioning (i.e., autonomic, motor, state, organizational, self regulatory, and attentional-interactional systems).

SUGGESTED OUTCOMES:

Child Development: 2 Months

Child Development: 4 Months

Child Development: 6 Months

Child Development: 12 Months

Muscle Function

Neurological Status

Sleep

Thermoregulation

Thermoregulation: Neonate

ADDITIONAL ASSOCIATED OUTCOMES:

Comfort Level   Pain: Disruptive Effects
Growth   Pain Level
Nutritional Status: Food & Fluid Intake

Infant Behavior, Potential for Enhanced, Organized

DEFINITION: A pattern of modulation of the physiologic and behavioral systems of functioning of an infant (i.e., autonomic, motor, state, organizational, self-regulatory, and attentional-interactional systems) that is satisfactory, but that can be improved, resulting in higher levels of integration in response to environmental stimuli.

SUGGESTED OUTCOMES:

Child Development: 2 Months

Child Development: 4 Months

Child Development: 6 Months

Child Development: 12 Months

Neurological Status

Sleep

Thermoregulation

Thermoregulation: Neonate

ADDITIONAL ASSOCIATED OUTCOMES:

Comfort Level
Pain Level

NANDA-NOC Linkages

Infant Behavior, Risk for Disorganized

DEFINITION: Risk for alteration in integration and modulation of the physiological and behavioral systems of functioning (i.e., autonomic, motor, state, organizational, self-regulatory, and attentional-interactional systems).

SUGGESTED OUTCOMES:

Child Development: 2 Months

Child Development: 4 Months

Child Development: 6 Months

Child Development: 12 Months

Comfort Level

Neurological Status

Pain Level

Sleep

ADDITIONAL ASSOCIATED OUTCOMES:

Muscle Function   Thermoregulation
Pain: Disruptive Effects   Thermoregulation: Neonate

Infant Feeding Pattern, Ineffective

DEFINITION: A state in which an infant demonstrates an impaired ability to suck or coordinate the suck-swallow response.

SUGGESTED OUTCOMES:

Breastfeeding Establishment: Infant

Breastfeeding: Maintenance

Muscle Function

Nutritional Status: Food & Fluid Intake

ADDITIONAL ASSOCIATED OUTCOMES:

Bowel Elimination   Nutritional Status: Biochemical Measures
Hydration   Nutritional Status: Body Mass
Neurological Status   Urinary Elimination

NANDA-NOC Linkages

Infection, Risk for

DEFINITION: The state in which an individual is at increased risk for being invaded by pathogenic organisms.

SUGGESTED OUTCOMES:

Immune Status

Knowledge: Infection Control

Risk Control

Risk Detection

ADDITIONAL ASSOCIATED OUTCOMES:

Immobility Consequences: Physiological

Nutritional Status

Risk Control: Sexually Transmitted Diseases (STD)

Tissue Integrity: Skin & Mucous Membranes

Treatment Behavior: Illness or Injury

Injury, Risk for

DEFINITION: A state in which the individual is at risk for injury as a result of environmental conditions interacting with the individual's adaptive and defensive resources.

SUGGESTED OUTCOMES:

Parenting: Social Safety

Risk Control

Safety Behavior: Fall Prevention

ADDITIONAL ASSOCIATED OUTCOMES:

Knowledge: Child Safety

Knowledge: Personal Safety

Safety Behavior: Home Physical Environment

Safety Behavior: Personal

Safety Status: Falls Occurrence

Safety Status: Physical Injury

Symptom Control Behavior

Intracranial Adaptive Capacity, Decreased

DEFINITION: A clinical state in which intracranial fluid dynamic mechanisms that normally compensate for increases in intracranial volumes are compromised, resulting in repeated disproportionate increases in intracranial pressure (ICP) in response to a variety of noxious and non-noxious stimuli.

SUGGESTED OUTCOMES:

Electrolyte & Acid/Base Balance

Fluid Balance

Neurological Status

Neurological Status: Consciousness

ADDITIONAL ASSOCIATED OUTCOMES:

Neurological Status: Autonomic

Neurological Status: Central Motor Control

Neurological Status: Cranial Sensory/Motor Function

Neurological Status: Spinal Sensory/Motor Function

Knowledge Deficit (Specify)

DEFINITION: Absence or deficiency of cognitive information related to specific topic.

SUGGESTED OUTCOMES:

Knowledge: Diet

Knowledge: Disease Process

Knowledge: Energy Conservation

Knowledge: Health Behaviors

Knowledge: Health Resources

Knowledge: Infection Control

Knowledge: Medication

Knowledge: Personal Safety

Knowledge: Prescribed Activity

Knowledge: Substance Use Control

Knowledge: Treatment Procedure(s)

Knowledge: Treatment Regimen

ADDITIONAL ASSOCIATED OUTCOMES:

Cognitive Ability

Communication: Receptive Ability

Concentration

Information Processing

Memory

Loneliness, Risk for

DEFINITION: A subjective state in which an individual is at risk of experiencing vague dysphoria.

SUGGESTED OUTCOMES:

Grief Resolution

Social Interaction Skills

Social Involvement

Social Support

ADDITIONAL ASSOCIATED OUTCOMES:

Immobility Consequences: Psycho-Cognitive
Loneliness
Psychosocial Adjustment: Life Change

Memory, Impaired

DEFINITION: The state in which an individual experiences the inability to remember or recall bits of information or behavioral skills. Impaired memory may be attributed to pathophysiological or situational causes that are either temporary or permanent.

SUGGESTED OUTCOMES:

Child Development: 12 Months

Child Development: 2 Years

Child Development: 3 Years

Child Development: 4 Years

Child Development: 5 Years

Child Development: Middle Childhood (6-11 Years)

Child Development: Adolescence (12-17 Years)

Cognitive Orientation

Memory

Neurological Status: Consciousness

ADDITIONAL ASSOCIATED OUTCOMES:

Cardiac Pump Effectiveness	Electrolyte & Acid/Base Balance
Circulation Status	Respiratory Status: Gas Exchange
Cognitive Ability	Respiratory Status: Ventilation

Noncompliance (Specify)

DEFINITION: A person's informed decision not to adhere to a therapeutic recommendation.

SUGGESTED OUTCOMES:

Adherence Behavior

Compliance Behavior

Pain Level

Symptom Control Behavior

Treatment Behavior: Illness or Injury

ADDITIONAL ASSOCIATED OUTCOMES:

Comfort Level   Health Orientation
Health Beliefs   Symptom Severity

Nutrition: Less than Body Requirements, Altered

DEFINITION: The state in which an individual experiences an intake of nutrients insufficient to meet metabolic needs.

SUGGESTED OUTCOMES:

Nutritional Status

Nutritional Status: Food & Fluid Intake

Nutritional Status: Nutrient Intake

ADDITIONAL ASSOCIATED OUTCOMES:

Bowel Elimination   Nutritional Status: Body Mass
Endurance   Nutritional Status: Energy
Nutritional Status: Biochemical Measures

Nutrition: More than Body Requirements, Altered

DEFINITION: The state in which an individual is experiencing an intake of nutrients which exceeds metabolic needs.

SUGGESTED OUTCOMES:

Nutritional Status: Food & Fluid Intake

Nutritional Status: Nutrient Intake

ADDITIONAL ASSOCIATED OUTCOMES:

Nutritional Status
Nutritional Status: Body Mass

Nutrition: Potential for More than Body Requirements, Altered

DEFINITION: The state in which an individual is at risk of experiencing an intake of nutrients which exceeds metabolic needs.

SUGGESTED OUTCOMES:
Nutritional Status: Food & Fluid Intake

ADDITIONAL ASSOCIATED OUTCOMES:
Nutritional Status: Body Mass
Nutritional Status: Nutrient Intake

Oral Mucous Membrane, Altered

DEFINITION: The state in which an individual experiences disruptions in the tissue layers of the oral cavity.

SUGGESTED OUTCOMES:
Oral Health

Tissue Integrity: Skin & Mucous Membranes

ADDITIONAL ASSOCIATED OUTCOMES:
Hydration
Infection Status
Nutritional Status

Nutritional Status: Food & Fluid Intake
Self-Care: Oral Hygiene

Pain

DEFINITION: A state in which an individual experiences and reports the presence of severe discomfort or an uncomfortable sensation.

SUGGESTED OUTCOMES:
Comfort Level

Pain Control Behavior

Pain: Disruptive Effects

Pain Level

ADDITIONAL ASSOCIATED OUTCOMES:
Symptom Control Behavior
Symptom Severity
Well-Being

Pain, Chronic

DEFINITION: A state in which the individual experiences pain that continues for more than six months in duration.

SUGGESTED OUTCOMES:

Comfort Level

Pain Control Behavior

Pain: Disruptive Effects

Pain Level

ADDITIONAL ASSOCIATED OUTCOMES:

Quality of Life	Well-Being
Symptom Control Behavior	Will to Live
Symptom Severity	

Parental Role Conflict

DEFINITION: The state in which the parent experiences role confusion and conflict in response to crises.

SUGGESTED OUTCOMES:

Caregiver Adaptation to Patient Institutionalization

Caregiver Home Care Readiness

Coping

Parenting

Psychosocial Adjustment: Life Change

Role Performance

ADDITIONAL ASSOCIATED OUTCOMES:

Caregiver Physical Health
Caregiver Stressors

Parent/Infant/Child Attachment, Risk for Altered

DEFINITION: Disruption of the interactive process between parent/significant other and infant that fosters the development of a protective and nurturing reciprocal relationship.

SUGGESTED OUTCOMES:

Caregiver Adaptation to Patient Institutionalization

Caregiver Performance: Direct Care

Child Development: 2 Months

Child Development: 4 Months

Child Development: 6 Months

Child Development: 12 Months

Child Development: 2 Years

Child Development: 3 Years

Child Development: 4 Years

Child Development: 5 Years

Parent-Infant Attachment

Parenting

ADDITIONAL ASSOCIATED OUTCOMES:

Cognitive Ability

Coping

Distorted Thought Control

Social Interaction Skills

NANDA-NOC Linkages

Parenting, Altered

DEFINITION: The state in which a nurturing figure(s) experiences an inability to create an environment which promotes the optimum growth and development of another human being.

SUGGESTED OUTCOMES:

Child Development: 2 Months

Child Development: 4 Months

Child Development: 6 Months

Child Development: 12 Months

Child Development: 2 Years

Child Development: 3 Years

Child Development: 4 Years

Child Development: 5 Years

Child Development: Middle Childhood (6-11 Years)

Child Development: Adolescence (12-17 Years)

Parent-Infant Attachment

Parenting

Parenting: Social Safety

Role Performance

Safety Behavior: Home Physical Environment

Social Support

ADDITIONAL ASSOCIATED OUTCOMES:

Abuse Cessation

Abuse Protection

Abusive Behavior Self-Control

Cognitive Ability

Coping

Knowledge: Child Safety

Neglect Recovery

Psychosocial Adjustment: Life Change

Social Interaction Skills

Parenting, Risk for Altered

DEFINITION: The state in which a nurturing figure(s) is at risk to experience an inability to create an environment which promotes the optimum growth and development of another human being.

SUGGESTED OUTCOMES:

Abuse Recovery: Emotional

Caregiver Stressors

Coping

Parent-Infant Attachment

Parenting

Risk Control: Unintended Pregnancy

ADDITIONAL ASSOCIATED OUTCOMES:

Abuse Recovery: Physical

Abuse Recovery: Sexual

Abusive Behavior Self-Control

Aggression Control

Caregiver Emotional Health

Caregiver Physical Health

Caregiver Well-Being

Decision Making

Distorted Thought Control

Social Interaction Skills

Perioperative Positioning Injury, Risk for

DEFINITION: A state in which the client is at risk for injury as a result of the environmental conditions found in the perioperative setting.

SUGGESTED OUTCOMES:

Body Positioning: Self-Initiated

Circulation Status

Cognitive Ability

Cognitive Orientation

Muscle Function

Tissue Perfusion: Peripheral

ADDITIONAL ASSOCIATED OUTCOMES:

Immune Status

Neurological Status

Nutritional Status

Nutritional Status: Body Mass

Respiratory Status: Gas Exchange

Respiratory Status: Ventilation

Peripheral Neurovascular Dysfunction, Risk for

DEFINITION: A state in which an individual is at risk of experiencing a disruption in circulation, sensation or motion of an extremity.

SUGGESTED OUTCOMES:

Circulation Status

Neurological Status

Neurological Status: Cranial Sensory/Motor Function

Neurological Status: Spinal Sensory/Motor Function

Tissue Perfusion: Peripheral

ADDITIONAL ASSOCIATED OUTCOMES:

Joint Movement: Active
Mobility Level
Muscle Function

Personal Identity Disturbance

DEFINITION: Inability to distinguish between self and nonself.

SUGGESTED OUTCOMES:

Identity

ADDITIONAL ASSOCIATED OUTCOMES:

Distorted Thought Control

Physical Mobility, Impaired

DEFINITION: A state in which the individual experiences a limitation of ability for independent physical movement.

SUGGESTED OUTCOMES:

Ambulation: Walking

Ambulation: Wheelchair

Joint Movement: Active

Mobility Level

Self-Care: Activities of Daily Living (ADL)

Transfer Performance

ADDITIONAL ASSOCIATED OUTCOMES:

Balance	Mood Equilibrium
Cognitive Ability	Muscle Function
Immobility Consequences: Physiological	Neurological Status
Immobility Consequences: Psycho-Cognitive	Pain Level

Poisoning, Risk for

DEFINITION: Accentuated risk for accidental exposure to or ingestion of drugs or dangerous products in doses sufficient to cause poisoning.

SUGGESTED OUTCOMES:

Knowledge: Medication

Risk Control

Risk Control: Drug Use

Risk Detection

ADDITIONAL ASSOCIATED OUTCOMES:

Safety Behavior: Home Physical Environment
Self-Care: Non-Parenteral Medication

Self-Care: Parenteral Medication
Suicide Self-Restraint

Post-Trauma Response

DEFINITION: The state of an individual experiencing a sustained painful response to an overwhelming traumatic event(s).

SUGGESTED OUTCOMES:

Abuse Cessation

Abuse Protection

Abuse Recovery: Emotional

Abuse Recovery: Sexual

Coping

Impulse Control

Self-Mutilation Restraint

ADDITIONAL ASSOCIATED OUTCOMES:

Anxiety Control
Body Image
Cognitive Ability
Distorted Thought Control

Grief Resolution
Quality of Life
Sleep

Powerlessness

DEFINITION: Perception that one's own actions will not significantly affect an outcome; perceived lack of control over a current situation or immediate happening.

SUGGESTED OUTCOMES:

Health Beliefs

Health Beliefs: Perceived Ability to Perform

Health Beliefs: Perceived Control

Health Beliefs: Perceived Resources

Participation: Health Care Decisions

ADDITIONAL ASSOCIATED OUTCOMES:

Health Orientation	Social Involvement
Social Interaction Skills	Social Support

Protection, Altered

DEFINITION: The state in which an individual experiences a decrease in the ability to guard the self from internal or external threats such as illness or injury.

SUGGESTED OUTCOMES:

Abuse Protection

Immune Status

ADDITIONAL ASSOCIATED OUTCOMES:

Cognitive Orientation	Neurological Status: Consciousness
Coping	Nutritional Status
Endurance	Wound Healing: Primary Intention
Infection Status	Wound Healing: Secondary Intention

Rape-Trauma Syndrome

(Includes Rape Trauma, Compound Reaction, Silent Reaction)

DEFINITION: Forced, violent sexual penetration against the victim's will and consent. The trauma syndrome that develops from this attack or attempted attack includes an acute phase of disorganization of the victim's lifestyle and a long-term process of reorganization of lifestyle.

SUGGESTED OUTCOMES:

Abuse Cessation

Abuse Protection

Abuse Recovery: Emotional

Abuse Recovery: Sexual

Coping

Impulse Control

Self-Mutilation Restraint

ADDITIONAL ASSOCIATED OUTCOMES:

Anxiety Control	Grief Resolution
Body Image	Quality of Life
Cognitive Ability	Sleep
Distorted Thought Control	

Relocation Stress Syndrome

DEFINITION: Physiological and/or psychosocial disturbances as a result of transfer from one environment to another.

SUGGESTED OUTCOMES:

Child Adaptation to Hospitalization

Coping

Psychosocial Adjustment: Life Change

Quality of Life

ADDITIONAL ASSOCIATED OUTCOMES:

Caregiver Adaptation to Patient Institutionalization	Grief Resolution
Caregiver Home Care Readiness	Social Support

Role Performance, Altered

DEFINITION: Disruption in the way one perceives one's role performance.

SUGGESTED OUTCOMES:

Caregiver Lifestyle Disruption

Psychosocial Adjustment: Life Change

Role Performance

ADDITIONAL ASSOCIATED OUTCOMES:

Caregiver Adaptation to Patient Institutionalization

Caregiver Home Care Readiness

Caregiver Performance: Direct Care

Caregiver Performance: Indirect Care

Parent-Infant Attachment

Self Care Deficit: Bathing/Hygiene

DEFINITION: A state in which the individual experiences an impaired ability to perform or complete bathing/hygiene activities for oneself.

SUGGESTED OUTCOMES:

Self-Care: Activities of Daily Living (ADL)

Self-Care: Bathing

Self-Care: Hygiene

ADDITIONAL ASSOCIATED OUTCOMES:

Anxiety Control

Child Development: 12 Months

Child Development: 2 Years

Child Development: 3 Years

Child Development: 4 Years

Child Development: 5 Years

Child Development: Middle Childhood (6-11 Years)

Cognitive Ability

Comfort Level

Endurance

Energy Conservation

Mobility Level

Mood Equilibrium

Muscle Function

Neurological Status

Pain Level

Self Care Deficit: Dressing/Grooming

DEFINITION: A state in which the individual experiences an impaired ability to perform or complete dressing and grooming activities for oneself.

SUGGESTED OUTCOMES:

Self-Care: Activities of Daily Living (ADL)

Self-Care: Dressing

Self-Care: Grooming

Self-Care: Hygiene

ADDITIONAL ASSOCIATED OUTCOMES:

Cognitive Ability	Mood Equilibrium
Comfort Level	Muscle Function
Endurance	Neurological Status
Energy Conservation	Pain Level
Mobility Level	

Self Care Deficit: Feeding

DEFINITION: A state in which the individual experiences an impaired ability to perform or complete feeding activities for oneself.

SUGGESTED OUTCOMES:

Self-Care: Activities of Daily Living (ADL)

Self-Care: Eating

ADDITIONAL ASSOCIATED OUTCOMES:

Anxiety Control	Mood Equilibrium
Cognitive Ability	Muscle Function
Endurance	Neurological Status: Central Motor Control
Joint Movement: Active	Pain Control Behavior
Mobility Level	

Self Care Deficit: Toileting

DEFINITION: A state in which the individual experiences an impaired ability to perform or complete toileting activities for oneself.

SUGGESTED OUTCOMES:

Self-Care: Activities of Daily Living (ADL)

Self-Care: Toileting

ADDITIONAL ASSOCIATED OUTCOMES:

Anxiety Control	Mood Equilibrium
Cognitive Ability	Muscle Function
Comfort Level	Neurological Status
Endurance	Pain Level
Energy Conservation	Transfer Performance
Mobility Level	

Self Esteem, Chronic Low

DEFINITION: Long standing negative self evaluation/feelings about self or self capabilities.

SUGGESTED OUTCOMES:

Self-Esteem

ADDITIONAL ASSOCIATED OUTCOMES:

Body Image	Role Performance
Hope	Social Interaction Skills
Mood Equilibrium	

Self Esteem Disturbance

DEFINITION: Negative self evaluation/feelings about self or self capabilities, which may be directly or indirectly expressed.

SUGGESTED OUTCOMES:

Child Development: 2 Years

Child Development: 3 Years

Child Development: 4 Years

Child Development: 5 Years

Child Development: Middle Childhood (6-11 Years)

Child Development: Adolescence (12-17 Years)

Self-Esteem

ADDITIONAL ASSOCIATED OUTCOMES:

Body Image   Role Performance
Hope   Social Interaction Skills
Mood Equilibrium

Self Esteem, Situational Low

DEFINITION: Negative self evaluation/feelings about self which develop in response to a loss or change in an individual who previously had a positive self evaluation.

SUGGESTED OUTCOMES:

Decision Making

Self-Esteem

ADDITIONAL ASSOCIATED OUTCOMES:

Abuse Recovery: Emotional   Psychosocial Adjustment: Life Change
Grief Resolution   Role Performance

Self-Mutilation, Risk for

DEFINITION: A state in which an individual is at risk to perform an act upon the self to injure, not kill, which produces tissue damage and tension relief.

SUGGESTED OUTCOMES:

Aggression Control

Impulse Control

Risk Detection

Self-Mutilation Restraint

ADDITIONAL ASSOCIATED OUTCOMES:

Abuse Recovery: Emotional   Distorted Thought Control
Abuse Recovery: Physical   Mood Equilibrium
Abuse Recovery: Sexual

Sensory/Perceptual Alterations (Specify)
(Visual, Auditory, Kinesthetic, Gustatory, Tactile, Olfactory)

DEFINITION: A state in which an individual experiences a change in the amount or patterning of incoming stimuli accompanied by a diminished, exaggerated, distorted, or impaired response to such stimuli.

SUGGESTED OUTCOMES:

Anxiety Control

Body Image

Cognitive Ability

Cognitive Orientation

Distorted Thought Process

Energy Conservation

ADDITIONAL ASSOCIATED OUTCOMES:

Electrolyte & Acid/Base Balance   Neurological Status
Endurance   Rest
Fluid Balance   Sleep

Sexual Dysfunction

DEFINITION: The state in which an individual experiences a change in sexual function that is viewed as unsatisfying, unrewarding, inadequate.

SUGGESTED OUTCOMES:

Abuse Recovery: Sexual

Child Development: Adolescence (12-17 Years)

Physical Aging Status

Risk Control: Sexually Transmitted Diseases (STD)

ADDITIONAL ASSOCIATED OUTCOMES:

Abuse Cessation	Endurance
Abuse Recovery: Emotional	Role Performance
Abuse Recovery: Physical	Self-Esteem
Body Image	Social Interaction Skills

Sexuality Patterns, Altered

DEFINITION: The state in which an individual expresses concern regarding his/her sexuality.

SUGGESTED OUTCOMES:

Abuse Recovery: Sexual

Body Image

Child Development: Middle Childhood (6-11 Years)

Child Development: Adolescence (12-17 Years)

Role Performance

Self-Esteem

ADDITIONAL ASSOCIATED OUTCOMES:

Abuse Cessation	Physical Maturation: Female
Anxiety Control	Physical Maturation: Male
Endurance	Psychosocial Adjustment: Life Change
Loneliness	Risk Control: Sexually Transmitted Diseases (STD)
Physical Aging Status	Well-Being

Skin Integrity, Impaired

DEFINITION: State in which the individual's skin is adversely altered.

SUGGESTED OUTCOMES:

Tissue Integrity: Skin & Mucous Membranes

Wound Healing: Primary Intention

Wound Healing: Secondary Intention

ADDITIONAL ASSOCIATED OUTCOMES:

Fluid Balance
Immobility Consequences: Physiological
Knowledge: Treatment Regimen
Nutritional Status
Self-Care: Hygiene

Thermoregulation
Thermoregulation: Neonate
Tissue Perfusion: Peripheral
Treatment Behavior: Illness or Injury

Skin Integrity, Risk for Impaired

DEFINITION: A state in which the individual's skin is at risk of being adversely altered.

SUGGESTED OUTCOMES:

Child Development: Adolescence (12-17 Years)

Immobility Consequences: Physiological

Nutritional Status

Risk Control

Self-Mutilation Restraint

Tissue Perfusion: Peripheral

ADDITIONAL ASSOCIATED OUTCOMES:

Nutritional Status: Biochemical Measures
Physical Aging Status
Tissue Integrity: Skin & Mucous Membranes

Wound Healing: Primary Intention
Wound Healing: Secondary Intention

Sleep Pattern Disturbance

DEFINITION: Disruption of sleep time causes discomfort or interferes with desired lifestyle.

SUGGESTED OUTCOMES:

Comfort Level

Pain Level

Psychosocial Adjustment: Life Change

Quality of Life

Rest

Sleep

Well-Being

ADDITIONAL ASSOCIATED OUTCOMES:

Anxiety Control	Pain Control Behavior
Bowel Elimination	Respiratory Status: Gas Exchange
Leisure Participation	Respiratory Status: Ventilation
Loneliness	Symptom Control Behavior
Mood Equilibrium	Urinary Elimination

Social Interaction, Impaired

DEFINITION: The state in which an individual participates in an insufficient or excessive quantity or ineffective quality of social exchange.

SUGGESTED OUTCOMES:

Child Development: 2 Months

Child Development: 4 Months

Child Development: 6 Months

Child Development: 12 Months

Child Development: 2 Years

Child Development: 3 Years

Child Development: 4 Years

Child Development: 5 Years

Child Development: Middle Childhood (6-11 Years)

Child Development: Adolescence (12-17 Years)

Play Participation

Role Performance

Social Interaction Skills

Social Involvement

ADDITIONAL ASSOCIATED OUTCOMES:

Communication Ability	Immobility Consequences: Psycho-Cognitive
Distorted Thought Control	Self-Esteem

Social Isolation

DEFINITION: Aloneness experienced by the individual and perceived as imposed by others and as a negative or threatened state.

SUGGESTED OUTCOMES:

Loneliness

Mood Equilibrium

Play Participation

Social Interaction Skills

Social Involvement

Social Support

Well-Being

ADDITIONAL ASSOCIATED OUTCOMES:

Aggression Control
Body Image
Leisure Participation

Spiritual Distress (Distress of the Human Spirit)

DEFINITION: Disruption in the life principle which pervades a person's being and which integrates and transcends one's biological and psychosocial nature.

SUGGESTED OUTCOMES:

Dignified Dying

Hope

Spiritual Well-Being

ADDITIONAL ASSOCIATED OUTCOMES:

Anxiety Control   Suicide Self-Restraint
Grief Resolution   Well-Being
Psychosocial Adjustment: Life Change   Will to Live
Quality of Life

Spiritual Well-Being, Potential for Enhanced

DEFINITION: Spiritual well-being is the process of an individual's developing/unfolding of mystery through harmonious interconnectedness that springs from inner strengths.

SUGGESTED OUTCOMES:

Hope

Quality of Life

Spiritual Well-Being

Well-Being

ADDITIONAL ASSOCIATED OUTCOMES:

Dignified Dying
Grief Resolution
Psychosocial Adjustment: Life Change

Suffocation, Risk for

DEFINITION: Accentuated risk of accidental suffocation (inadequate air available for inhalation).

SUGGESTED OUTCOMES:

Knowledge: Personal Safety

Risk Detection

Safety Behavior: Home Physical Environment

Substance Addiction Consequences

ADDITIONAL ASSOCIATED OUTCOMES:

Mobility Level   Neurological Status: Consciousness
Muscle Function   Respiratory Status: Gas Exchange

Swallowing, Impaired

DEFINITION: The state in which an individual has decreased ability to voluntarily pass fluids and/or solids from the mouth to the stomach.

SUGGESTED OUTCOMES:

Muscle Function

Neurological Status: Consciousness

Neurological Status: Cranial Sensory/Motor Function

Self-Care: Eating

ADDITIONAL ASSOCIATED OUTCOMES:

Cognitive Ability   Energy Conservation
Endurance   Infection Status

Thermoregulation, Ineffective

DEFINITION: The state in which the individual's temperature fluctuates between hypothermia and hyperthermia.

SUGGESTED OUTCOMES:

Thermoregulation

Thermoregulation: Neonate

ADDITIONAL ASSOCIATED OUTCOMES:

Vital Signs Status

Thought Processes, Altered

DEFINITION: A state in which an individual experiences a disruption in cognitive operations and activities.

SUGGESTED OUTCOMES:

Cognitive Ability

Cognitive Orientation

Concentration

Decision Making

Distorted Thought Control

Identity

Information Processing

Memory

Neurological Status: Consciousness

ADDITIONAL ASSOCIATED OUTCOMES:

Communication Ability
Electrolyte & Acid/Base Balance
Fluid Balance
Parenting: Social Safety
Respiratory Status: Gas Exchange
Risk Control: Alcohol Use

Risk Control: Drug Use
Safety Behavior: Fall Prevention
Safety Behavior: Home Physical Environment
Safety Behavior: Personal
Thermoregulation

Tissue Integrity, Impaired

DEFINITION: A state in which an individual experiences damage to mucous membrane, corneal, integumentary or subcutaneous tissue.

SUGGESTED OUTCOMES:

Tissue Integrity: Skin & Mucous Membranes

Wound Healing: Primary Intention

Wound Healing: Secondary Intention

ADDITIONAL ASSOCIATED OUTCOMES:

Fluid Balance
Immobility Consequences: Physiological
Knowledge: Treatment Regimen
Nutritional Status
Self-Care: Hygiene

Thermoregulation
Thermoregulation: Neonate
Tissue Perfusion: Peripheral
Treatment Behavior: Illness or Injury

NANDA-NOC Linkages

Tissue Perfusion, Altered: Cardiopulmonary

DEFINITION: The state in which an individual experiences a decrease in nutrition and oxygenation at the cellular level due to a deficit in capillary blood supply.

SUGGESTED OUTCOMES:

Cardiac Pump Effectiveness

Circulation Status

Tissue Perfusion: Cardiac

Tissue Perfusion: Peripheral

Vital Signs Status

ADDITIONAL ASSOCIATED OUTCOMES:

Electrolyte & Acid/Base Balance
Fluid Balance
Pain Level

Tissue Perfusion, Altered: Cerebral

DEFINITION: The state in which an individual experiences a decrease in nutrition and oxygenation at the cellular level due to a deficit in capillary blood supply.

SUGGESTED OUTCOMES:

Circulation Status

Cognitive Ability

Neurological Status

Tissue Perfusion: Peripheral

ADDITIONAL ASSOCIATED OUTCOMES:

Cognitive Orientation   Concentration
Communication Ability   Information Processing
Communication: Expressive Ability   Memory
Communication: Receptive Ability

Tissue Perfusion, Altered: Gastrointestinal

DEFINITION: The state in which an individual experiences a decrease in nutrition and oxygenation at the cellular level due to a deficit in capillary blood supply.

SUGGESTED OUTCOMES:

Bowel Elimination

Circulation Status

Electrolyte & Acid/Base Balance

Fluid Balance

Hydration

Nutritional Status

ADDITIONAL ASSOCIATED OUTCOMES:

Nutritional Status: Biochemical Measures
Nutritional Status: Body Mass
Nutritional Status: Energy

Tissue Perfusion, Altered: Peripheral

DEFINITION: The state in which an individual experiences a decrease in nutrition and oxygenation at the cellular level due to a deficit in capillary blood supply.

SUGGESTED OUTCOMES:

Fluid Balance

Muscle Function

Tissue Integrity: Skin & Mucous Membranes

Tissue Integrity: Peripheral

ADDITIONAL ASSOCIATED OUTCOMES:

Electrolyte & Acid/Base Balance

NANDA-NOC Linkages

Tissue Perfusion, Altered: Renal

DEFINITION: The state in which an individual experiences a decrease in nutrition and oxygenation at the cellular level due to a deficit in capillary blood supply.

SUGGESTED OUTCOMES:

Circulation Status

Electrolyte & Acid/Base Balance

Fluid Balance

Hydration

Urinary Elimination

ADDITIONAL ASSOCIATED OUTCOMES:

Blood Transfusion Reaction Control
Cardiac Pump Effectiveness

Trauma, Risk for

DEFINITION: Accentuated risk of accidental tissue injury e.g., wound, burn, fracture.

SUGGESTED OUTCOMES:

Risk Control

Safety Behavior: Fall Prevention

ADDITIONAL ASSOCIATED OUTCOMES:

Balance
Knowledge: Personal Safety
Safety Behavior: Home Physical Environment

Safety Status: Falls Occurrence
Safety Behavior: Personal
Safety Status: Physical Injury

Unilateral Neglect

DEFINITION: A state in which an individual is perceptually unaware of, and inattentive to one side of the body.

SUGGESTED OUTCOMES:

Body Image

Body Positioning: Self-Initiated

Self-Care: Activities of Daily Living (ADL)

ADDITIONAL ASSOCIATED OUTCOMES:

Balance
Joint Movement: Active
Joint Movement: Passive
Neurological Status

Safety Behavior: Home Physical Environment
Safety Behavior: Personal
Self-Care: Instrumental Activities of Daily Living (IADL)
Transfer Performance

Urinary Elimination, Altered

DEFINITION: The state in which the individual experiences a disturbance in urine elimination.

SUGGESTED OUTCOMES:

Knowledge: Medication

Urinary Continence

Urinary Elimination

ADDITIONAL ASSOCIATED OUTCOMES:

Knowledge: Disease Process

Knowledge: Treatment Regimen

Muscle Function

Neurological Status

Self-Care: Toileting

Self-Esteem

Social Involvement

Symptom Control Behavior

Symptom Severity

Tissue Integrity: Skin & Mucous Membranes

Treatment Behavior: Illness or Injury

Urinary Retention

DEFINITION: The state in which the individual experiences incomplete emptying of the bladder.

SUGGESTED OUTCOMES:

Urinary Continence

Urinary Elimination

ADDITIONAL ASSOCIATED OUTCOMES:

Cognitive Ability

Infection Status

Knowledge: Disease Process

Knowledge: Medication

Knowledge: Treatment Regimen

Neurological Status

Symptom Control Behavior

Symptom Severity

Treatment Behavior: Illness or Injury

Ventilation, Inability to Sustain Spontaneous

DEFINITION: A state in which the response pattern of decreased energy reserves results in an individual's inability to maintain breathing adequate to support life.

SUGGESTED OUTCOMES:

Endurance

Muscle Function

Neurological Status: Central Motor Control

Vital Signs Status

ADDITIONAL ASSOCIATED OUTCOMES:

Electrolyte & Acid/Base Balance
Energy Conservation
Neurological Status: Consciousness

Respiratory Status: Gas Exchange
Respiratory Status: Ventilation

Ventilatory Weaning Response, Dysfunctional

DEFINITION: A state in which a patient cannot adjust to lowered levels of mechanical ventilator support, which interrupts and prolongs the weaning process.

SUGGESTED OUTCOMES:

Respiratory Status: Gas Exchange

Respiratory Status: Ventilation

Vital Signs Status

ADDITIONAL ASSOCIATED OUTCOMES:

Cognitive Ability
Electrolyte & Acid/Base Balance
Knowledge: Treatment Procedure(s)

Muscle Function
Neurological Status: Consciousness
Symptom Severity

Violence, Risk for: Self-Directed
or Directed at Others

DEFINITION: A state in which an individual experiences behaviors that can be physically harmful either to the self or others.

SUGGESTED OUTCOMES:

Abusive Behavior Self-Control

Aggression Control

Impulse Control

Self-Mutilation Restraint

Suicide Self-Restraint

ADDITIONAL ASSOCIATED OUTCOMES:

Distorted Thought Control

Quality of Life

Risk Control: Alcohol Use

Risk Control: Drug Use

Risk Detection

Care Plans

Appendix B contains two standardized care plans. The first is a critical path for patients with acute myocardial infarction, and the second is a standardized teaching plan for patients with respiratory problems. The critical path is modified from a critical path Sue Gettman, RN, MSN, developed as part of her program of study for a master's degree in nursing at the University of Iowa College of Nursing. Diagnostic tests and medications originally on the critical path have not been included, and the outcomes have been made consistent with the NOC language. The teaching plan was developed by a committee of nurses at a regional hospital where the NOC outcomes are being implemented. The teaching plan also was modified for inclusion in this volume. The original plan included assessment of learning readiness and columns to fill in for identifying whether instruction is needed, the date taught, the resources used, whether reinforcement is needed, and for caregiver signatures. The columns were eliminated to simplify the format of the plan for publication in this text. The reader should note that the plan's authors have elected to use one scale for all of the outcomes rather than the scales suggested with the Self-Care: Non-Parenteral Medication outcome; this presents no problem since the five-point scale was retained throughout the plan. The authors of the teaching plan are: Patricia Moore, RN, MSN, CDE; Deborah Rapp, RN, MSN; and Judy Maupin, RN, MSN. Other members of the organization who contributed to the development of the teaching plan are Jean Bandos, RN, BS; Sandra Beatty, RN; Helen Carter, MSN, RNC; Cherona Hajewski, RN, MSN; Patricia Jackson, RN, BSN; and Dan Spartz, BSN, RRT. Mary Campbell, a secretary, formatted the plan.

We thank these individuals for allowing us to include their work in this volume. We believe these plans provide the reader with some excellent examples of the use of NOC outcomes.

Critical Pathway
Acute MI

	Day 1	Day 2	Day 3
Actual/ Potential Patient Problems	**Days 1 through 6** • Decreased cardiac output • Tissue perfusion altered, cardiopulmonary • Pain • Fluid volume excess • Anxiety • Home maintenance management, impaired • Knowledge deficit—procedures		
Nursing Activities	**Day 1** • **Admission Care** Orient patient/family/significant other (SO) to immediate environment **Days 1 through 6** • **Anxiety Reduction** Provide factual information concerning diagnosis, treatment, prognosis • **Cardiac Care: Acute** Evaluate chest pain Monitor intake/output, urine output, and daily weight Monitor the effectiveness of oxygen therapy Maintain an environment conducive to rest/healing • **Intravenous Therapy** Administer IV fluids at room temperature • **Vital Signs Monitoring** Monitor blood pressure, pulse, temperature, respiratory status • **Environmental Management** Create a safe environment for the patient • **Visitation Facilitation** Discuss visiting policy with family/SO		
Diet	**Days 1 through 6** 1. Low sodium 2. Small, frequent meals 3. Limited intake of caffeine, cholesterol, foods high in fat		
Activity	• Bed rest—explain reasons for bed rest • Bedside commode—instruct patient on avoiding Valsalva's maneuver	Chair	
Discharge Planning	1. Develop data base— assess home care situation 2. Coordinate referrals relevant to linkages among HCPs (health care providers) 3. Develop/document written plan that considers the health care, social, financial needs of patient	1. Coordinate discharge efforts 2. Identify patient's under- standing of knowledge/ skills required post- discharge 3. Identify patient teaching needed for postdischarge care	1. Assist patient/SO in planning for supportive environment 2. Arrange for caregiver support as needed

Day 4	Day 5	Day 6

Days 4 through 6
- Knowledge deficit—heart diseases, medications

Days 4 through 6
- **Cardiac Care: Rehabilitation**
  Instruct the patient and family/SO on cardiac risk factor modification
- **Embolus Precautions**
  Administer prophylactic low-dose anticoagulant and/or antiplatelet medication

- Increase gradually per cardiac rehabilitation
- Monitor activity tolerance

Day 4	Day 5	Day 6
1. Encourage self-care as appropriate 2. Formulate a maintenance plan for postdischarge follow-up	1. Monitor readiness for discharge 2. Evaluate need for further cardiac rehabilitation	1. Complete discharge instructions and review with patient/SO 2. Arrange for postdischarge evaluation as appropriate

Continued.

Critical Pathway—cont'd
Acute MI

Patient outcomes	Day 1	Day 3	Day 6
Days 1 through 6 **Cardiac Pump Effectiveness** BP IER* Heart rate IER Activity tolerance IER Peripheral pulses strong Skin color Neck vein distension not present Dysrhythmia not present Abnormal heart sounds not present Peripheral edema not present	1 2 3 4 5	1 2 3 4 5	1 2 3 4 5
Tissue Perfusion: Cardiac Angina not present Profuse diaphoresis not present Nausea not present ECG WNL* Cardiac enzymes WNL	1 2 3 4 5	1 2 3 4 5	1 2 3 4 5
Fluid Balance Orthostatic hypotension not present 24-hour intake and output balanced Adventitious breath sounds not present Body weight stable Confusion not present Serum electrolytes WNL	1 2 3 4 5	1 2 3 4 5	1 2 3 4 5
Anxiety Control Seeks information to reduce anxiety Uses effective coping strategies Uses relaxation techniques to reduce anxiety Maintains concentration Reports adequate sleep	1 2 3 4 5	1 2 3 4 5	1 2 3 4 5
Pain Control Behavior Recognized pain onset Reports pain controlled Reports pain level Recognizes symptoms of pain Reports symptoms to health care professional	1 2 3 4 5	1 2 3 4 5	1 2 3 4 5

Definition of Scales	1	2	3	4	5
Patient Outcome Cardiac Pump Effectiveness Tissue Perfusion: Cardiac Fluid Balance	Extremely compromised	Substantially compromised	Moderately compromised	Mildly compromised	Not compromised
Anxiety Control Pain Control Behavior	Never demonstrated	Rarely demonstrated	Sometimes demonstrated	Often demonstrated	Consistently demonstrated

*BP = Blood pressure; IER = in expected range; ECG = electrocardiogram; WNL = within normal limits.

Patient outcomes	Day 1	Day 3	Day 6
Days 1 through 6—cont. **Knowledge: Treatment Procedure(s)** Description of treatment procedure Explanation of purpose of procedure Description of restrictions related to procedure Description of potential side effects	1 2 3 4 5	1 2 3 4 5	

	Day 4	Day 5	Day 6
Closer to discharge (days 4 through 6) **Health Beliefs: Perceived Resources** Perceived adequacy of personal finances Perceived access to transportation Perceived access to physical assistance	1 2 3 4 5		1 2 3 4 5
Knowledge: Disease Process Description of disease process Description of risk factors Description of signs and symptoms Description of measures to minimize disease progression	1 2 3 4 5		1 2 3 4 5

Knowledge: Treatment Regimen
Description of rationale for treatment regimen
Description of self-care responsibilities for ongoing
  treatment
Description of self-care responsibilities for
  emergency situations
Description of prescribed diet
Description of prescribed medication
Description of prescribed activity
Performance of self-monitoring techniques
Description of plan for follow-up care
	1 2 3 4 5		1 2 3 4 5

Definition of Scales	1	2	3	4	5
Patient Outcome Knowledge: Treatment Procedures	None	Limited	Moderate	Substantial	Extensive
Health Belief: Perceived Resources	Very weak	Weak	Moderate	Strong	Very strong
Knowledge: Disease Process Knowledge: Treatment Regimen	None	Limited	Moderate	Substantial	Extensive

COLUMBUS REGIONAL HOSPITAL
Patient Education Plan

Patient Problems: Ineffective Airway Clearance R/T Pneumonia
                    Ineffective Breathing Pattern R/T Pneumonia

Scale Descriptors:

1 = NONE, Dependent for all information
2 = LIMITED, Requires assistive person and resource(s)
3 = MODERATE, Requires assistive resource(s)
4 = SUBSTANTIAL, Independent with minimal cues
5 = EXTENSIVE, Independently verbalizes/demonstrates information without cues

Learning needs assessment	Interventions/ activities*
1. Tell me what you know about pneumonia	*Teaching: Disease Process* • Appraise the patient's level of knowledge related to specific disease process • Explain the pathophysiology of the disease and how it relates to the anatomy and physiology, as appropriate • Describe common signs and symptoms of the disease, as appropriate • Provide information about available diagnostic measures, as appropriate • Identify possible etiologic factors, as appropriate
2. Tell me what you know about the treatment of pneumonia	*Teaching: Disease Process* • Discuss therapy/treatment options • Describe rationale behind management/therapy/treatment recommendations *Airway Management* • Instruct how to cough effectively • Teach patient how to use prescribed inhalers, as appropriate • Instruct patient on correct positioning to alleviate dyspnea *Oxygen Therapy* • Instruct patient about importance of leaving on oxygen delivery device • Instruct patient and family about use of oxygen at home
	Teaching Prescribed Medication • Instruct the patient on the purpose and action of each medication • Instruct the patient on the dosage, route, and duration of each medication • Instruct the patient on possible adverse side effects of each medication

Iowa Intervention Project (1996). Nursing Interventions Classification (NIC). (2nd ed.). St. Louis: Mosby.
†Iowa Outcomes Project: Nursing-sensitive Outcomes Classification (NOC).

Outcome indicators	Indicator scale 1 2 3 4 5	Outcome/discharge status†
Patient/family care provider describes: • Disease process • Cause or contributing factors • Signs & symptoms • Usual disease course	1 2 3 4 5 1 2 3 4 5 1 2 3 4 5 1 2 3 4 5	*Knowledge: Disease Process* (Pneumonia) • Extent of understanding conveyed about the specific disease process Outcome Met Scale: 1 2 3 4 5 Continue at DC (discharge): ___Yes ___No Comments:
Patient/family care provider describes: • Prescribed procedures • Rationale for treatment regimen • Self-care responsibilities for ongoing treatment • Expected effects of treatment • Performs treatment procedure	1 2 3 4 5 1 2 3 4 5 1 2 3 4 5 1 2 3 4 5 1 2 3 4 5	*Knowledge: Treatment Regimen* • Extent of understanding and skills conveyed about a specific treatment regimen Outcome Met Scale: 1 2 3 4 5 Continue at DC (discharge): ___Yes ___No Comments:
Patient/family care provider will demonstrate understanding of the medication regimen: • Informs health provider of all medications being taken • Uses correct medication name • Describes actions of medications • Describes side effects of medications	1 2 3 4 5 1 2 3 4 5 1 2 3 4 5 1 2 3 4 5	*Knowledge: Medication* • Extent of understanding conveyed about safe use of medication Outcome Met Scale: 1 2 3 4 5 Continue at DC (discharge): ___Yes ___No Comments:

Continued.

COLUMBUS REGIONAL HOSPITAL
Patient Education Plan—cont'd

Learning needs assessment	Interventions/ activities
	Teaching Prescribed Medication—cont'd • Provide the patient with written information about the action, purpose, side effects, etc., of medications • Instruct the patient on the proper care of devices used for administration
3. Tell me what you know about preventing the complications of pneumonia	*Teaching: Disease Process* • Discuss lifestyle changes that may be required to prevent further complications and/or control the disease process • Instruct the patient on which signs and symptoms to report to health care provider, as appropriate • Provide the phone number(s) to call if complications occur • Reinforce information provided by other health care team members, as appropriate • Identify possible etiologic factors, as appropriate
4. Tell me what you can do to prevent pneumonia	*Teaching: Disease Process* • Discuss lifestyle changes that may be required to prevent future complications and/or control the disease process • Identify possible etiologic factors, as appropriate *Immunization/Vaccination Administration* • Provide immunization information in written form • Identify latest recommendations about use of immunizations
	Health System Guidance • Inform patient of appropriate community resources and contact persons • Give written instructions for purpose & location of post-hospitalizations/outpatient activities, as appropriate

Outcome indicators	Indicator scale 1 2 3 4 5	Outcome/discharge status†
• Describes correct administration of medication • Describes proper care of administration devices • Administers medication correctly	1 2 3 4 5 1 2 3 4 5 1 2 3 4 5	*Self-Care: Non-Parenteral Medication* • Ability to administer oral and topical medications to meet therapeutic goals Outcome Met Scale: 1 2 3 4 5 Continue at DC (discharge): ___Yes ___No Comments:
Patient/family care provider describes: • Measures to minimize disease progression • Complications • Signs and symptoms of complications • Precautions to prevent complications • Risk factors • Cause or contributing factors	 1 2 3 4 5 1 2 3 4 5 1 2 3 4 5 1 2 3 4 5 1 2 3 4 5 1 2 3 4 5	*Knowledge: Disease Process* • Extent of understanding conveyed about the specific disease process Outcome Met Scale: 1 2 3 4 5 Continue at DC (discharge): ___Yes ___No Comments:
Patient/family care provider describes: • Strategies to eliminate unhealthy behavior • Strategies to maximize health	 1 2 3 4 5 1 2 3 4 5	*Adherence Behavior* • Self-initiated action taken to promote wellness, recovery, and rehabilitation Outcome Met Scale: 1 2 3 4 5 Continue at DC (discharge): ___Yes ___No Comments:
Patient/family care provider describes: • Need for follow-up care • Plan for follow-up care • When to contact a health professional • How to connect with needed services • Community resources available for assistance	 1 2 3 4 5 1 2 3 4 5 1 2 3 4 5 1 2 3 4 5 1 2 3 4 5	*Knowledge: Health Resources* • Extent of understanding and skills conveyed about health care resources Outcome Met Scale: 1 2 3 4 5 Continue at DC (discharge): ___Yes ___No Comments:

Case Study

Cindy A. Scherb

T he case study presented in Appendix C was developed by Cindy Scherb, MS, RN, while she was a research assistant on the Nursing Outcomes Classification grant during her studies as a doctoral student at the University of Iowa College of Nursing. The study describes a patient situation and identifies and discusses possible nursing diagnoses, interventions, and outcomes for the patient. The outcomes selected for the patient with all of the possible indicators are provided first, and then the indicators selected for this particular patient are provided in the patient scores postdischarge sections.

The team believes this example will be particularly useful for educators and practitioners. The team thanks Cindy Scherb for allowing us to include her work in this volume.

Woman Recovering from Fractured Hip

Alice is a 68-year-old female who has been in the hospital for 5 days after having a hip replacement due to fracturing her hip when she slipped on a throw rug in her dining room. Alice's plan of care during hospitalization has been centered around monitoring for any postoperative complications and getting her walking as quickly as possible. Alice has been going to physical therapy twice a day and has progressed within the limits of her hip replacement. Alice is able to transfer herself from the bed to a chair with minimal assistance. She understands the use of the assistive devices introduced to assist her with activities of daily living, but remains clumsy with her use of them. Alice's postoperative recovery has been progressing without any significant delays or difficulty. The discharge plan is that she will be released from the hospital within the next 3 days. Alice has stated since admission that she plans to return to her home after discharge. A home health case manager has been assigned to Alice and will follow her care through the remainder of the hospitalization and after her discharge to home.

The case manager gathered information from Alice about her plans to return to home and factors that will help or impede this process. Alice has three children. One daughter has been at the hospital with her since the day after surgery, but lives over 500 miles away and must return home within 1 week. The other two children also live quite a distance from Alice and are not able to come and help her at this time. She states that she will be able to care for herself with assistance from her daughter until she has to leave and then with assistance from a neighbor.

Alice lives alone in a rural community of approximately 1000 people, which is 30 miles from the hospital in which she is currently hospitalized. Alice lives in a two-story home with a bedroom and a bathroom on the first floor. She has four steps to climb to get into her home, but no other steps if she stays on the main floor. Alice had been married for 40 years but her husband passed away 2 years ago. She never worked outside the home, but is active in church and community events. Alice has many friends, but often speaks of not wanting to be a burden on anyone.

Alice has a history of arthritis and hypertension. Her hypertension is controlled with the medications furosemide (Lasix) and metoprolol (Lopressor). She does experience painful movement of her joints at the wrists, fingers, and knees due to the arthritis. She takes medication for her arthritis as necessary (an over-the-counter anti-inflammatory 2 to 3 times per day).

In reviewing the chart, consulting with the staff nurses, discussing her care with physical therapy and talking with the physician, the case manager elicits information about the proposed health care that Alice will need upon discharge. Alice will be sent home on the medications Lasix, Lopressor, and propoxyphene (Darvocet). She is familiar with the Lasix and the Lopressor, but the Darvocet is new to her. The nurses in the hospital have completed medication teaching, and Alice is able to verbalize knowledge about the medication. She will need to return to the hospital for physical therapy after discharge—once a day for the first week and then 3 days a week the following 2 weeks, with the goal of Alice being able to care for herself without assistance at that time. She will need to return to see the surgeon in 1 week.

In collaboration with Alice and her daughter, the case manager has developed the following plan of care:

NURSING DIAGNOSIS: IMPAIRED PHYSICAL MOBILITY

Nursing outcome	Nursing interventions
Ambulation: Walking	Exercise Therapy: Ambulation Fall Prevention Teaching: Prescribed Activity/Exercise
Mobility Level	Body Mechanics Promotion Exercise Therapy: Joint Mobility Exercise Therapy: Muscle Control

NURSING DIAGNOSIS: RISK FOR INJURY

Nursing outcome	Nursing interventions
Safety Behavior: Fall Prevention	Environmental Management: Safety Home Maintenance Assistance Surveillance: Safety
Symptom Control Behavior	Infection Protection Skin Surveillance Teaching: Disease Process

Other nursing diagnoses that could also apply to this case study are Home Maintenance Management, Impaired; Individual Management of Therapeutic Regimen, Effective; Self-Care Deficit: Bathing/Hygiene; Self-Care Deficit: Dressing/Grooming; Chronic Pain; and Knowledge Deficit: Medication.

•   •   •

The case manager visited Alice at least once a week during the first 3 weeks postdischarge. An evaluation of the plan of care was completed at each of these visits. Her daughter had gone home after 1 week as originally planned, so after 1 week Alice was living alone in her home. Friends and neighbors had been helping Alice by taking her to physical therapy once a day and checking on her frequently by stopping by to visit.

Alice was not having trouble moving around her own home since adjustments had been made (i.e., moving needed items within reach, removing throw rugs, rearranging furniture) in the environment to accommodate her decreased mobility and her risk for falls. Alice still preferred someone to be with her if she was doing any walking outside her home.

Alice was able to bathe, groom, and dress herself with the use of assistive devices and some minor difficulty. If she was not able to complete something herself, she asked one of her friends for assistance. Alice denied any pain from the hip surgery 2 weeks postdischarge and was back on her routine of medicine for her arthritis. She stated that she had a better understanding of arthritis and interventions she could do to lessen the pain. Alice's Darvocet had been discontinued.

OUTCOME
Ambulation: Walking

DEFINITION: Ability to walk from place to place

AMBULATION: WALKING	Dependent, does not participate 1	Requires assistive person & device 2	Requires assistive person 3	Independent with assistive device 4	Completely independent 5
INDICATORS:					
Bears weight	1	2	3	4	5
Walks with effective gait	1	2	3	4	5
Walks at slow pace	1	2	3	4	5
Walks at moderate pace	1	2	3	4	5
Walks at fast pace	1	2	3	4	5
Walks up steps	1	2	3	4	5
Walks down steps	1	2	3	4	5
Walks up inclines	1	2	3	4	5
Walks down inclines	1	2	3	4	5
Walks short distance (<1 block)	1	2	3	4	5
Walks moderate distance (>1 block <5 blocks)	1	2	3	4	5
Walks long distance (5 blocks or >)	1	2	3	4	5
Other _____ Specify	1	2	3	4	5

Patient Outcome Scores Postdischarge

AMBULATION: WALKING	Day of discharge 2	2 days post-discharge 2	6 days post-discharge 4	8 days post-discharge 4	15 days post-discharge 4	22 days post-discharge 4
INDICATORS:						
Bears weight	2	2	4	4	4	5
Walks with effective gait	2	2	4	4	4	5
Walks at slow pace	2	2	4	4	4	5
Walks at moderate pace	1	1	2	2	4	4
Walks up steps	2	2	4	4	4	4
Walks down steps	2	2	4	4	4	4
Walks up inclines	2	2	4	4	4	5
Walks down inclines	2	2	4	4	4	5
Walks short distance (<1 block)	2	2	4	4	4	5
Walks moderate distance (> 1 block <5 blocks)	1	1	2	4	4	5

OUTCOME
Mobility Level

DEFINITION: Ability to move purposefully					
MOBILITY LEVEL	Dependent, does not participate **1**	Requires assistive person & device **2**	Requires assistive person **3**	Independent with assistive device **4**	Completely independent **5**
INDICATORS:					
Balance performance	1	2	3	4	5
Body positioning performance	1	2	3	4	5
Muscle movement	1	2	3	4	5
Joint movement	1	2	3	4	5
Transfer performance	1	2	3	4	5
Ambulation: walking	1	2	3	4	5
Ambulation: wheelchair	1	2	3	4	5
Other _____ Specify	1	2	3	4	5

Patient Outcome Scores Postdischarge

MOBILITY LEVEL	Day of discharge **2**	2 days postdischarge **2**	6 days postdischarge **4**	8 days postdischarge **4**	15 days postdischarge **4**	22 days postdischarge **4**
INDICATORS:						
Muscle movement	2	2	4	4	4	5
Joint movement	2	2	5	5	5	5
Ambulation: walking	2	2	4	4	4	4

OUTCOME
Safety Behavior: Fall Prevention

DEFINITION: Individual or caregiver actions to minimize risk factors that might result in falls

SAFETY BEHAVIOR: FALL PREVENTION	Not adequate 1	Slightly adequate 2	Moderately adequate 3	Substantially adequate 4	Totally adequate 5
INDICATORS:					
Correct use of assistive devices	1	2	3	4	5
Provision of personal assistance	1	2	3	4	5
Placement of barriers to prevent falls	1	2	3	4	5
Use of restraints as needed	1	2	3	4	5
Placement of handrailings as needed	1	2	3	4	5
Elimination of clutter, spills, glare from floors	1	2	3	4	5
Tacking down rugs	1	2	3	4	5
Arrangement for removal of snow and ice from walking surfaces	1	2	3	4	5
Appropriate use of stools/ladders	1	2	3	4	5
Use of well-fitting, tied shoes	1	2	3	4	5
Adjustment of toilet height as needed	1	2	3	4	5
Adjustment of chair height as needed	1	2	3	4	5
Adjustment of bed height as needed	1	2	3	4	5
Use of rubber mats in tub/shower	1	2	3	4	5
Use of grab bars	1	2	3	4	5
Agitation and restlessness controlled	1	2	3	4	5
Use of precautions when taking medications that increase risk for falls	1	2	3	4	5
Use of vision-correcting devices	1	2	3	4	5
Use of safe transfer procedure	1	2	3	4	5
Compensation for physical limitations	1	2	3	4	5
Other _____ Specify	1	2	3	4	5

Patient Outcome Scores Postdischarge

SAFETY BEHAVIOR: FALL PREVENTION	Day of discharge 2	2 days post-discharge 3	6 days post-discharge 4	8 days post-discharge 4	15 days post-discharge 5	22 days post-discharge 5
INDICATORS:						
Correct use of assistive devices	3	3	3	4	5	5
Provision of personal assistance	5	5	5	5	5	5
Placement of barriers to prevent falls	1	1	5	5	5	5
Placement of handrailings as needed	1	1	5	5	5	5
Elimination of clutter, spills, glare from floors	1	3	5	5	5	5
Tacking down rugs	1	3	5	5	5	5
Use of well-fitting, tied shoes	5	5	5	5	5	5
Use of safe transfer procedure	3	3	3	4	5	5

OUTCOME
Symptom Control Behavior

DEFINITION: Personal actions to minimize perceived adverse changes in physical and emotional functioning

SYMPTOM CONTROL BEHAVIOR	Never demonstrated 1	Rarely demonstrated 2	Sometimes demonstrated 3	Often demonstrated 4	Consistently demonstrated 5
INDICATORS:					
Recognizes symptom onset	1	2	3	4	5
Recognizes symptom persistence	1	2	3	4	5
Recognizes symptom severity	1	2	3	4	5
Recognizes symptom frequency	1	2	3	4	5
Recognizes symptom variation	1	2	3	4	5
Uses preventive measures	1	2	3	4	5
Uses relief measures	1	2	3	4	5
Uses warning signs to seek health care	1	2	3	4	5
Uses available resources	1	2	3	4	5
Uses symptom diary	1	2	3	4	5
Reports controlling symptoms	1	2	3	4	5
Other _____ Specify	1	2	3	4	5

Patient Outcome Scores Postdischarge

SYMPTOM CONTROL BEHAVIOR	Day of discharge 3	2 days post-discharge 3	6 days post-discharge 4	8 days post-discharge 4	15 days post-discharge 5	22 days post-discharge 5
INDICATORS:						
Recognizes symptom onset	3	3	4	4	5	5
Recognizes symptom persistence	3	3	4	4	5	5
Recognizes symptom severity	3	3	4	4	5	5
Uses preventive measures	3	3	4	4	5	5
Uses warning signs to seek health care	3	3	4	4	5	5
Uses available resources	5	5	5	5	5	5
Reports controlling symptoms	5	5	5	5	5	5

Nursing-sensitive Outcomes Classification Review Form

The Nursing-sensitive Outcomes Classification (NOC) research team is interested in feedback and submission of outcomes for review and potential addition to the NOC. Suggestions and submissions may be sent by letter or e-mail and should be addressed to:

Lori Penaluna
Project Director
Nursing-sensitive Outcomes Classification
412 NB, College of Nursing
The University of Iowa
Iowa City, Iowa 52242
E-mail: lori-penaluna@uiowa.edu
Phone: (319)353-5414
FAX: (319)335-7106

A. GENERAL COMMENTS ABOUT THE CLASSIFICATION

Comments about the classification in general are welcome.

B. FEEDBACK ON A PARTICULAR OUTCOME:

If the submission is a revision of an existing NOC outcome, provide a paragraph clearly describing the rationale for changes, and note the changes on a copy of the existing outcome. Suggestions can include changes in the definition, indicators, or scale. Additional indicators also can be suggested.

C. GUIDELINES FOR OUTCOME SUBMISSION

All submissions should be typed. Three copies of all materials should be submitted. Background readings/references should be typed in American Psychological Association format. Each submission of a proposed outcome must include a label, a definition, indicators, and a short list of references that support the outcome and indicators. You also may suggest a scale to use with the outcomes (see Chapter 4). A brief paragraph describing the rationale for adding the outcome to the NOC should be included. The rationale should note how the proposed outcome is different from outcomes already included in the NOC.

General Principles for Developing Outcomes

1. Define the outcome as a variable patient or family caregiver state, behavior, or perception that is responsive to nursing intervention(s).
2. Labels should be concise, stated in five or fewer words.

3. Colons can be used to make broader concepts more specific.
4. Labels should describe concepts that can be measured along a continuum.
5. Labels should be neutral and **not** stated as goals.
6. A group of indicators, more specific than the outcome, must be listed that are used to determine the status of the outcome.
7. The definition should be a brief phrase that defines the concept and encompasses the indicators.

Index

A

Abdominal organs, perfusion of, 293-294, 371
Abuse, drug; *see* Chemical dependency
Abuse cessation, 67
Abuse prevention; *see also* Caregiver *entries*
  abuse cessation, 67
  abuse protection, 68
  abusive behavior self-control, 73-74
  aggression control, 78-79
  impulse control, 174-175
  parenting, 229-231
  safety behavior: falls prevention, 258
  safety behavior: home physical environ-
    ment, 259
  safety behavior: personal, 260
Abuse protection, 68
Abuse recovery
  emotional, 69
  financial, 70
  neglect recovery, 207-208
  physical, 71
  sexual, 72
Abusive behavior self-control, 73-74
Acceptance
  acceptance: health status, 75
  adherence behavior, 76
  compliance behavior, 132-133
  hope, 162
  loneliness, 200-201
  social interactions skills, 279
  social involvement, 280
  social support, 281
Accident prevention; *see* Safety
Acid-base balance
  electrolyte and acid/base balance, 143-144
  fluid balance, 148-149
  hydration, 163
  respiratory status: gas exchange, 240
  urinary elimination, 304-305
Acquired immunodeficiency syndrome
  grief resolution, 150-151
  immune hypersensitivity control, 168-169
  immune status, 170-171
  infection status, 176-177

Acquired immunodeficiency syndrome—
  cont'd
  knowledge: disease process, 186
  knowledge: health behaviors, 188
  knowledge: health resources, 189
  knowledge: infection control, 190
  knowledge: medication, 191-192
  knowledge: treatment procedures, 196
  knowledge: treatment regimen, 197
  risk control: sexually transmitted diseases,
    250-251
  treatment behavior, 300-301
Activities of daily living, 263; *see also* Self-
  care *entries*
  ambulation: walking, 80
  ambulation: wheelchair, 81
  body positioning: self-initiated, 87
  instrumental, 269-270
    self-care: non-parenteral medication, 271
    self-care: parenteral medication, 273
  transfer performance, 299
Activity
  ambulation: walking, 80
  ambulation: wheelchair, 81
  diversional
    leisure participation, 199
    play participation, 237
    social involvement, 280
  endurance, 145
  energy conservation, 146
  knowledge: energy conservation, 187
  knowledge: prescribed activity, 194
  leisure participation, 199
  mobility level, 203
  play participation, 237
Activity deficit, diversional, 330
Activity intolerance, 318
Adaptation, psychosocial
  acceptance: health status, 75
  adherence behavior, 76
  caregiver adaptation of patient institution-
    alization, 100-101
  caregiver lifestyle disruption, 104
  child adaptation to hospitalization, 112
  compliance behavior, 132-133

Adaptation, psychosocial—cont'd
  coping, 136-137
  psychosocial adjustment: life change, 238
Adaptive capacity, intracranial, 346
Addiction consequences, 284
Adherence behavior, 76
Adjustment; *see* Adaptation, psychological
  impaired, 319
  psychosocial, life change, 238
Adolescence
  body image, 86
  child development: adolescence, 122
  growth, 152
  health beliefs, 153-157
  health promoting behavior, 159
  knowledge: personal safety, 193
  nutritional status: body mass, 219
  nutritional status: food and fluid intake,
    221
  physical maturation, 235, 236
  risk control, 244-255
  safety behavior: personal, 260
  self-esteem, 275-276
Advance directives
  decision-making, 138
  dignified dying, 139-140
  health beliefs: perceived control, 155
  participation: health care decisions, 232-
    233
Adverse reaction, blood transfusion, 85
Affective disorder, 204-205
Aged patient; *see also* Abuse; Caregiver *en-*
    tries; Mobility
  acceptance: health status, 75
  bowel continence, 89
  bowel elimination, 90-91
  grief resolution, 150-151
  knowledge: health behavior, 188
  knowledge: health resources, 189
  knowledge: personal safety, 193
  physical aging status, 234
  safety behavior: fall prevention, 258
  safety behavior: home physical environ-
    ment, 259
  safety status: falls occurrence, 261
  urinary continence, 302-303
  urinary elimination, 304-305
Age-related changes; *see also* Child develop-
    ment
  growth, 152
  physical aging status, 234
  physical maturation, 235, 236
Aggression control, 78-79
AIDS; *see* Acquired immunodeficiency syn-
    drome
Airway
  respiratory status: gas exchange, 240
  respiratory status: ventilation, 241-242
  tissue perfusion: pulmonary, 298
Airway clearance, ineffective, 319
  patient education for, 382-385
Alcohol abuse; *see* Chemical dependency

Alcohol use, 246-247
Allergy
  immune hypersensitivity control, 168-169
  knowledge: treatment regimen, 197
  risk control, 244
Altered body temperature, 321
Ambulation; *see also* Activity; Safety behav-
    ior *entries*
  balance, 84
  mobility level, 204
  walking, 80
  wheelchair, 81
Anesthesia recovery; *see also* Perfusion
  pain level, 226
  physical injury, 262
  respiratory status, 240-242
  safety status: falls occurrence, 261
  thermoregulation, 289-291
  vital signs status, 306
Anger management
  abusive behavior self-control, 73-74
  aggression control, 78-79
  impulse control, 174-175
  self-mutilation restraint, 277
  suicide self-restraint, 285
Anorexia; *see* Eating disorder
Anticipatory grieving, 334
Anxiety, 320
  anxiety control, 82-83
  fear control, 147
Aphasia; *see* Communication *entries*
Apnea
  neurological status, 209
  neurological status: autonomic, 211-212
  respiratory status: gas exchange, 240
  respiratory status: ventilation, 241-242
Arterial blood gases
  electrolyte and acid/base balance, 143-144
  respiratory status: gas exchange, 240
  urinary elimination, 304-305
Aspiration; *see also* Airway
  neurological status: cranial sensory/motor
    function, 215
  self-care: eating, 266
Aspiration, risk for, 320
Atherosclerosis; *see* Perfusion
Attachment, parent-infant, 227-228, 351; *see*
    also Bonding
Attention, 134
Attitude
  acceptance: health status, 75
  caregiver-patient relationship, 105
  health beliefs, 153-157
  health orientation, 158
  hope, 162
  participation: health care decisions, 232-
    233
  will to live, 308
Autoimmune disorder
  immune hypersensitivity control, 168
  immune status, 170-171
Autonomic neurological status, 211-212

Autonomy
  adherence behavior, 76
  dignified dying, 139-140
  participation: health care decisions, 232-233

B

Balance, 84
  acid-base, 143-144
  fluid, 148-149, 163, 332
Bathing
  self-care: activities of daily living, 263
  self-care: bathing, 264
  self-care: hygiene, 268
  self-care: oral hygiene, 272
Battering; *see* Abuse *entries*
Bed rest
  body positioning: self-initiated, 87
  immobility consequences, 166, 167
  mood equilibrium, 204-205
  tissue integrity: skin and mucous membranes, 292
Behavior
  adherence behavior, 76
  compliance behavior, 132-133
  compulsive; *see* Compulsive behavior
  health promoting behavior, 159
  health seeking behavior, 160-161, 336
  immunization behavior, 172-173
  impulse control, 174-175
  leisure participation, 199
  nurturing; *see* Nurturing behavior
  pain control behavior, 224
  risk control, 244-255
  role performance behavior, 257
  safety behavior: fall prevention, 258
  safety behavior: home physical environment, 259
  safety behavior: personal, 260
  self-destructive; *see* Self-destructive behavior
  sick role
    child adaptation to hospitalization, 112
    role performance, 257
    treatment behavior: illness or injury, 300-301
  social interaction skills, 279
  social involvement, 280
  suicide self-restraint, 285
  symptom control, 287
  treatment, illness or injury, 300-301
Belief, health, 153-157
Bereavement
  dignified dying, 136-140
  grief resolution, 150-151
Biochemical measures, of nutritional status, 218
Bipolar disorder, 204-205
Birth control
  knowledge: health behavior, 188
  risk control: unintended pregnancy, 254-255

Birth weight, 219
Bladder control
  self-care: hygiene, 268
  self-care: toileting, 274
  urinary continence, 302-303
  urinary elimination, 304-305
Blood pressure
  circulation status, 123-124
  fluid balance, 148-149
  hydration, 163
  vital signs status, 306
Blood transfusion reaction control, 85
Body image, 86
Body image disturbance, 321
Body mass, 219
  growth, 152
  nutritional status: body mass, 219
  physical aging status: growth, 234
Body positioning, self-initiated, 87
Body temperature; *see* Thermoregulation
Bonding
  caregiver-patient relationship, 105
  parent-infant attachment, 277-278
  parenting, 229-230
Bone healing, 88
Bottle-feeding; *see* Feeding, bottle
Bowel continence, 89
Bowel elimination, 90-91
  constipation, 327
  diarrhea, 329
Bowel incontinence, 338
Brain, cerebral perfusion, 296
Brain death; *see* Cognitive status
Breastfeeding
  effective, 322
  ineffective, 322
  interrupted, 323
  knowledge about, 181-182
Breastfeeding establishment
  infant, 92
  maternal, 93-94
Breastfeeding maintenance, 95
Breastfeeding weaning, 96-97
Breathing pattern, ineffective, 323; *see also* Respiratory status
Bulimia; *see* Eating disorder
Burn; *see also* Nutritional status; Pain
  body image, 86
  electrolyte and acid/base balance, 143-144
  fluid balance, 148-149
  infection status, 176-177
  knowledge: infection control, 190
  leisure participation, 199
  muscle function, 206
  self-esteem, 275-276
  tissue integrity: skin and mucous membranes, 292

C

Caloric intake
  growth, 152
  nutritional status, 218-222

Cardiac function
  cardiac pump effectiveness, 98-99
  circulation status, 123-124
  energy conservation, 146
  health seeking behavior, 160-161
  knowledge: diet, 184-185
  knowledge: disease process, 186
  knowledge: energy conservation, 187
  knowledge: medication, 191-192
  knowledge: prescribed activity, 194
  knowledge: substance use control, 195
  knowledge: treatment regimen, 196
  risk control: tobacco use, 252-253
  treatment behavior: illness or injury, 300-
    301
  vital signs status, 306
Cardiac pump effectiveness, 98-99
Caregiver adaptation to patient institutional-
    ization, 100-101
Caregiver emotional health, 102
Caregiver home care readiness, 103
Caregiver lifestyle disruption, 104
Caregiver performance
  direct care, 106
  indirect care, 107
Caregiver physical health, 108
Caregiver role strain, 324, 325
Caregiver stressors, 109
Caregiver well-being, 110
Caregiver-patient relationship, 105
Caregiving endurance potential, 111
Case study on fractured hip, 388-396
Catheterization, urinary
  infection status, 176-177
  knowledge: infection control, 190
  knowledge: treatment procedure, 196
  urinary elimination, 304-305
Central motor control, 213
Cerebral perfusion, 296; *see also* Mobility;
    Neurological status
  altered, 370
Change, life, 238
Chemical dependency
  health promoting behavior, 159
  impulse control, 174-175
  knowledge: medication, 191-192
  knowledge: substance use control, 195
  risk control: alcohol use, 246-247
  risk control: drug use, 248-249
  substance addiction consequences, 284
Child; *see also* Infant
  growth, 152
  parent-infant attachment, 227-228, 351
Child abuse; *see* Abuse
Child adaptation to hospitalization, 112
Child development
  2 months, 113
  4 months, 114
  6 months, 115
  12 months, 116
  2 years, 117
  3 years, 118

Child development—cont'd
  4 years, 119
  5 years, 120
  adolescence (12-17 years), 122
  altered, 335
  middle childhood (6-11 years), 121
Child health; *see also* Nutritional status; Par-
    enting
  growth, 152
  immunization status, 170-171
  oral health, 223
  rest, 243
  self-esteem, 275-276
  sleep, 278
Child safety, knowledge about, 183
Childproofing
  safety behavior: home physical environ-
    ment, 259
  safety behavior: personal, 260
Chronic pain; *see* Pain
Circulation status, 123-124
  immobility consequences: physiological,
    166
  tissue perfusion: peripheral, 297
Classification, 12-13, 41-64
  definition of, 41-45
  future work with, 63-64
  implementation of, 48-63
    indicator and, 49-50
    measurement scales and, 50-51
    outcome and, 48-49
    questions about, 51
  measurement scales used in, 52-61
  outcomes classification review form, 397-
    398
  structure of, 27, 43
  uses of, 46-48
Clinical innovation, 12
Cognitive ability, 125-126
Cognitive orientation, 127
Cognitive status; *see also* Neurological status
  cognitive ability, 125-126
  cognitive orientation, 127
  concentration, 134
  decision making, 138
  distorted thought control, 141-142
  information processing, 178-179
  memory, 202
Colonic constipation, 327
Coma, 209, 214
Comfort level, 128
Communicable disease; *see* Infection
Communication
  expressive ability, 130
  impaired verbal, 325
  receptive ability, 131
Communication ability, 129
Compliance behavior, 132-133
Comprehension; *see* Knowledge *entries*
Compulsive behavior
  abusive behavior self-control, 73-74
  aggression control, 78-79

Compulsive behavior—cont'd
    impulse control, 174-175
    knowledge: substance use control, 195
    risk control: alcohol use, 246-247
    risk control: drug use, 248-249
    self-mutilation restraint, 277
    suicide self-restraint, 285
Computerized nursing information systems, 9
Concentration, 134
Condition-specific outcomes, 7
Conflict
    decisional, 328
    parental role, 350
Confusion, acute or chronic, 326; *see also* Cognitive status
Consciousness, level of, 209, 214
Conservation, energy, 146
    knowledge about, 187
Constipation, 327
    bowel elimination, 90-91
    immobility consequences: physiological, 166
    mobility level, 203
    nutritional status: food and fluid intake, 221
Continence
    bowel, 89
    bowel continence, 89
    self-care: toileting, 274
    urinary, 302-303
Contraception
    knowledge: health behavior, 188
    risk control: unintended pregnancy, 254-255
Control
    aggression, 78-79
    anxiety, 82-83
    central motor, 213
    fear, 147
    immune hypersensitivity, 168-169
    impulse, 174-175
    infection, 190
    pain, 224
    perceived, 155
    risk, 244-245
        alcohol use, 246-247
        drug use, 248-249
        sexually transmitted diseases, 250-251
        tobacco use, 252-253
        unintended pregnancy, 254-255
    substance use, 195
    symptom, 287
    thought, distorted, 141-142
Coping, 136-137; *see also* Abuse *entries;* Adaptation, psychological; Stress
    acceptance: health status, 75
    anxiety control, 82-83
    caregiver well-being, 110
    defensive, 328
    dignified dying, 139-140
    hope, 162

Coping—cont'd
    ineffective, 341
    spiritual well-being, 282-283
    will to live, 308
Coronary disease; *see* Cardiac function
Cranial sensory/motor function, 215
Crisis
    emotional
        abuse protection, 68
        abusive behavior self-control, 73-74
        aggression control, 78-79
        caregiver lifestyle disruption, 104
        coping, 136-137
        fear control, 147
        impulse control, 174-175
        self-mutilation restraint, 277
        suicide self-restraint, 285
    physiological
        blood transfusion reaction control, 85
        cardiac pump effectiveness, 98-99
        circulation status, 123-124
        electrolyte and acid/base balance, 143-144
        neurological status, 209
        thermoregulation, 289-291
        vital signs status, 306
Critical path, 60
    for myocardial infarction, 378-381

D

Data base management, 34
Data set, 9-10
Data source
    rating of, 32-33
    selection of, 25, 26, 28
Death; *see also* Hospice
    dignified dying, 136-140
    grief resolution, 150-151
Decision making, 48, 138
    information processing, 178-179
    participation: health care decisions, 232-233
Decisional conflict, 328
Decubitus ulcer; *see also* Nutritional status
    body positioning: self-initiated, 87
    immobility consequences: physiological, 166
    self-care: non-parenteral medication, 271
    tissue integrity: skin and mucous membranes, 292
    tissue perfusion: peripheral, 297
    wound healing: second intention, 310
Defecation, 89-91
Defensive coping, 328
Dehydration; *see* Hydration
Delirium; *see* Cognitive status
Delusion, 141-142
Dementia; *see* Cognitive status
Denial, ineffective, 329
Denominator, 47
Dental care; *see* Oral *entries*

Dependency, chemical; *see* Chemical dependency
Depression, 204-205
Development; *see* Age-related changes; Child development
Diagnosis, nursing, 12-14
  outcomes vs, 45
  resolution of, 24
Diagnosis-specific outcomes, 7
Diarrhea, 329
  bowel elimination, 90-91
  hydration, 163
  knowledge: diet, 184-185
  knowledge: treatment regimen, 197
  treatment behavior: illness or injury, 300-301
Diet; *see also* Feeding; Nutritional status
  knowledge: diet, 184-185
  self-care: eating, 266
Dignified dying, 139-140; *see also* Hospice
Direct care by caregiver, 106
Discharge planning; *see also* Knowledge *entries*; Self- care *entries*
  caregiver home care readiness, 103
  health beliefs: perceived resources, 156
  safety behavior: fall prevention, 258
  safety behavior: home physical environment, 259
Discipline; *see* Parenting
Discipline-specific outcomes, 7
Discomfort; *see* Pain
Disease; *see also* Infection
  infection control, 190
  infection status, 176-177
  knowledge about, 186
  myocardial infarction, 378-381
  pneumonia, 382-385
  sexually transmitted, 250-251
  treatment behavior, 300-301
Disease prevention
  adherence behavior, 76
  health promoting behavior, 159
  health seeking behavior, 160-161
  immunization behavior, 172-173
Disfigurement
  body image, 86
  psychosocial adjustment: life change, 238
  self-esteem, 275-276
  self-mutilation control, 277
Disorganized infant behavior, 343, 344
Disorientation; *see* Cognitive status; Neurological status
Distorted thought control, 141-142
Disuse syndrome, risk for, 330
Diversional activity
  leisure participation, 199
  play participation, 237
  social involvement, 280
Diversional activity deficit, 330
Do Not Resuscitate orders; *see* Advance directives
Domestic violence; *see* Violence management

Drainage management, 309-310
Dressing
  self-care: activities of daily living, 263
  self-care: dressing, 265
  self-care: grooming, 267
Drug abuse; *see* Chemical dependency
Drugs
  knowledge: medication, 191-192
  self-care: non-parenteral medication, 271
  self-care: parenteral medication, 273
Durable power of attorney; *see* Advance directives
Dying; *see also* Hospice
  dignified, 139-140
  grief resolution, 150-151
Dyspnea; *see* Respiratory status
Dysreflexia, 331

E

Eating; *see* Feeding; Nutritional status
Eating disorder
  body image, 86
  energy conservation, 146, 187
  growth, 152
  impulse control, 174-175
  knowledge: diet, 184-185
  knowledge: energy conservation, 187
  nutritional status, 217-222
  oral health, 223
  physical maturation, 235, 236
  risk control, 244
  safety behavior: personal, 260
  self-esteem, 275-276
Edema
  cardiac pump effectiveness, 98-99
  circulation status, 123-124
  fluid balance, 148-149
  hydration, 163
  respiratory status, 240-242
  tissue integrity: skin and mucous membranes, 292-293
Education; *see also* Knowledge
  adherence behavior, 76
  caregiver performance: direct care, 106
  caregiver performance: indirect care, 107
  compliance behavior, 132-133
  health promoting behavior, 159
  health seeking behavior, 160-161
  nursing, 48
  patient, for pneumonia, 382-385
  risk control, 244-255
  treatment behavior: illness or injury, 300-301
Elderly; *see* Abuse *entries*; Aged patient; Caregiver *entries*; Mobility
Electrolyte and acid-base balance, 143-144
Elimination
  bowel, 90-91
    constipation, 327
    diarrhea, 329
  toileting, 274
  urinary, 304-305
    altered, 373

Emotional abuse; *see* Abuse *entries*
Emotional well-being; *see* Abuse *entries*; Psychological status; Well-being
Encopresis, 89-91
Endurance, 145
    caregiving endurance potential, 111
Energy
    endurance, 145
    energy conservation, 146, 187
    nutritional status: energy, 220
    rest, 243
    sleep, 278
Energy, nutritional status and, 220
Energy conservation, 146
    knowledge about, 187
Energy field disturbance, 331
Enuresis, 302-305
Environment; *see also* Safety *entries*
    caregiver adaptation to hospitalization, 100-101
    child adaptation to institutionalization, 112
    self-care: instrumental activities of daily living, 269-270
    social support, 281
Environment, home, 259
Environmental interpretation syndrome, impaired, 331
Equilibrium, 84
Equilibrium, mood, 204-205
Equipment
    caregiver: home care readiness, 103
    knowledge: treatment procedure(s), 196
    safety behavior: home physical environment, 259
    treatment behavior: illness or injury, 300-301
Euvolia; *see* Hydration
Exchange, gas, 240
Exercise; *see also* Activity; Fitness
    adherence behavior, 76
    cardiac pump effectiveness, 98-99
    endurance, 145
    health promoting behavior, 159
    joint movement, 179-180
    knowledge: health behavior, 188
    knowledge: treatment regimen, 197
    leisure participation, 199
    muscle function, 206
    nutritional status: energy, 220
    risk control, 244
    treatment behavior: illness or injury, 300-301
    vital signs status, 306
Exercise tolerance
    endurance, 145
    energy conservation, 148, 187
Expressive ability, communication, 130

F

Falls occurrence, 261
Falls prevention, 258
Family; *see* Parenting

Family violence; *see* Abuse; Violence management
Fatigue, 332; *see also* Activity; Energy
Fear, 332
Fear control, 147
Fecal impaction; *see* Impaction, fecal
Feedback, 64
Feeding; *see also* Nutritional status
    bottle
        growth, 152
        nutritional status: body mass, 219
        nutritional status: food and fluid intake, 221
        parent-infant attachment, 227-228
    breastfeeding, 92-97, 181-182
    caregiver performance: direct care, 106
    infant, ineffective, 344
    self-care: parenteral medication, 273
Female physical maturation, 235
Fertility control
    knowledge: health behavior, 188
    risk control: unintended pregnancy, 254-255
Fever
    hydration, 163
    infection status, 176-177
    knowledge: infection status, 190
    thermoregulation, 289-291
    vital signs status, 306
Field testing of outcomes, 29-30, 39-40
Financial issues
    abuse recovery: financial, 70
    health beliefs: perceived resources, 156
    psychosocial adjustment: life change, 238
Financial recovery, abuse, 70
Fitness; *see* Exercise
Fluid and electrolytes
    electrolyte and acid/base balance, 143-144
    fluid balance, 148-149
    hydration, 163
    nutritional status: food and fluid intake, 221
Fluid balance, 148-149
Fluid status
    hydration, 163
    nutritional status: fluid and food intake, 221
Fluid volume deficit, 332-333
Fluid volume excess, 333
Focus group concept analysis, 35-39
Food; *see* Eating disorder; Feeding; Nutritional status
Food intake, 221
Foot care
    self-care: grooming, 267
    self-care: hygiene, 268
    tissue integrity: skin and mucous membranes, 292
    tissue perfusion: peripheral, 297
Fractured hip, case study on, 388-396

Functional status; *see also* Cognitive status; Self-care *entries*
  ambulation: walking, 80
  ambulation: wheelchair, 81
  balance, 84
  body positioning: self-initiated, 87
  immobility consequences, 166-167
  joint movement, 179-180
  mobility level, 203
  muscle function, 206
  transfer performance, 299

G

Gait
  ambulation: walking, 80
  neurological status: central motor control, 213
Gas exchange, 240, 333
  impaired, 333
Gastric feeding; *see* Nutritional status
Gastrointestinal function; *see also* Nutritional status
  knowledge: diet, 184-185
  tissue perfusion: abdominal organs, 293-294
Geriatric patient; *see* Abuse; Aged patient; Caregiver *entries*; Mobility
Grief resolution, 150-151
  dignified dying, 139-140
Grieving
  anticipatory, 334
  dysfunctional, 334
  grief resolution, 150-151
  hope, 162
  loneliness, 200-201
  mood equilibrium, 204-205
Grooming, 267; *see* Self-care *entries*
Growth, 152; *see* Age-related changes
  altered, 335
  female physical maturation, 235
  male physical maturation, 236

H

Hair care, 263, 267
Hallucinations, 141-142
Hay fever, 168-169
Head injury; *see* Neurological deficits
Healing, bone, 88
Health, oral, 223
  self-care: hygiene, 268
  self-care: oral hygiene, 272
Health beliefs, 153-157
  perceived ability to perform, 154
  perceived control, 155
  perceived resources, 156
  perceived threat, 157
Health care decisions, 232-233
Health care system, outcome development in, 3-15
Health knowledge; *see* Knowledge
Health maintenance, altered, 336

Health orientation, 158
Health promoting behavior, 159
Health promotion
  adherence behavior, 76
  health orientation, 158
  health promoting behavior, 159
  health seeking behavior, 160-161
  immunization behavior, 172-173
  knowledge: health behaviors, 188
  risk control, 244-255
Health resources, knowledge about, 189
Health screening; *see also* Risk control
  health seeking behavior, 160-161
  risk detection, 256, 276
Health seeking behavior, 160-161, 336
Health status
  acceptance: health status, 75
  caregiver: emotional health, 102
  caregiver: physical health, 108
  caregiver: stressors, 109
  caregiver: well-being, 110
  well-being, 307
Health status acceptance, 75
Hearing
  communication: receptive ability, 131
  neurological status: cranial sensory/motor function, 215
  safety behavior: personal, 260
Heart; *see* Cardiac function
Heart rate, 306
Heat production; *see* Thermoregulation
Hemodynamic status
  cardiac pump effectiveness, 98-99
  circulation status, 123-124
  fluid balance, 148-149, 163
  immobility consequences: physiological, 166
Hip fracture, case study on, 388-396
Holistic care
  quality of life, 239
  well-being, 307
    spiritual, 282-283
Home care; *see* Caregiver *entries*; Discharge planning; Self-care *entries*
Home care readiness of caregiver, 103
Home maintenance management, impaired, 337
Home physical environment, 259
Hope, 162
  spiritual well-being, 282-283
  will to live, 308
Hopelessness, 337
Hospice; *see also* Caregiver *entries*; Pain *entries*
  acceptance: health status, 75
  dignified dying, 139-140
  grief resolution, 150-151
  quality of life, 239
  spiritual well-being, 282-283
  treatment behavior: illness or injury, 300-301

Hospitalization
  caregiver adaptation to patient institution-
    alization, 100-101
  child adaptation to hospitalization, 112
Housekeeping
  safety behavior: home physical environ-
    ment, 259
  self-care: instrumental activities of daily
    living, 269-270
Human immunodeficiency virus infection;
    see Acquired immunodeficiency syn-
    drome
Hydration, 163
  fluid balance, 148-149
  nutritional status: food and fluid intake,
    221
Hygiene, 268; *see also* Self-care *entries*
  oral, 272
Hyperalimentation; *see* Nutrition, total par-
    enteral
Hypersensitivity; *see* Allergy
Hypersensitivity control, immune, 168-169
Hyperthermia, 338; *see* Fever
Hypotension; *see* Blood pressure
Hypothermia
  thermoregulation, 289-291
  vital signs status, 308

I

ICU psychosis; *see also* Cognitive status
  immobility consequences: psycho-cogni-
    tive, 167
  sleep, 278
Identity, 164-165
  personal identity disturbance, 354
Illness, treatment behavior, 300-301; *see also*
    Disease
Illness behavior
  compliance behavior, 132-133
  treatment behavior: illness or injury, 300-
    301
Image, body, 86
Immobility consequences; *see also* Mobility
  physiological, 166
  psycho-cognitive, 167
Immune hypersensitivity control, 168-169
Immune status, 170-171
  blood transfusion reaction control, 85
Immunization behavior, 172-173
Immunodeficiency; *see* Acquired immunode-
    ficiency syndrome
Impaction, fecal
  bowel elimination, 90-91
  immobility consequences: physiological,
    166
  mobility level, 203
  nutritional status: food and fluid intake,
    221
Implementation of classification, 48-63; *see
    also* Classification, implementation of

Impulse control, 174-175; *see also* Compulsive
    behavior
Incision healing, 309-310
Incontinence; *see also* Continence
  bowel, 338
  functional, 339
  reflex, 339
  stress, 340
  total, 340
  urge, 341
Independence; *see* Activities of daily living
Indicator
  definition of, 36
  initial list of, 29
  outcome labels vs, 62
  validation of, 25-27, 29-30
Indirect care by caregiver, 107
Individual coping, ineffective, 341
Infant; *see also* Breastfeeding *entries*; Feeding;
    Parenting
  bowel elimination, 90-91
  breastfeeding establishment by, 92
  caregiver home care readiness, 103
  disorganized behavior, 343, 344
  growth, 152
  hydration, 163
  ineffective feeding pattern, 344
  muscle function, 206
  neurological status, 209-216
  nutritional status: body mass, 219
  nutritional status: food and fluid intake, 221
  parent/infant/child attachment, 227-228,
    351
  role performance, 257
  sleep, 278
  social support, 281
  thermoregulation, 291
  thermoregulation in, 291
  urinary elimination, 304-305
  vital signs status, 306
Infarction, myocardial, critical pathway for,
    378-381
Infection; *see also* Disease prevention; Risk
    control
  human immunodeficiency virus; *see* Ac-
    quired immunodeficiency syndrome
  immune status, 170-171
  immunization behavior, 172-173
  infection status, 176-177
  knowledge: health behaviors, 188
  knowledge: infection control, 190
  nosocomial
    respiratory status: gas exchange, 240
    respiratory status: ventilation, 241-242
    urinary elimination, 304-305
  risk control: sexually transmitted diseases,
    250-251
  risk for, 345
  sexually transmitted, 250-251
  thermoregulation, 289-291

Infection—cont'd
    vital signs status, 306
Infection control, knowledge about, 190
Infection status, 176-177
Information processing, 178-179
Information systems, computerized, 9
Infusion therapy, 273
Injury; *see* Abuse *entries*; Violence management
    head; *see* Neurological deficits
    perioperative positioning, 353
    physical, 262; *see also* Safety *entries*
    post-trauma response, 355
    risk for, 345, 372
    self-inflicted
        impulse control, 174-175
        self-mutilation restraint, 277
        suicide self-restraint, 285
    treatment behavior, 300-301
Injury prevention; *see also* Safety *entries*
    abuse protection, 68
    knowledge: personal safety, 193
    parenting: social safety, 231
    risk control, 244-255
Innovations, evaluation of, 12
Inoculation, 172-173
Institutionalization; *see* Adaptation, psychological
    caregiver adaptation to patient institutionalization, 100-101
    child adaptation to hospitalization, 112
Instrumental activities of daily living; *see* Activities of daily living
Intake and output; *see also* Hydration
    circulation status, 123-124
    nutritional status: food and fluid intake, 221
    nutritional status: nutrient intake, 222
Interaction
    caregiver-patient relationship, 105
    communication, 129-131
    parent-infant attachment, 227-228
    parenting, 229-230
    social, 279
        impaired, 365
    social interaction skills, 279
    social involvement, 280
    social support: involvement, 281
Interpersonal relations; *see* Interaction
Interpretation, environmental, impaired, 331
Intervention, classification and, 13
Intolerance, activity, 318
Intracranial adaptive capacity, decreased, 346
Intracranial pressure; *see* Neurological status
Intramuscular medication
    knowledge: medication, 191-192
    self-care: parenteral medication, 273
Intravenous medication
    knowledge: medication, 191-192
Intubation; *see* Airway
Ischemia; *see* Perfusion

J
Joint Commission on Accreditation of Healthcare Organizations, 21
Joint movement
    active, 179
    passive, 180

K
Knowledge
    breastfeeding, 181-182
    child safety, 183
    diet, 184-185
    disease process, 186
    energy conservation, 187
    health behaviors, 188
    health resources, 189
    infection control, 190
    medication, 191-192
    nursing, development of, 12-14
    personal safety, 193
    prescribed activity, 194
    substance use control, 195
    treatment procedures, 196
    treatment regimen, 197-198
Knowledge deficit, 346

L
Label, outcome, 32-34
Lactation; *see* Breastfeeding *entries*
Language
    communication ability, 129
    nursing, 8-9, 43
Laxative, 89-91
Learning; *see* Knowledge
Legal issues; *see* Advance directives
Leisure participation, 199
Level of consciousness, 209, 214
Life change, 238
Life changes; *see also* Adaptation, psychological
    caregiver lifestyle disruption, 104
    caregiver well-being, 110
    dignified dying, 139-140
    parenting, 229-230
    physical aging status, 234
    psychosocial adjustment: life change, 238
    role performance, 257
Lifestyle; *see also* Risk control
    caregiver lifestyle disruption, 104
    psychosocial adjustment: life change, 238
    quality of life, 239
Linkages, NANDA-NOC, 315-375
Living will; *see* Advance directives
Loneliness, 200-201
    risk for, 347
Loss
    dignified dying, 139-140
    grief resolution, 150-151
    psychosocial adjustment: life change, 238
Lung, perfusion of, 298
Lung disease, 240-242

M

Maintenance
  of breastfeeding, 95
  health, altered, 336
  home, impaired, 337
Male physical maturation, 236
Management innovation, 12
Manic depressive psychosis, 204-205
Mass, body, 219
Maternal behavior; *see* Parenting
Maternal breastfeeding establishment, 93-94
Maturation, physical; *see also* Age-related
        changes
  female, 235
  male, 236
Meal preparation
  self-care: eating, 266
  self-care: instrumental activities of daily
        living, 269-270
Measure, outcome, 47-48
Measurement scale, 52-61
Medical Outcomes Study, 4
Medication; *see* Drugs
Membrane, mucous
  integrity of, 292
  oral, 439
Memory, 202
  impaired, 347
Mental status; *see also* Neurological status
  cognitive ability, 125-126
  cognitive orientation, 127
  concentration, 134
  confusion, 326
  decision making, 138
  distorted thought control, 141-142
  information processing, 178-179
  memory, 202
  psycho-cognitive consequences of immo-
        bility, 167
Middle childhood, 121
Minimum nursing data set, 9-10
Mobility
  ambulation: walking, 80
  ambulation: wheelchair, 81
  balance, 84
  body positioning: self-initiated, 87
  endurance, 145
  energy conservation, 146, 187
  immobility consequences, 166, 167
  joint movement, 179-180
  knowledge: prescribed activity, 194
  mobility level, 203
  muscle function, 206
  transfer performance, 299
Mobility, impaired physical, 354
Mobility level, 203
Mood equilibrium, 204-205
Motor control, central, 213
Motor function
  cranial, 215
  spinal, 216
Mourning; *see* Grief; Grieving

Mouth care, 272; *see* Oral *entries*
Movement; *see* Mobility
Mucous membranes
  integrity of, 292
  oral, 439
Multidisciplinary outcomes, 7
Muscle function, 206
Mutilation of self
  restraint from, 277
  risk for, 362
Myocardial infarction, critical pathway for,
        378-381

N

NANDA-NOC linkages, 315-375
  how to use, 316-317
  methodology used in development of, 315-
        316
  specific, 318-375
National data set, 10
Neglect, unilateral, 372; *see also* Abuse *entries*
Neglect recovery, 207-208
Neonatal care; *see* Infant
Neonate, thermoregulation in, 291; *see also*
        Infant
Neurological deficits; *see also* Neurological
        status
  balance, 84
  communication, 129-131
  immobility consequences: physiological,
        166
  tissue perfusion: cerebral, 296
Neurological status, 209-216
  autonomic, 211-212
  central motor control, 213
  cerebral perfusion, 296
  consciousness, 214
  cranial sensory/motor function, 215
  dysreflexia, 331
  spinal sensory/motor function, 216
Neuropathy; *see also* Pain
  circulation status, 123-124
  neurological status: autonomic, 211-212
  neurological status: spinal sensory/motor
        function, 216
  tissue perfusion: peripheral, 297
Neurosis
  aggression control, 78-79
  anxiety control, 82-83
  decision making, 138
  fear control, 147
  self-esteem, 275-276
Neurovascular dysfunction, peripheral, 354
Newborn care; *see* Infant
Nipple; *see* Breastfeeding *entries*
Noncompliance, 348
Non-parenteral medication, 271
  knowledge: medication, 191-192
  self-care: non-parenteral medication, 271
Non-prescription drugs; *see* Drugs
Nonverbal communication; *see* Communica-
        tion

North American Nursing Diagnosis Association, 18, 45
    NANDA-NOC linkages, 315-375
Nosocomial infection; *see* Infection, nosocomial
Numerator, 47
Nursing, outcomes development in, 4-7
Nursing data set, 9-10
Nursing diagnosis
    NANDA-NOC linkages of, 315-375
    outcomes vs, 45
    resolution of, 24
Nursing information systems, computerized, 9
Nursing innovations, evaluation of, 12
Nursing language, 8-9
Nursing-sensitive outcomes classification; *see*
    Classification; Outcomes
Nursing-sensitive outcomes classification review form, 397-398
Nurturing behavior
    breastfeeding establishment: infant, 92
    breastfeeding maintenance, 95
    caregiver performance: direct care, 106
    caregiver performance: indirect care, 107
    caregiver-patient relationship, 105
    parent-infant attachment, 227-228
    parenting, 229-230
Nutrient intake, 222
Nutrition, total parenteral
    knowledge: medication, 191-192
    nutritional status: food and fluid intake, 221
    nutritional status: nutrient intake, 222
    self-care: parenteral medication, 273
Nutritional status, 217-222; *see also* Eating disorder
    altered
      less than body requirements, 348
      more than body requirements, 348, 439
    biochemical measures, 218
    body mass, 219
    energy, 220
    food and fluid intake, 221
    nutrient intake, 222
    self-care: eating, 266

O

Older patient; *see* Abuse *entries*; Aged patient; Caregiver *entries*; Mobility
Oral administration of drug, 271
Oral airway; *see* Airway
Oral health, 223
    self-care: hygiene, 268
    self-care: oral hygiene, 272
Oral mucous membranes, altered, 439
Organized infant behavior, 343
Orientation
    cognitive, 127
    health, 158
Ostomy
    bowel continence, 89
    bowel elimination, 90-91

Ostomy—cont'd
    self-care: toileting, 274
    tissue integrity: skin and mucous membranes, 292
    treatment behavior: illness or injury, 300-301
    urinary elimination, 304-305
Outcome development, 3-14
    history of, 3-7
    methods for, 32-40
    standardization of, 8-14
Outcomes
    categories of, 6
    classification of, 41-64; *see also* Classification
    current evaluation of, 6-7
    definition of, 36
    field testing of, 29-30, 39-40
    initial list of, 32-34
    NANDA-NOC linkages and, 315-375
    standardization of, 8-14, 23
    terminology of, 22
Outcomes classification review form, 397-398
Outcomes research, 18-30
    development of, 3-7
    development of initial list in, 29
    methodologic strategies in, 25-29
    preliminary work in, 19-20
    purpose and significance of, 18-19
    resolution of issues in, 20-24
    team development for, 20
    validation of, 29-30
Oxygenation; *see* Respiratory status

P

Pain, 349
    chronic, 350
    disruptive effects, 225
Pain control behavior, 224
Pain level, 226
Parental role conflict, 350
Parenteral drug
    knowledge: medication, 191-192
    self-care: parenteral medication, 273
Parenteral medication, 273
Parent-infant attachment, 227-228
    risk for altered, 351
Parenting, 229-230; *see also* Caregiver *entries*
    altered, 352, 353
    breastfeeding; *see* Breastfeeding *entries*
    immunization behavior, 172-173
    knowledge: personal safety, 193
    parent-infant attachment, 227-228
    play participation, 237
    role performance, 257
    safety behavior: home physical environment, 259
    safety behavior: personal, 260
    social safety, 231
    social support, 281
Participation; *see also* Interaction
    caregiver well-being, 110

Participation—cont'd
  dignified dying, 139-140
  health care decisions, 232-233
  leisure, 199
  leisure participation, 199
  play, 237
  play participation, 237
  quality of life, 239
  social involvement, 280
  well-being, 307
Passive joint movement, 180
Patient
  in classification, 42
  definition of, 20
Patient education plan for pneumonia, 382-
      385; see also Knowledge entries
Patient-controlled analgesia
  knowledge: medication, 191-192
  self-care: parenteral medication, 273
Pediatric patient; see Adolescence; Child en-
      tries; Infant
Perceived ability to perform, 154
Perceived constipation, 327
Perceived control, 155
Perceived resources, 156
Perceived threat, 157
Perfusion, tissue
  abdominal organs, 293-294
  altered, 370-372
  cardiac, 295
  cerebral, 296
  peripheral, 297
  pulmonary, 298
Perioperative positioning injury, 353
Peripheral neurovascular dysfunction, 354
Peripheral tissue perfusion, 297, 371
Personal identity disturbance, 354
Personal safety, knowledge about, 193
Personal safety behavior, 260
Physical abuse; see Abuse entries; Violence
      management
Physical aging status, 234
Physical environment, home, 259
Physical fitness; see Exercise; Fitness
Physical health of caregiver, 108
Physical injury, 262
Physical maturation
  female, 235
  male, 236
Physical mobility, impaired, 354
Physical recovery, abuse, 71
Physical status
  endurance, 145
  passive joint movement, 180
Physiology, immobility consequences, 166
Play
  leisure participation, 199
  play participation, 237
Pneumonia, patient education plan for, 382-
      385
Poisoning, risk for, 355
Poisoning prevention, 259

Policy formulation, 48
Positioning
  perioperative, 353
  self-initiated, 87
Post-trauma response, 355
Power of attorney; see Advance directives
Powerlessness, 356
Pregnancy
  knowledge: health behaviors, 188
  risk control: unintended pregnancy, 254-255
Pregnancy, unintended, 254-255
Premature infant; see Infant
Prescribed activity, knowledge about, 194
Prescription drug; see Drugs
Pressure ulcer; see Decubitus ulcer
Prevention; see Abuse entries; Health promo-
      tion; Risk control
Primary intention, healing by, 309
Problem solving; see Decision making
Procedures, treatment, 196
Processing, information, 178-179
Protection
  abuse, 68
  altered, 356
Psycho-cognitive consequences of immobil-
      ity, 167
Psychological status; see Adaptation, psy-
      chosocial; Emotional status; Well-being
  acceptance: health status, 75
  aggression control, 78-79
  body image, 86
  caregiver emotional health, 102
  caregiver stressors, 109
  caregiver well-being, 110
  cognitive ability, 125-126
  cognitive orientation, 127
  cognitive status; see Cognitive status
  communication, 129-131
  concentration, 134
  coping, 136-137
  decision making, 138
  dignified dying, 139-140
  distorted thought control, 141-142
  fear control, 147
  grief resolution, 150-151
  hope, 162
  identity, 164-165
  immobility consequences: psycho-cogni-
      tive, 167
  impulse control, 174-175
  information processing, 178
  loneliness, 200-201
  memory, 202
  mood equilibrium, 204-205
  neurological status: consciousness, 214
  parent-infant attachment, 227-228
  psychosocial adjustment: life change, 238
  quality of life, 239
  self-esteem, 275-276
  self-mutilation restraint, 277
  spiritual well-being, 282-283
  suicide restraint, 285

Psychosis; *see also* Cognitive status
distorted thought control, 141-142
ICU
immobility consequences: psycho-cognitive, 167
sleep, 278
identity, 164-165
manic depressive, 204-205
mood equilibrium, 204-205
Psychosocial adjustment: life change, 238
Puberty; *see* Adolescence
Pulmonary perfusion, 298
Pulse rate, 306
Pump, cardiac, effectiveness of, 98-99

Q

Quality of care, 10-12
Quality of life, 239

R

Range of motion, 179-180
Rape, 72
Rape-trauma syndrome, 357
Reaction, blood transfusion, 85
Receptive ability, communication, 131
Recovery
abuse
emotional, 69
financial, 70
physical, 71
sexual, 72
neglect, 207-208
Reflex incontinence, 339
Regimen, treatment
effective management of, 342
knowledge about, 197-198
Relationship, caregiver-patient, 105
Relocation stress syndrome, 357
Renal perfusion, 372
Resolution, grief, 150-151
Resources
health, knowledge about, 189
perceived, 156
Respiratory status
dysfunctional weaning response, 374
education plan for pneumonia, 382-385
gas exchange, 240, 333
inability to sustain spontaneous ventilation, 374
ineffective breathing pattern, 323
pulmonary tissue perfusion, 298
risk for aspiration, 320
ventilation, 241-242
Responsibility
adherence behavior, 76
compliance behavior, 132-133
decision making, 138
health promoting behavior, 159
participation: health care decisions, 232-
233
risk control, 244-255
risk detection, 256

Rest, 243
Restraint
self-mutilation, 277
suicide, 285
Retention, urinary, 373
Risk control, 244-255
alcohol use, 246-247
drug use, 248-249
sexually transmitted diseases, 250-251
tobacco use, 252-253
unintended pregnancy, 254-255
Risk detection, 256
Role conflict, parental, 350
Role performance, 257
altered, 358

S

Safety; *see also* Risk control; Safety behavior
abuse cessation, 67
aggression control, 78-79
aggressive behavior self-control, 73-74
immune status, 170-171
impulse control, 174-175
infection status, 176-177
knowledge: personal safety, 193
knowledge about
for child, 183
personal, 193
parenting, 229-231
self-mutilation restraint, 277
social, 231
suicide self-restraint, 285
Safety behavior
fall prevention, 258
home physical environment, 259
personal, 260
Safety status
falls occurrence, 261
physical injury, 262
Scale, measurement, 52-61
Screening; *see also* Risk control
health seeking behavior, 160-161
risk detection, 256, 276
Secondary intention, healing by, 310
Sedation
rest, 243
sleep, 278
Seizure
neurological status, 209
neurological status: central motor control,
213
neurological status: consciousness, 214
Self-awareness
body image, 86
self-esteem, 275-276
Self-care
activities of daily living, 263
instrumental, 269-270
bathing, 264
dressing, 265
eating, 266
grooming, 267

Self-care—cont'd
  hygiene, 268
  non-parenteral medication, 271
  oral hygiene, 272
  parenteral medication, 273
  toileting, 274
Self-care deficit
  bathing/hygiene, 358
  dressing/grooming, 359
  feeding, 359
  toileting, 360
Self-control; *see* Abuse *entries*; Control; Self-
      destructive behavior
  abusive behavior, 73-75
  aggression behavior, 78-79
  self-mutilation restraint, 277
  suicide self-restraint, 285
Self-destructive behavior
  impulse control, 174-175
  knowledge: substance use control, 195
  risk control: alcohol use, 246-247
  risk control: drug use, 248-249
  self-mutilation restraint, 277
  suicide self-restraint, 285
Self-esteem, 275-276
  body image, 86
  chronic low, 360
  disturbance, 361
  situational low, 361
Self-image
  body image, 86
  self-esteem, 275-276
Self-initiated body positioning, 87
Self-mutilation, risk for, 362
Self-mutilation restraint, 277
Self-responsibility; *see* Responsibility
Sensitivity, nursing, criteria for, 24
Sensory function
  neurological status, 215-216
  tissue perfusion: peripheral, 297
Sensory/motor function
  cranial, 215
  spinal, 216
Sensory/perceptual alterations, 362
Sexual abuse, 72
Sexual abuse recovery, 72
Sexual dysfunction, 363
Sexuality patterns, altered, 363
Sexually transmitted diseases, 250-251
  infection status, 176-177
  knowledge: infection control, 190
  risk control: sexually transmitted diseases,
      250-251
Shock; *see also* Cardiac function
  hydration, 163
  thermoregulation, 289-291
Shower; *see* Bathing
Sick role behavior
  child adaptation to hospitalization, 112
  role performance, 257
  treatment behavior: illness or injury, 300-
      301

Similarity-dissimilarity analysis, 27
Skin integrity, 292
  immobility consequences: physiological,
      166
  impaired, 364
  tissue integrity: skin and mucous mem-
      branes, 292
  wound healing, 309-310
Sleep, 278
Sleep disorder
  abuse recovery: emotional, 69
  abuse recovery: sexual, 72
  immobility consequences: psycho-cogni-
      tive, 167
  rest, 243
  sleep, 278
Sleep pattern disturbance, 365
Smoking
  knowledge: substance use control, 195
  risk control: tobacco use, 252-253
  substance addiction consequences, 284
Social activities
  leisure participation, 199
  quality of life, 239
  social involvement, 280
Social interaction, impaired, 365
Social interaction skills, 279
Social involvement, 280
Social isolation, 366
Social network
  social involvement, 280
  social support, 281
  well-being, 307
Social safety, 231
Social status
  caregiver lifestyle disruption, 104
  caregiver-patient relationship, 105
  leisure participation, 199
  loneliness, 200-201
  parent-infant attachment, 227-228
  parenting, 229-230
  play participation, 237
  quality of life, 239
  role performance, 257
  social interaction skills, 279
  social involvement, 280
  social support, 281
  well-being, 307
Social support, 281
Socialization
  leisure participation, 199
  play participation, 237
  quality of life, 239
  social interaction skills, 279
  social involvement, 280
  well-being, 307
Source, data
  rating of, 32-33
  selection of, 25, 26, 28
Speech deficit; *see* Communication
Spinal cord injury; *see* Neurological status
Spinal sensory/motor function, 216

Spiritual distress, 366
Spiritual well-being, 282-283, 367
    dignified dying, 139-140
    grief resolution, 150-151
Spouse abuse; *see* Abuse *entries*
Standardization of outcomes
    reasons for, 8-14, 60-61
    rules for, 23
Statement, outcome, 33
Stoma; *see* Ostomy
Strength
    endurance, 145
    energy conservation, 146
Stress; *see also* Abuse *entries*; Adaptation, psy-
        chological
    anxiety control, 82-83
    caregiver lifestyle disruption, 104
    caregiver stressor, 109
    fear control, 147
    mood equilibrium, 204-205
    pain: disruptive effects, 225
    pain level, 226
    symptom control behavior, 287
    will to live, 308
Stress, relocation, 357
Stress incontinence, 340
Stressors, on caregiver, 109
Subcutaneous medication, 191, 273
Substance abuse; *see* Chemical dependency
Substance addiction consequences, 284
Suffocation, risk for, 367
Suicide self-restraint, 285
Support system; *see also* Caregiver *entries*
    grief resolution, 150-151
    health beliefs: perceived resources, 156
    loneliness, 200-201
    social involvement, 280
    social support, 281
    spiritual well-being, 282-283
Survey, 37-39
Swallowing
    impaired, 368
    neurological status, 209
    neurological status: cranial sensory/motor
        function, 215
    nutritional status: food and fluid intake,
        221
    self-care: eating, 266
Symptom control behavior, 287
Symptom severity, 288
System-specific outcomes, 7

T

Tachypnea; *see* Apnea
Task performance, 106-107
Taxonomy, 22
Teaching; *see* Education
Team, research, 20
Temperature; *see* Thermoregulation
Terminal care; *see* Hospice
Terminology, 22

Thermoregulation, 289-290; *see also* Fever
    altered body temperature, 321
    hyperthermia, 338
    hypothermia, 338
    ineffective, 368
    neonate, 291
Thinking; *see* Cognitive *entries*
Thought control, distorted, 141-142
Thought process, altered, 368
Threat, perceived, 157
Tissue integrity
    immobility consequences: physiological,
        166
    impaired, 368
    skin and mucous membranes, 292
    wound healing, 309-310
Tissue perfusion
    abdominal organs, 293-294
    altered
        cardiopulmonary, 370
        cerebral, 370
        gastrointestinal, 371
        peripheral, 371
        renal, 372
    cardiac, 295
    cerebral, 296
    peripheral, 297
    pulmonary, 298
Tobacco use, 252-253; *see* Smoking
Toileting, 274; *see* Elimination
Toothbrushing; *see* Oral health
Total incontinence, 340
Transfer performance, 299
Transfusion reaction control, 85
Translation; *see* Communication
Transportation
    ambulation: wheelchair, 81
    self-care: instrumental activities of daily
        living, 269-270
Trauma, rape, 357; *see also* Injury
Treatment behavior, illness or injury, 300-301
Treatment procedures, knowledge about, 196
Treatment regimen
    effective management of, 342
    knowledge about, 197-198
Tube feeding; *see* Nutritional status
Turning
    body positioning: self-initiated, 87
    immobility consequences: physiological,
        166

U

Ulcer, pressure; *see* Decubitus ulcer
Unconsciousness, 209, 214
Uniform nursing data sets, 9-10
Unilateral neglect, 372
Unintended pregnancy, 254-255
Urge, incontinence, 341
Urinary cauterization; *see* Catheterization,
    urinary
Urinary continence, 302-303

Urinary control
   self-care: hygiene, 268
   self-care: toileting, 274
   urinary continence, 302-303
   urinary elimination, 304-305
Urinary elimination, 304-305
   altered, 373
Urinary incontinence, 341
Urinary retention, 373

V

Vaccination, 172-173
   immune status, 170-171
   immunization behavior, 172-173
Validation
   focus group concept analysis in, 35-39
   of outcomes, 25-26, 29-30
Values
   acceptance: health status, 75
   decision making, 138
   health beliefs, 153-157
   health orientation, 153-158
   parenting, 229-230
   spiritual well-being, 282-283
   well-being, 307
Venereal disease; *see* Sexually transmitted
      diseases
Ventilation, 241-242
   body positioning: self-initiated, 87
   inability to sustain spontaneous, 374
   respiratory status: ventilation, 241-242
Verbal communication; *see* Communication
Violence, risk for, 375
Violence management
   abuse cessation, 67
   abusive behavior self-control, 73-74
   aggression control, 78-79
   impulse control, 174-175
   parenting: social safety, 231
   self-mutilation restraint, 277
   suicide self-restraint, 285
Vision
   neurological status: cranial sensory/motor
      function, 215
   safety behavior: home physical environ-
      ment, 259
   safety behavior: personal, 260
Vital signs status, 306

W

Walking, 78-79
Walking, ambulation, 80
Weakness, 206
Weaning; *see also* Airway
   breastfeeding, 96-97
   breastfeeding: weaning, 96-97
   nutritional status: food and fluid intake,
      221
   ventilatory, 374
Weight control; *see also* Nutritional status
   adherence behavior, 76
   compliance behavior, 132-133
   health promoting behavior, 159
   knowledge: diet, 184-185
   knowledge: health behaviors, 188
Well-being, 307
   of caregiver, 110
   comfort level, 128
   emotional
      caregiver emotional health, 102
      caregiver lifestyle disruption, 104
      caregiver stressors, 109
      caregiver well-being, 110
      caregiver-patient relationship, 105
      caregiving endurance potential, 111
      dignified dying, 139-140
      hope, 162
      loneliness, 200-201
      quality of life, 239
      will to live, 308
   endurance, 145
   spiritual, 282-283
      dignified dying, 139-140
      grief resolution, 150-151
   symptom severity, 288
Wellness; *see* Health promotion; Risk control
Wheelchair
   ambulation: wheelchair, 81
   transfer performance, 299
Wheelchair ambulation, 81
Will to live, 308
Wound healing
   primary intention, 309
   secondary intention, 310

Y

Youth; *see* Adolescence